Management of Epilepsy

Management of Epilepsy

Sudhansu Chokroverty, M.D.

Professor of Neurology, Robert Wood Johnson Medical School, New Brunswick, New Jersey; Adjunct Professor of Neurology, New York Medical College, Valhalla, New York; Chief of Neurology, Veterans Affairs Medical Center, Lyons, New Jersey; Associate Chairman of Neurology, Saint Vincent's Hospital and Medical Center of New York, New York

Foreword by

Ernst Niedermeyer, M.D.

Professor Emeritus of Neurology and Neurosurgery, Johns Hopkins University School of Medicine and Johns Hopkins Hospital, Baltimore, Maryland

Butterworth–Heinemann

Boston•Oxford•Johannesburg•Melbourne•New Delhi•Singapore

Every effort has been made to ensure that the drug dosage schedules within this text are accurate and conform to standards accepted at the time of publication. However, as treatment recommendations vary in the light of continuing research and clinical experience, the reader is advised to verify drug dosage schedules herein with information found on product information sheets. This is especially true in cases of new or infrequently used drugs.

Library of Congress Cataloging-in-Publication Data

Management of epilepsy / [edited by] Sudhansu Chokroverty ; foreword by Ernst Niedermeyer.
    p.   cm.
    Includes bibliographical references and index.
    ISBN 0-7506-9754-7 (alk. paper)
    1. Epilepsy   I. Chokroverty, Sudhansu.
    [DNLM: 1. Epilepsy--therapy.   2. Anticonvulsants--therapeutic use.
    3. Convulsions--therapy.   WL 385M2658 1996]
    RC372.M26   1996
    616.8'53--dc20
    DNLM/DLC
    for Library of Congress   96-16864
                                       CIP

British Library Cataloguing-in-Publication Data
A catalogue record for this book is available from the British Library.

The publisher offers discounts on bulk orders of this book.
For information, please contact:

Manager of Special Sales
Butterworth–Heinemann
313 Washington Street
Newton, MA 02158–1626
Tel: 617-928-2500
Fax: 617-928-2620

For information on all medical publications available, contact our World Wide Web home page at http://www.bh.com/bh/

10 9 8 7 6 5 4 3 2 1

Printed in the United States of America

*To my parents, Debendranath and Ashalata Chakrabarti;
my wife, Manisha; and our daughters, Linda and Keka*

Contents

Contributing Authors

Thomas R. Browne, M.D.
Professor and Vice Chairman, Department of Neurology, Boston University School of Medicine, Boston, Massachusetts; Associate Chief, Neurology Service, Department of Neurology, Department of Veterans Affairs Medical Center, Boston

Gregory D. Cascino, M.D.
Professor of Neurology, Mayo Medical School, Rochester, Minnesota; Consultant, Department of Neurology, Mayo Clinic and Mayo Foundation, Rochester

Sudhansu Chokroverty, M.D.
Professor of Neurology, Robert Wood Johnson Medical School, New Brunswick, New Jersey; Adjunct Professor of Neurology, New York Medical College, Valhalla, New York; Chief of Neurology, Veterans Affairs Medical Center, Lyons, New Jersey; Associate Chairman of Neurology, Saint Vincent's Hospital and Medical Center of New York, New York

Stephen D. Collins, M.D., Ph.D.
Assistant Professor of Neurology and Neurosciences, Case Western Reserve University School of Medicine, Cleveland, Ohio; Director, Epilepsy Center and EEG Laboratory, Department of Neurology, University Hospitals of Cleveland, Cleveland

Fritz E. Dreifuss, M.B., F.R.C.P., F.R.A.C.P.
Professor of Neurology, University of Virginia School of Medicine, Charlottesville; Director, Comprehensive Epilepsy Program, Department of Neurology, University of Virginia Health Sciences Center, Charlottesville

Robert R. Goodman, M.D., Ph.D.
Assistant Professor of Neurological Surgery, Columbia University College of Physicians and Surgeons, New York, New York; Attending Physician, Department of Neurological Surgery, Columbia-Presbyterian Medical Center, New York

W. Allen Hauser, M.D.
Professor of Neurology and Public Health and Associate Director, G. H. Sergievsky Center, Columbia University College of Physicians and Surgeons, New York, New York; Attending Neurologist, Columbia- Presbyterian Medical Center, New York

Gregory L. Holmes, M.D.
Associate Professor of Neurology, Harvard Medical School, Boston, Massachusetts; Director, Division of Clinical Neurophysiology and Epilepsy, Department of Neurology, Children's Hospital, Boston

Peter W. Kaplan, M.B., B.S., F.R.C.P.
Associate Professor of Neurology, Johns Hopkins University School of Medicine, Baltimore, Maryland; Chairman, Department of Neurology, Johns Hopkins Bayview Medical Center, Baltimore

Douglas R. Labar, M.D., Ph.D.
Director, Comprehensive Epilepsy Center, Department of Neurology, New York Hospital-Cornell Medical Center, New York, New York

Ronald P. Lesser, M.D.
Professor of Neurology, Johns Hopkins University School of Medicine, Baltimore, Maryland; Director, Johns Hopkins Epilepsy Center and EEG Laboratories, Department of Neurology, Johns Hopkins Hospital, Baltimore

Timothy A. Pedley, M.D.
Professor and Vice Chairman, Department of Neurology, Columbia University College of Physicians and Surgeons, New York, New York;

Director, Comprehensive Epilepsy Center and Associate Director, Neurology Service, Columbia-Presbyterian Medical Center and the Neurological Institute of New York

Norman L. Pflaster, M.D.
Assistant Professor of Neurology, Columbia University College of Physicians and Surgeons, New York, New York; Assistant Attending Physician, Department of Neurology, Harlem Hospital, New York

Roger J. Porter, M.D.
Adjunct Professor of Neurology, University of Pennsylvania School of Medicine, Philadelphia; Vice President, Department of Clinical Pharmacology, Wyeth-Ayerst Research, Radnor, Pennsylvania

Venkat Ramani, M.D.
Professor of Neurology and Associate Professor of Psychiatry, Albany Medical College, Albany, New York; Attending Neurologist, Albany Medical Center Hospital, Albany

Rajesh C. Sachdeo, M.D.
Associate Professor of Clinical Neurology and Director, New Jersey Comprehensive Epilepsy Center, Robert Wood Johnson Medical School and University Hospital, New Brunswick, New Jersey

Carl E. Stafstrom, M.D., Ph.D.
Associate Professor of Pediatrics and Neurology, Tufts University School of Medicine, Boston, Massachusetts; Director, Epilepsy Center for Children, Division of Pediatric Neurology, New England Medical Center, Boston

Thaddeus S. Walczak, M.D.
Assistant Professor of Neurology, Columbia University College of Physicians and Surgeons, New York, New York; Head, Epilepsy Monitoring Unit, Comprehensive Epilepsy Center, The Neurological Institute of New York, Columbia-Presbyterian Medical Center, New York

Mark S. Yerby, M.D., M.P.H.
Associate Clinical Professor, Departments of Public Health, Neurology, and Obstetrics-Gynecology, Oregon Health Sciences University, Portland

Foreword

It is a great pleasure and honor to write these heralding lines for the book of my highly regarded colleague, Dr. Sudhansu Chokroverty, who has become widely recognized as a leading clinical neurologist and neurophysiologist. In his work, Dr. Chokroverty has always been a voice of reason and common sense: a highly experienced practicing neurologist with deep insights into the scientific foundations of neurologic thinking.

Epileptology has become one of the most hotly debated fields in neurology. Notwithstanding the considerable number of books written on this subject, Dr. Chokroverty has been able to inspire a work of his own with the assistance of extremely able and prestigious contributors. Dr. Chokroverty and his team have emphasized the therapeutic segment of the field and limited the topics to the essential clinical problems to produce a concise new work.

May this book be helpful to physicians and patients in the daily struggle with difficult cases of epileptic seizure disorders—may it be a guiding beacon of light whenever therapeutic problems seem insurmountable.

Ernst Niedermeyer

Preface

The first pharmacologically active agent against epilepsy was used in the middle of the nineteenth century. As we approach the twenty-first century, we still do not have an ideal antiepileptic drug (AED). An ideal AED is one that controls the seizures or probably cures a patient with epilepsy and does not produce undesirable side effects. An ideal AED should also be easy to administer without any compliance problems and should effectively eradicate the basic fundamental mechanisms for epileptogenesis.

Despite the unavailability of an ideal AED, there is cause for optimism. The recent development of pharmacotherapy of epilepsy based on cellular and neurotransmitter mechanisms and the emergence of many newer AEDs (some are already available for general use and many are undergoing active clinical trials) have resparked the hope that we may have an ideal AED during the first quarter of the next century. Until then, however, the physicians responsible for the day-to-day care of epilepsy patients must use the old as well as the newer AEDs in a rational manner to effectively control seizures. This is sometimes a daunting and challenging task, and some physicians are at a loss in treating such patients.

The goal of this book is to provide a comprehensive, step-by-step approach toward managing a patient with epilepsy. This is neither a comprehensive textbook of epilepsy nor an encyclopedic tome dealing with the pharmacologic and therapeutic aspects of epilepsy. We did not attempt to discuss the pathophysiology of epilepsy but instead have emphasized practical management. This volume should be useful to practicing physicians and those in training. There are repetitions in different chapters that are necessary to make a point and to reiterate the practical aspects of management.

A chapter on classification of epilepsies and epileptic syndromes is an essential prerequisite for treatment. We also discuss the role of electroencephalography, the single most important diagnostic test in epilepsy, for a physician must comprehend it with all its limitations before attempting to treat a patient with a seizure disorder. This book also emphasizes certain special circumstances (e.g., pregnant patients with epilepsy) that require special attention to management. It is important to remember as well that management of epilepsy involves not only pharmacotherapy and occasionally surgery but also psychosocial, vocational, legal, and ethical aspects.

The contributors to this volume are all nationally and internationally known for their work on epilepsy and their dedication to patients with epilepsy. I am most grateful to them for their scholarly and very practical contributions.

I am indebted to Susan Pioli, Director of Medical Publishing at Butterworth-Heinemann, for her thoughtfulness and professionalism, and for agreeing to publish the work speedily. I thank Scott Snell for the photographs of the electroencephalograms and Lena Theusen for typing and retyping many of the chapters. I express my gratitude to the authors, editors, and publishers who granted permission to reproduce some of the illustrations for Chapter 5 that were first published in other books and journals.

Finally, I express my appreciation to my wife, Manisha Chokroverty, M.D., for her unfailing support, patience, and forbearance during the prolonged, arduous, and often frustrating months of preparation of this monograph.

Sudhansu Chokroverty, M.D.

Management of Epilepsy

1

Introduction

Sudhansu Chokroverty

Epilepsy has been known since antiquity. In the fifth century B.C., Hippocrates recognized that epilepsy originated in the brain; thus, in the hippocratic era the disease was referred to as "the sacred disease."[1] The Greek physician Galen classified epilepsy into "idiopathic" or "symptomatic" types,[1] which is remarkably similar to the modern classification of epilepsy. In fact, the English word "epilepsy" is derived from the Greek word "epilepsia," meaning "to take hold of" or "seize."

Knowledge about epilepsy advanced slowly from antiquity and the hippocratic and galenic eras through the middle ages. There are numerous references to epilepsy in various religious writings in which it is shrouded in mysticism, magical powers, and demonic spirits. Those who believed in supernatural forms as the cause of epilepsy advised exorcism to get rid of the demonic spirits that supposedly possessed epileptics. Physicians often prescribed "shotgun" medications consisting of both animal and vegetable materials.[1] Treatments included agents that qualify as bizarre and fantastic, such as human blood; dragon's blood; powdered human skull; wolf's liver; and liquor made from the juices of shrubs mixed with a hawk's intestine, stag's horn, hair of a corpse, and the burned flesh of a mole.[1] Other remedies in the ancient days included purging, blood letting, vomiting, and the use of diuretics to get rid of the poisons in the body thought to be responsible for the seizures.[1] Ancient surgical treatment was as bizarre as the medical treatment. Trephining of the skull with a hot iron cautery was often practiced to release the evil spirits or morbid secretions from the brain.[1] Classic accounts of the history of epilepsy can be found in Temkin's *The Falling Sickness*[2] and the two volumes on epilepsy by Lennox.[1] The brief introduction in this chapter on epilepsy and its treatment is largely derived from these volumes.

After centuries of ignorance and superstitious beliefs, the treatment of epilepsy entered the modern age, and recent advances in the management of epilepsy have seen an explosive growth. John Hughlings Jackson is considered the father of modern epileptology. In 1861, he defined epilepsy as a sudden, excessive discharge from the gray matter of the cerebral cortex.[3] The era of pharmacotherapy of epilepsy began in 1857 with the serendipitous observation that bromides helped patients with epilepsy.[4] The modern era of medical treatment began in 1912 with the discovery of phenobarbital by Hauptmann.[5] This was followed a quarter of a century later by the discovery of phenytoin by Merritt and Putnam.[6] Subsequently, several other antiepileptic drugs (AEDs) were introduced.[7] These included trimethadione (1946), mephenytoin (1947), paramethadione (1949), phenacemide (1951), phensuximide (1953), primidone (1954), methsuximide (1957), ethotoin (1957), ethosuximide (1960), diazepam (1968), carbamazepine (1974), clonazepam (1975), and valproic acid (1978). In the United States, no new AEDs were introduced between 1978 and 1993. Since that time, four promising new drugs have been tested[8] (see Chapters 14 and 19); two of these (felbamate or Felbatol and gabapentin or Neurontin) were introduced for use in late 1993 and the beginning of 1994. Use of felbamate, however, was restricted recently because of an increasing incidence of aplastic anemia and liver failure. A third drug, lamotrigine (Lamictal), became available in February of 1995; and a fourth drug, vigabatrin (GVG), is still not available for general use. The future of pharmacotherapy for epilepsy appears promising and exciting with the possibility of the development of ideal AEDs based on cellular and neurotransmitter mechanisms. Recent advances in the surgical treatment of epilepsy, which is indicated in a small percentage of patients with refractory epilepsy, also hold great promise for further improvement and refinement in the localization of the epileptic foci and surgical intervention.

References

1. Lennox WG. Epilepsy and Related Disorders. Boston: Little, Brown, 1960.
2. Temkin O. The Falling Sickness (2nd ed). Baltimore: Johns Hopkins University Press, 1971.
3. Jackson JH. On the Anatomical, Physiological and Pathological Investigation of Epilepsies. West Riding Lunatic Asylum Medical Reports 3:315–332, 1873. In J Taylor (ed), Selected Writings of John Hughlings Jackson. I. London: Hodder and Stoughton, 1931.
4. Sieveking EH. Analysis of 52 cases of epilepsy observed by the author. Lancet 1857;1:528.
5. Hauptmann A. Luminal bei epilepsia. Munch Med Wochenschr 1912;59:1907.
6. Merritt HH, Putnam TJ. A new series of anticonvulsant drugs tested by experiments on animals. Arch Neurol Psychiatr 1938;39:1003.
7. Uthman BM, Wilder BJ. Less Commonly Used Antiepileptic Drugs. In E Wyllie (ed), The Treatment of Epilepsy: Principles and Practice. Philadelphia: Lea & Febiger, 1993;959.
8. Fisher RS. Emerging antiepileptic drugs. Neurology 1993;43(Suppl 5):S12.

2

Classification of Epileptic Seizures and the Epilepsies

Fritz E. Dreifuss

Introduction

As long ago as 175 A.D., Galen[1] classified epilepsies as idiopathic or symptomatic. The reason for this classification was the identification of underlying causes, the removal of which, Galen understood, would ameliorate epilepsy. This utilitarian purpose was elaborated with the development of antiepileptic drugs and their increasing sophistication. Initially, when bromides and barbiturates were the only drugs available, they were used regardless of the nature of the epileptic seizures or the underlying process. The modern era of antiepileptic drug development was ushered in with the increased understanding of the pathophysiology of individual epileptic seizures. Since then, specific antiepileptic drugs have been developed for their particular physiologic effect, which in turn is reflected in their use for particular seizure types. Thus, drugs such as phenytoin and carbamazepine appear to act predominantly at the level of the sodium channel and benzodiazepines and valproate at the level of the chloride channel. Calcium channel activity and N-methyl-D-aspartate (NMDA) receptor-blocking activity, as well as enhancement or depression of putative neurotransmitters, are the subjects of intensive pharmacotherapeutic research.

With this increased attention to the mechanisms of action of antiepileptic drugs, it has become essential to accurately classify individual epileptic seizure types so that the most appropriate therapeutic agent can be chosen. The realization that all antiepileptic drugs are potentially toxic and the fact that antiepileptic drugs must be administered for a very prolonged period of time have mandated diagnostic accuracy. Examples of specific seizure types that mandate specific therapeutic responses include the distinction between absence seizures and complex partial seizures. This is potentially one of the more difficult differential diagnoses in epileptology, as complex partial seizures may present with only a blank stare and absence seizures may present with quite elaborate automatisms. Repeated absence seizures may give the impression of postictal confusion, and immediate return of consciousness, which usually characterizes absence seizures, may also be seen in complex partial seizures of frontal lobe origin. The penalty of mistaking the diagnosis is that a patient may be given inappropriate antiepileptic drugs for prolonged periods of time, such as ethosuximide for complex partial seizures or carbamazepine or phenytoin for absence seizures. The classification of epilepsy in current use is summarized in Table 2-1.[2]

A further reason for the classification of epileptic seizures is the need for clear communication between physicians in order to facilitate patient management and clinical research.[3] The development of objective methods of documenting seizures, including prolonged electroencephalographic (EEG) recording and the use of video tape, has resulted in a more accurate description of individual seizure types. Moreover, it is recognized that the patient with epilepsy may show a progression from one type of seizure to another during the evolution of the epileptic process, such as may happen in a progression of a simple partial seizure to a complex partial seizure and ultimately to a secondary generalized tonic-clonic seizure.

Epilepsy Syndromes

The evaluation of a person with a history of a seizure disorder includes verification of whether the seizures represent epilepsy; identification of the individual seizure type, which forms the basis for the choice of the most appropriate anticonvulsant regimen; and the elucidation, where possible, of the underlying cause, which may lead to the correction of the process responsible for the epilepsy. It is increas-

Table 2-1. Types of Seizures

I. **Partial (focal, local) seizures**

Partial seizures are those in which, in general, the first clinical and electroen-cephalographic changes indicate activation of a system of neurons limited to part of one cerebral hemisphere. A partial seizure is classified primarily on the basis of whether or not consciousness is impaired during the attack. When consciousness is not impaired, the seizure is classified as a simple partial seizure. When consciousness is impaired, the seizure is classified as a complex partial seizure. Impairment of consciousness may be the first clinical sign, or simple partial seizures may evolve into complex partial seizures. In patients with impaired consciousness, aberrations of behavior (automatisms) may occur. A partial seizure may not terminate but instead may progress to a generalized motor seizure. Impaired consciousness is defined as the inability to respond normally to exogenous stimuli by virtue of altered awareness and/or responsiveness.

There is considerable evidence that simple partial seizures usually have unilateral hemispheric involvement and only rarely have bilateral hemispheric involvement; complex partial seizures, however, frequently have bilateral hemispheric involvement.

Partial seizures can be classified into of the following three fundamental groups:

A. Simple partial seizures (consciousness not impaired)

   1. With motor symptoms

   2. With somatosensory or special sensory symptoms

   3. With autonomic symptoms

   4. With psychic symptoms

B. Complex partial seizures (with impairment of consciousness)

   1. Beginning as simple partial seizures and progressing to impairment of consciousness

     a. With no other features

     b. With features as in A. 1–4

     c. With automatisms

   2. With impairment of consciousness at onset

     a. With no other features

     b. With features as in A. 1–4

     c. With automatisms

C. Partial seizures secondarily generalized

Table 2-1. *(continued)*

II.   **Generalized seizures (convulsive or nonconvulsive)**

Generalized seizures are those in which the first clinical changes indicate initial involvement of both hemispheres. Consciousness may be impaired; this impairment may be the initial manifestation. Motor manifestations are bilateral. The ictal electroencephalographic patterns initially are bilateral and presumably reflect neuronal discharge, widespread in both hemispheres.

   A.   Absence seizures

      1.   Typical absence seizures

      2.   Atypical absence seizures

   B.   Myoclonic seizures

   C.   Clonic seizures

   D.   Tonic seizures

   E.   Tonic-clonic seizures

   F.   Atonic seizures

III.   **Unclassified epileptic seizures**

Unclassified epileptic seizures include all seizures that cannot be classified because of inadequate or incomplete data and some that defy classification in hitherto described categories, including some neonatal seizures (e.g., rhythmic eye movements, chewing, and swimming movements).

---

ingly apparent that the cause of a seizure disorder is of primary importance. Whereas the seizure type is the product of the area of the nervous system involved, causative factors have implications that reach into areas of genetics, higher cortical function, and intelligence, and they determine a prognosis, response to medication, and natural history. The seizure is only the symptom that brings the patient to the physician. The epileptic syndrome[4] of which the seizure is a symptom determines the prognosis and is the product of the underlying disease. Thus, family history, age of onset, rate of progression, presence or absence of neurologic abnormalities, presence or absence of interictal electroencephalographic (EEG) abnormalities, and the response to medication all contribute to the diagnosis of the syndrome. Identification and classification of etiologic factors, apart from their usefulness in communication, are essential for appropriate therapy, not only in terms of using the most appropriate antiepileptic agent, but also in gauging the natural history of the condition under consideration in order to be able to prognosticate regarding the duration of therapy or to determine whether antiepileptic drugs are essential for the management of the particular condition under consideration. Moreover, the identification of individual syndromes has allowed molecular biology to be applied to the ultimate elucidation of the so-called idiopathic epilepsies; syndromes can on occasion be sufficiently discretely identified that their genetic localization can be determined on the human genome.[5,6]

The epilepsies may be classified according to seizure type and EEG findings—that is, either partial or generalized or according to etiology (idiopathic [genetic] or symptomatic). They may also be anatomically localized, for example, into frontal lobe, rolandic, occipital, or temporal epilepsy; finally, they may be classified into precipitating factors. There are two major dichotomies in the present classification of the epilepsies and epileptic syndromes. The first major dichotomy is between epilepsies characterized by seizures that are partial in onset and those that are generalized. The second dichotomy is between seizures that are idiopathic and those that are symptomatic; this usually devolves into those that have a genetic predisposition and those that are determined by a structural or lesional cause.

The present classification of the epilepsies and epileptic syndromes adopted by the International League Against Epilepsy in 1989[4] is summarized in Table 2-2.

Many childhood epilepsies may be classified in an age-related manner. Thus, childhood epilepsies include neonatal seizures; early myoclonic encephalopathy; infantile spasms; febrile seizures; astatic myoclonic epilepsy; pyknoleptic petit mal; benign childhood partial epilepsy (rolandic); juvenile myoclonic epilepsy; epilepsia partialis continua; and the anatomically determined syndromes characterized by partial seizures, such as those of temporal lobe, frontal lobe, parietal lobe, and occipital lobe epilepsy. Most of these categories consist of two main syndromic subgroups, namely, the primary epilepsies and the secondary, lesional or symptomatic epilepsies. Primary epilepsies are unassociated with an underlying pathologic condition, there is frequently a positive family history of a similar seizure type, and the patient has usually progressed normally up to the time of the development of the epilepsy, which is often self-limited and responds to medication if appropriately used. Secondary (lesional or symptomatic) epilepsies have an anatomicopathologic substrate, there are frequently associated neurologic abnormalities, and there is frequently abnormal neurologic development. The seizures are often difficult to control. Examples of

Table 2-2. International Classification of Epilepsies (ICE), Epileptic Syndromes, and Related Seizure Disorders

1. Localization-related (focal, local, partial)
    1.1 Idiopathic (primary)
        Benign childhood epilepsy with centrotemporal spike
        Childhood epilepsy with occipital paroxysms
        Primary reading epilepsy
    1.2 Symptomatic (secondary)
        Temporal lobe epilepsies
        Frontal lobe epilepsies
        Parietal lobe epilepsies
        Occipital lobe epilepsies
        Chronic progressive epilepsia partialis continua of childhood
        Syndromes characterized by seizures with specific modes of precipitation
    1.3 Cryptogenic, defined by the following:
        Seizure type (see International Classification of Epileptic Seizures [ICES])
        Clinical features
        Etiology
        Anatomic localization
2. Generalized
    2.1 Idiopathic
        Benign neonatal familial convulsions
        Benign neonatal convulsions
        Benign myoclonic epilepsy in infancy
        Childhood absence epilepsy (pyknolepsy)
        Juvenile absence epilepsy
        Juvenile myoclonic epilepsy (impulsive petit mal)
        Epilepsies with grand mal seizures, generalized tonic-clonic seizures (GTCS) on awakening
        Other generalized idiopathic epilepsies
        Epilepsies with seizures precipitated by specific modes of activation
    2.2 Cryptogenic or symptomatic
        West's syndrome (infantile spasms, Blitz-Nick-Salaam-Krämpfe)
        Lennox-Gastaut syndrome

       Epilepsy with myoclonic-astatic seizures

       Epilepsy with myoclonic absences

2.3.1 Nonspecific etiology

       Early myoclonic encephalopathy

       Early infantile epileptic encephalopathy with suppression bursts

       Other symptomatic generalized epilepsies

2.3.2 Specific syndromes

       Epileptic seizures may complicate many disease states

3. Undetermined epilepsies

  3.1   With both generalized and focal seizures

       Neonatal seizures

       Severe myoclonic epilepsy in infancy

       Epilepsy with continuous spike waves during slow wave sleep

       Acquired epileptic aphasia (Landau-Kleffner syndrome)

       Other undetermined epilepsies

  3.2   Without unequivocal generalized or focal features

4. Special syndromes

  4.1   Situation-related seizures (Gelegenheitsanfälle)

       Febrile convulsions

       Isolated seizures or isolated status epilepticus

       Seizures occurring only when there is an acute or toxic event due to factors such as alcohol, drugs, eclampsia, or nonketotic hyperglycemia

Source: Adapted from Commission on Classification and Terminology of the International League Against Epilepsy. Proposal for revised classification of epilepsies and epileptic syndromes. Epilepsia 1989;30:389.

well-recognized epileptic syndromes and their cardinal features[7] are illustrated in Table 2-1.

    Fejerman and Medina[8] have incorporated in one table (Table 2-3) the features of the individual syndromes and those of the seizures that represent the symptoms of the individual epilepsies. In doing this they have largely clarified the relationships of the different classifications, thereby obviating some of the misunderstandings arising out of the need to deal with separate publications that do not sufficiently stress the interrelationships.

Table 2-3. Epilepsies and Epileptic Seizures

Identified Syndromes	Principal Type of Epileptic Seizures	Most Typical Electroencephalographic Pattern
Generalized epilepsies		
Epileptic encephalopathies (cryptogenic)		
Early myoclonic epileptic encephalopathy	Fragmentary or massive myoclonies; erratic partial seizures	Suppression-burst
West's syndrome	Infantile spasms	Hypsarrhythmia
Lennox-Gastaut syndrome	Atypical absences, tonic seizures, and atonic seizures	Slow spike waves, discharges of bilateral rapid rhythms, multifocal spike bursts of polyspike or polyspike wave poorly structured background rhythm
Myoclonic and myoclonic-atonic epilepsies (idiopathic)		
Benign myoclonic epilepsy of infancy	Cephalic or massive myoclonies	Bursts of generalized spike waves or polyspike waves
Cryptogenic myoclonic epilepsy	Massive myoclonic seizures	Fast spike waves and polyspike waves
Myoclonic-atonic (astatic) epilepsy	Drop attacks	Brief generalized bursts of polyspike waves
Juvenile myoclonic epilepsy	Myoclonies in upper limbs on awakening, generalized tonic-clonic seizures	Fast polyspike waves and spike wave
Generalized tonic-clonic epilepsies		
Epilepsy with generalized convulsive seizures in childhood	Loss of consciousness and tonic or clonic or hypnotic seizures	Generalized discharges, focal spikes, or both
Classic "grand mal" epilepsy	Loss of consciousness and tonic seizure followed by clonic seizures	Generalized discharges, focal spikes, or both

Identified Syndromes	Principal Type of Epileptic Seizures	Most Typical Electroencephalographic Pattern
Awakening "grand mal" seizures in adolescence	Loss of consciousness and tonic seizure followed by clonic seizures	Generalized spike wave discharges and vegetative signs on awakening
Petit mal epilepsies		
Childhood absence epilepsy	Pure absences or absences with other signs (clonic, tonic, atonic or vegetative phenomena: automatisms, etc.)	Symmetric generalized 3-per-second spike wave discharges
Epilepsy with myoclonic absences	Absences with rhythmic diffuse myoclonies	Symmetric generalized 3-per-second spike wave discharges
Juvenile absence epilepsy	Absences associated with tonic-clonic and/or myoclonic seizures	Generalized 3.5- to 4.0-per-second spike wave discharges
Miscellaneous		
Febrile convulsions	Loss of consciousness and clonic, tonic or hypnotonic seizures	Normal; hypnagogic spike wave bursts in 20% of cases
Epilepsy with continuous spike waves during slow sleep	Atypical absences	Continuous diffuse spike waves during slow sleep
Partial epilepsies		
Benign partial epilepsies (BPE) (idiopathic)		
BPE with rolandic (or midtemporal) spikes	Unilateral tonic or clonic seizures in face or arm, speech arrest, paresthesias in mouth or tongue	Rolandic (or midtemporal) spikes
BPE with affective symptomatology	Fear or terror seizures, autonomic phenomena	Temporal spikes
BPE with occipital paroxysms	Visual seizures (transitory amaurosis, flashing lights)	Occipital spikes, spike wave, or both

Table 2-3. *(continued)*

Identified Syndromes	Principal Type of Epileptic Seizures	Most Typical Electroencephalographic Pattern
BPE with occipital paroxysms *(continued)*	hemiclonic seizures, migrainous headaches	
Atypical BPE	Motor partial seizures, myoclonic or myoclonic-atonic seizures	Generalized spike waves, focal spikes
Simple partial epilepsies (SPE) (symptomatic)		
SPE with motor signs	Motor partial seizures (with or without jacksonian march) other seizures: versive, rotatory, postural, etc.	Focal spikes or spike waves
SPE with autonomic symptoms	Vomiting, abdominal, pain, pallor, flushing, sweating, etc.	Focal spikes or spike waves
SPE with somatosensory or special sensory symptoms	Paresthetic, vertiginous, visual, auditory, gustatory, olfactory, etc.	Focal spikes or spike waves
SPE with disturbance of higher cerebral function (psychic symptoms)	Gelastic, affective, dysphasic, dysmnesic, cognitive, etc.	Focal spikes or spike waves
Complex partial epilepsies (CPE) (symptomatic)		
CPE with temporolimbic symptoms	Temporal absences, automatisms, psychic symptoms	Temporal spikes or spike waves
CPE with frontal symptoms	Temporal absence, gestural or postural automatisms	Focal frontal abnormalities
Hemiconvulsion-hemiplegia-epilepsy syndrome	Unilateral clonic status	Postictal electroencephalographic tracing: contralateral continuous delta activity with or without spikes

Identified Syndromes	Principal Type of Epileptic Seizures	Most Typical Electroencephalographic Pattern
Miscellaneous		
Classic Kojewnikow syndrome	Motor partial status, partial myoclonies	Central spikes
Progressive continuous partial epilepsy	Motor partial status, myoclonies with variable topography	Diffuse delta activity, poorly structured background rhythm
Syndromes not deter-mined whether partial or generalized		
Severe myoclonic epilepsy of infancy	Clonic seizures (with or without fever) myoclonic seizures-partial seizures	Fast spike wave and polyspike wave, generalized bursts, focal spikes and spike waves
Acquired epileptic aphasia (Landau-Kleffner syndrome epilepsies with generalized and partial features not comprising identifiable syndromes)	Persistent aphasia clonic or myoclonic seizures, atypical absences	Spike and spike waves discharges, generalized or dominant over lateral regions

Source: Reprinted with permission from N Fejerman, CS Medina. Convulsiones en la Infancia (2nd ed). Buenos Aires: El Ateneo, 1986.

Idiopathic Epilepsies with Partial Seizures

Idiopathic epilepsies with partial seizures have in common the absence of a neurologic or intellectual deficit, a frequent family history of benign epilepsy, onset after 18 months of age, and seizures that are usually relatively brief without a prolonged postictal deficit. The EEG shows normal background interictal activity, frequently shows focal epileptic discharges, and sometimes shows bursts of generalized spike and wave discharges. Focal abnormalities frequently increase during sleep.

Two principal syndromes are described under this rubric: benign childhood epilepsy with centrotemporal spikes[9,10] and idiopathic generalized epilepsy syndromes.

Benign Childhood Epilepsy with Centrotemporal Spikes

In benign childhood epilepsy with centralized spikes the seizures consist of brief hemifacial motor seizures frequently with associated somatosensory systems, usually occur at night, and sometimes become generalized. The onset is between 3 and 13 years of age, and as a rule, spontaneous recovery occurs during adolescence. There is often a genetic predisposition, and the EEG shows blunt high-voltage centrotemporal spikes often followed by slow waves that are activated by sleep. Occasionally, these discharges shift from side to side. Symptoms of childhood migraine with headaches or abdominal complaints frequently coexist with benign partial epilepsies.

Childhood epilepsies with occipital paroxysms were first described by Gastaut[11] and share some characteristics with the centrotemporal spike epilepsies, including age of onset, proclivity to migraine, and relative benignity, although the prognosis is in general not as favorable as in centrotemporal spike epilepsy. The seizures usually begin with visual symptoms (unilateral or bilateral loss of vision, teichopsia or hallucinations), followed by hemiclonic seizures or automatisms. The EEG is characterized by high-amplitude spikes or sharp waves that rhythmically occur in posterior head regions but are seen only with the eyes closed.

Idiopathic Generalized Epilepsy Syndromes

Idiopathic generalized epilepsy syndromes generally show an age relationship. Although many syndromes occurring in childhood have been described,[12] a few idiopathic generalized epilepsy syndromes are described here in detail to stress the characteristics of the syndromes and also because some of these symptoms tend to overlap. With increasing age, some symptoms become relatively de-emphasized, and others emerge.

Benign Neonatal Familial Convulsions

Although the syndrome of benign neonatal familial convulsions is relatively rare, it does demonstrate a dominant inheritance and represents one of the very few benign forms of neonatal seizures.[13] Recent interest in this syndrome has been rekindled because of the finding that there appears to be a gene locus on chromosome 20 associated with this condition.[6] There are no specific EEG criteria. About 14% of infants with benign neonatal familial convulsions develop a generalized epilepsy later in life.

Benign Myoclonic Epilepsy in Infancy

Benign myoclonic epilepsy in infancy begins with myoclonus during the first or second year of life on the background of a family history. The

EEG background is normal but shows bursts of generalized spike and wave or polyspike and wave occurring during the early stages of sleep. Seizures are easily controlled with appropriate therapy.[14]

Pyknoleptic Petit Mal (Childhood Absence) Epilepsy
Pyknoleptic petit mal epilepsy represents the paradigm of nonconvulsive generalized epilepsy. The peak incidence is between 6 and 7 years of age, there is a strong genetic predisposition, and there is a female preponderance. Attacks occur many times a day (*pyknos* refers to crowding). The EEG is characterized by bilateral synchronous, symmetric, three-cycle-per-second spikes and waves with a normal interictal background. Generalized tonic-clonic seizures may occur, particularly during adolescence. In older children, absence status may be seen, although the prognosis is characteristically for resolution of the seizures by puberty. Absence attacks may be precipitated or augmented by hyperventilation and hypoglycemia, and there is occasionally photic sensitivity. The individual seizures are characterized by cessation of ongoing activities, a blank stare, a brief upward rotation of the eyes and sometimes changes in postural tone, the association of mild clonic components, and frequently automatism.[15, 16]

Juvenile Absence Epilepsy
The individual seizures in juvenile absence epilepsy are the same as in pyknolepsy, but the age at manifestation is around puberty, and the seizure frequency is considerably lower, with absences occurring less frequently than every day. An association with generalized tonic-clonic seizures is frequent, and these may precede the manifestation of absence. Characteristically, the convulsive seizures occur near the time of awakening from sleep. The spike and wave bursts seen on EEG are frequently at a rate more rapid than three per second.[17]

Juvenile Myoclonic Epilepsy
One of the chief interests in the syndrome of juvenile absence is that there appears to be a considerable overlap between it, juvenile myoclonic epilepsy (the syndrome of Janz), and generalized tonic-clonic convulsions near the time of awakening. These conditions occur together quite frequently, but the age at which these manifestations occur tends to vary, with juvenile absence occurring early in adolescence, juvenile myoclonic epilepsy occurring later in adolescence, and generalized convulsions on awakening occurring at any age but more often later, when this syndrome occurs in isolation. The EEG manifestations are similar in the three conditions. If familial photic sensitivity epilepsy, with its female preponderance, is excluded, both sexes are affected equally.[18, 19, 20]

In juvenile myoclonic epilepsy, the invariable symptom is myoclonic seizures that frequently occur in the mornings. The myoclonus is particularly prominent in the upper extremities and upper trunk. Many patients complain of morning jitters or clumsiness because of the myoclonus, which is often contributed to by sleep deprivation and emotional stress.[21] Whereas the response to appropriate drug therapy is excellent, medication is probably required on a lifelong basis, because there is a tendency for recurrence when medication is discontinued.

One of the intriguing investigative aspects of this condition is the place it has in the human genome. There is evidence favoring the sixth chromosome as the genomic localization for this condition.[5]

The Cryptogenic Generalized Epilepsies

West's Syndrome (Infantile Spasms)   Classically, West's syndrome[22] begins between the ages of 4 and 7 months, affects boys more frequently than girls, and is characterized by the onset of infantile spasms, arrest of psychomotor development, and the EEG finding of hypsarrhythmia. In the truly cryptogenic group, prior neurologic development is normal, there is no evidence of a cause, and the condition usually responds to the administration of corticotropin, although the prognosis remains guarded.[23, 24]

Phenotypically similar seizures may be seen in a condition that begins early and frequently has a known associated cause, a less benign course after treatment, and a frequent progression into the Lennox-Gastaut syndrome. The severe and symptomatic variety is often referred to as "atypical West's syndrome."

Lennox-Gastaut Syndrome   Lennox-Gastaut syndrome[25, 26] is characterized by seizures that usually occur between the ages of 1 and 8 years. These seizures are typically axial tonic seizures, atypical absence with more severe and prolonged changes in postural tone than is usually seen with absence seizures, and frequent atonic or drop attacks. Generalized tonic-clonic seizures and partial seizures may also occur in these patients, whose attacks are characteristically extremely difficult to treat and frequently occur in the form of status epilepticus with stupor, myoclonia, and tonic and atonic seizures resistant to most presently available medications. The EEG characteristics are those of an abnormal, slow background with slow spike waves, diffuse anteriorly accentuated and frequently associated multifocal abnormalities. During sleep, bursts of fast rhythms occur. Mental retardation is the rule.

Symptomatic Epilepsies Characterized by Partial Seizures

The majority of epilepsies seen in association with focal brain lesions result in seizures whose characteristics are those resulting from lesions or irritations of the area of involvement. There are relatively few specific symptomatic epilepsy syndromes in that the syndromic characteristics are imparted by the disease under consideration rather than the specific epilepsy. One example is epilepsy partialis continua of the Rasmussen type, which is thought to be caused by chronic focal encephalitis; the seizures are characteristically partial seizures with motor phenomena that begin as focal fragmentary seizures and later become more diffuse, persisting during sleep, and associated with a progressive motor deficit and mental retardation.

Sometimes seizure symptomatology and anatomic site impart characteristics that are so specific and diagnostic as to warrant the appellation of syndrome. This is particularly true of temporal lobe epilepsy and frontal lobe epilepsy. The seizure types and patterns; the accompanying symptomatology; the frequent antecedent event, such as prolonged febrile seizures for temporal lobe epilepsy; and prognostic features render these identifiable syndromes and not individual seizure varieties.

Thus, temporal lobe epilepsy is characterized by simple or complex partial seizures with or without secondary generalization or a progression from one to the other. A history of febrile seizures is common; memory disturbances may occur; onset is frequently in childhood or young adulthood; and seizures occur periodically, in clusters, or randomly. On metabolic imaging studies, hypometabolism is frequently seen in the affected temporal lobe. The actual seizure content depends on anatomic involvement—that is, whether the amygdalohippocampal or the lateral temporal areas are predominantly involved.

Frontal lobe epilepsies are characterized by simple partial, complex partial, or secondarily generalized seizures. In frontal lobe epilepsies, partial seizures occur frequently, very rapidly, and generalize, or there may be a combination of these. Seizures frequently occur several times a day and may occur in sleep. Status epilepticus is particularly frequent. The seizures may be mistaken for psychogenic seizures. Postictally, confusion is less than with temporal lobe seizures. Again, the individual seizure symptoms vary with site of origin, whether cingulate, supplementary motor, frontopolar, orbitofrontal, or perirolandic. Other symptoms typical of lesions in the affected brain areas impart the remainder of the syndromic characteristics to the clinical picture.

Symptomatic Epilepsies with Generalized Seizures

Symptomatic epilepsies with generalized seizures result from specific brain diseases whose epileptic manifestations present as generalized seizures but whose prognosis and disease characteristics are predicated on the nature of the underlying condition. Examples of underlying conditions include the following:

1. *Malformations.* Aicardi syndrome,[27] which is confined to females, is associated with retinal lacunae, absence of corpus callosum, and infantile spasms with an EEG showing asynchronous hypsarrhythmia. Lissencephaly is characterized by axial hypotonia and infantile spasms, frequently by facial abnormalities, and by specific cerebral changes on imaging studies. The individual phacomatoses, particularly tuberous sclerosis, may be associated with hypsarrhythmia and infantile spasms.

2. *Metabolic disorders.* Metabolic abnormalities may manifest as infantile spasms or myoclonus, usually beginning in the first weeks or months of life and include the amino acidurias, the cerebral lipidoses, and ceroid lipofuscinosis.

3. *Progressive myoclonic epilepsies.* Progressive myoclonic epilepsy may be due to Lafora's disease, usually occurring between ages 6 and 19 years and characterized by generalized tonic-clonic seizures with frequent association of myoclonus, partial seizures with visual symptoms, and progressive mental deterioration.[28, 29] Unverricht-Lundborg disease occurs in a similar age group with rather prominent myoclonus-associated cerebellar ataxia and a progressive course that is rather slower than that of Lafora's disease.[30, 31] Dyssynergia cerebellaris myoclonica (Ramsey Hunt syndrome) occurs at a slightly later age, is less likely to be associated with convulsive seizures, and the myoclonus is characteristically a startle or action myoclonus. Mental deterioration is uncommon, and most of the neurologic manifestations are limited to the cerebellar signs. A neuraminidase deficiency leading to sialidosis behaves rather similarly; there is frequently amblyopia and the presence of a cherry red spot on funduscopic examination.

Some of the myoclonic epilepsies have a genetic basis characterized by female transmission and are associated with mitochondrial changes resulting from enzyme defects in the respiratory chain. They are diagnostically characterized by the presence of ragged-red fibers on muscle biopsy as a manifestation of the myoclonus epilepsy with ragged-red fibers (MERRF) syndrome.[32]

These examples illustrate the rationale for a syndromic classification that includes the pragmatic goal of furnishing a definitive treatment plan. Such a plan should include much more than the administration of the appropriate medication. It should include some inkling of whether one is dealing with a relatively benign condition such as febrile convulsions, benign childhood epilepsy, or pyknoleptic petit mal, all of which allow of an early discontinuation of medication, or whether one is dealing with a severe symptomatic or lesional epilepsy, in which life-long medication administration must be expected or the option of a surgical intervention entertained. The diagnosis of a juvenile myoclonic epilepsy, which carries a very good prognosis for response to medication, at the same time implies the need for continuing medication because of the high relapse rate despite the relatively benign outcome.

Analyses of this sort are particularly significant in circumstances where early termination of treatment may improve the outcome of pregnancy and where such decisions can be made on the basis of knowledge concerning the syndrome under treatment. Knowledge about the condition may also aid in genetic counseling and in the further elaboration of information that could potentially lead to localization of the epilepsy in the human genome. Any prediction of outcome is predicated on the nature of the underlying condition, of which the epileptic seizure is the symptom the patient brings to the physician.

References

1. Temkin O. The Falling Sickness: A History of Epilepsy from the Greeks to the Beginnings of Modern Neurology (2nd ed). Baltimore: Johns Hopkins University Press, 1971.
2. Commission on Classification and Terminology of the International League Against Epilepsy. Proposal for Revised Clinical and Electroencephalographic Classification of Epileptic Seizures. Epilepsia 1981;22:489.
3. Commission on Antiepileptic Drugs of the International League Against Epilepsy. Guidelines for Clinical Evaluation of Antiepileptic Drugs. Epilepsia 1989;30:400.
4. Commission on Classification and Terminology of the International League Against Epilepsy. Proposal for Revised Classification of Epilepsies and Epileptic Syndromes. Epilepsia 1989;30:389.
5. Greenberg DA, Delgado-Escueta AV, Maldonado HM, Widelitz H. Segregation analysis of juvenile myoclonic epilepsy. Genet Epidemiol 1988;5:81.

6. Leppert M, Anderson VE, Quattlebaum T, et al. Benign familial neonatal convulsions linked to genetic markers on chromosome 20. Nature 1988;337:647.
7. Roger J, Dravet C, Bureau M. In J Roger, C Dravet, M Bureau, et al. (eds), Epileptic Syndromes in Infancy, Childhood and Adolescence. London: John Libbey Eurotext, 1984.
8. Fejerman N, Medina CS. Convulsiones en la Infancia (2nd ed). Buenos Aires: El Ateneo, 1986.
9. Beaussart M. Benign epilepsy of children with rolandic (centro-temporal) paroxysmal foci: a clinical entity. Study of 221 cases. Epilepsia 1972;13:793.
10. Blom S, Heijbel J, Bergfass IG. Benign epilepsy of children with centrotemporal electrographic foci. Epilepsia 1972;13:609.
11. Gastaut H. A new type of epilepsy: benign partial epilepsy of childhood with occipital spike waves. Clin Electroencephalogr 1982;13:13.
12. Ogunyemi AO, Dreifuss FE. Syndromes of epilepsy in childhood and adolescence. J Child Neurol 1988;3:214.
13. Tibbles JAR. Dominant benign neonatal seizures. Devel Med Child Neurol 1980;22:664.
14. Dravet C, Bureau M, Roger J. Benign Myoclonic Epilepsy in Infants. In J Roger, C Dravet, M Bureau, et al. (eds), Epileptic Syndromes in Infancy, Childhood and Adolescence. London: John Libbey Eurotext, 1985.
15. Drury I, Dreifuss FE. Pyknoleptic petit mal. Acta Neurol Scand 1985;72:353.
16. Loiseau P. Childhood Absence Epilepsy. In J Roger, C Dravet, M Bureau, et al. (eds), Epileptic Syndromes in Infancy, Childhood and Adolescence. London: John Libbey Eurotext, 1985.
17. Wolf P. Juvenile Absence Epilepsy. In J Roger, C Dravet, M Bureau, et al. (eds), Epileptic Syndromes in Infancy, Childhood and Adolescence. London: John Libbey Eurotext, 1985;242.
18. Asconape J, Penry JK. Some clinical and EEG aspects of benign juvenile myoclonic epilepsy. Epilepsia 1984;25:108.
19. Delgado-Escueta AV, Enrile-Bascal F. Juvenile myoclonic epilepsy of Janz. Neurology 1984;34:285.
20. Janz D, Christian W. Impulsive-petit mal. Dtsch Z Nervenheilkd 1957;176:346.
21. Wolf P. Juvenile Myoclonic Epilepsy. In J Roger, C Dravet, M Bureau, et al. (eds), Epileptic Syndromes in Infancy, Childhood and Adolescence. London: John Libbey Eurotext, 1985.
22. West WJ. On a peculiar form of infantile convulsions. Lancet 1841;1:724.
23. Jeavons PM, Bower BD. Infantile Spasms. A Review of the Literature and a Study of 112 Cases. London: Heinemann, 1964.
24. Lacy JR, Penry JK. Infantile Spasms. New York: Raven, 1976.
25. Chevrie JJ, Aicardi J. Childhood epileptic encephalopathy with slow spike wave. A statistical study of 80 cases. Epilepsia 1972;13:259.
26. Gastaut H, Roger J, Soulayrol R, et al. Childhood epileptic encephalopathy with diffuse slow spike-waves (otherwise known as "petit mal variant" or Lennox syndrome). Epilepsia 1966;7:139.

27. Aicardi J. The Syndrome of Callosal Agenesis, Choroidal Lacunae and Infantile Spasms (Aicardi syndrome). In G Wise, M Blaw, PG Procopis (eds), Topics in Child Neurology (Vol. 2). New York: Spectrum, 1962;205.
28. Janeway R, Ravens JR, Pearce LA. Progressive myoclonic epilepsy with Lafora bodies: clinical, genetic, histopathological and biochemical study. Arch Neurol 1967;16:565.
29. Van Heycopten Ham MW, De Jager H. Progressive myoclonic epilepsy with Lafora bodies. Clinical and pathological features. Epilepsia 1963;4:95.
30. Koskiniemi M, Donner M, Majuri H, et al. Progressive myoclonus epilepsy: a clinical and histopathological study. Acta Neurol Scand 1974;50:307.
31. Koskiniemi M, Toivakka E, Donner M. Progressive myoclonus epilepsy: electroencephlographic findings. Acta Neurol Scand 1974;50:333.
32. Berkovic SF, Andermann F, Carpenter S, et al. Progressive myoclonus epilepsies. Specific causes and diagnosis. N Engl J Med 1986;315:296.

3

A Rational Approach to the Management of Epilepsy

Norman L. Pflaster and Timothy A. Pedley

Introduction

Current and future changes in the delivery of health care in the United States will surely affect patients with epilepsy. It is increasingly important to document that the management of patients with epilepsy, as other conditions, is based on medically sound, rational, and cost-effective considerations. Even with the enormous availability of technological devices now at our disposal, clinical data remain the cornerstones of diagnosis and management for patients with seizures and epilepsy.

This chapter provides an overview of one way of approaching patients with seizures or the possibility of a seizure disorder. Of course, it reflects our personal and institutional prejudices, and, while we hope it will be authoritative, is not meant to be authoritarian. We believe that the majority of patients with epilepsy can be initially managed with a minimum of costly measures. On the other hand, it is equally important to have criteria for identifying patients for more extensive testing and re-evaluation.

Is It a Seizure?

Not all paroxysmal events are epileptic in origin, and it is important to consider alternative diagnoses critically when confronted with a patient who has episodic symptoms that are equivocal for epilepsy.[1, 2] This is frequently the case, for example, when the history is ambiguous, incomplete, or open to different interpretations. Implicit in classifying an event as a seizure is the understanding that a given constellation of symptoms and signs is caused by a specific pathophysiologic mechanism: a (usually) self-limited, abnormally excessive, synchronous discharge of a population of cortical neurons and, to a variable degree, of the subcortical neurons to which they project. The clinical electrophysiologic correlates of these cerebral events can usually be recorded by an electroencephalogram (EEG).

In evaluating a patient with possible epilepsy, it is useful to consider other conditions that, depending on the patient's age and symptomatology, can be mistaken for seizures (Table 3-1). These other paroxysmal disorders may be difficult to distinguish from epilepsy on the basis of historical information alone, but awareness of them and of their most distinguishing characteristics assists in avoiding misdiagnosis.

Syncope is one of the most common causes of fading or complete loss of consciousness.[3] In all forms of syncope, symptoms result from a sudden and critical decrease in cerebral perfusion. Cardiovascular causes are most common and include hypotension (often from a failing myocardium), arrhythmias, and direct cardiac inhibition (carotid sinus syndrome, Valsalva-related). An especially common form of syncope (vasovagal, or neurocardiogenic, syncope) results when hypotension and bradycardia develop as abnormal responses from activation of myocardial mechanoreceptors.[4] Syncope can also occur when vasomotor tone is altered by emotional states, autonomic and peripheral neuropathies, peripheral vascular disease, postural changes, and a variety of medications. The nature of the patient's fall (typically more of a swoon or limp collapse) is usually easily distinguished from a generalized tonic-clonic seizure. Other important features that help differentiate syncope from an epileptic seizure are the character of prodromal symptoms, clinical evolution of the attack, and rate of recovery. At times, a few generalized clonic movements or brief tonic stiffening occur with syncopal episodes, so-called convulsive syncope,[5] and this juxtaposition can complicate the diagnostic problem.

Panic attacks (panic disorder) and *anxiety attacks* with hyperventilation (generalized anxiety disorder with autonomic hyperactivity) are

Table 3-1. Differential Diagnosis of Seizures and Epilepsy

Neonates and infants
    Jitteriness and benign myoclonus
    Apnea
    Shuddering attacks
    Gastroesophageal reflux
Young children
    Breathholding spells
    Infantile syncope
    Parasomnias
    Benign paroxysmal vertigo
    Tics and habit spasms
    Rage attacks
Adolescents and adults
    Movement disorders
        Myoclonus
        Paroxysmal choreoathetosis
    Migraine
        Confusional
        Vertebrobasilar
    Syncope and cardiac arrhythmias
    Hyperventilation syndrome
    Panic attacks
    Narcolepsy and sleep apnea
        Automatic behavior syndrome
        Partial cataplexy
    Transient global amnesia
    Transient ischemic attacks
    Acute confusional states
    Psychogenic seizures

Source: Reproduced with permission from TA Pedley. The Challenge of Intractable Epilepsy. In D Chadwick (ed), New Trends in Epilepsy Management: The Role of Gabapentin. Royal Society of Medicine Symposium Series No. 198. London: Royal Society of Medicine, 1993;3.

often unrecognized in our experience. In both conditions, symptoms can superficially mimic partial seizures with affective or special sensory symptoms. With panic attacks, patients commonly report "lack of oxygen" or a suffocating sensation, often with choking; dizziness; racing heart beat or palpitations; trembling or shaking; a feeling of detachment or depersonalization; fear, especially of dying or "going crazy"; and gastrointestinal discomfort, including nausea or cramping. Hyperventilation episodes can be similar, and the overbreathing may not be obvious unless specifically looked for. The most common complaints are of dizziness, a sense of floating or levitation, feelings of anxiety, epigastric or substernal discomfort, muscle twitching or spasms (tetany), flushing or chills, and blanking out ("my mind goes blank"). Symptoms can be reproduced by hyperventilation in the office or clinic. If sufficiently prolonged and intense, hyperventilation may result in syncope.

In epilepsy monitoring units, *psychogenic seizures* account for a significant number of admissions, perhaps 30% in some cases[6, 7] (TS Walczak, personal communication). Definitive diagnosis of psychogenic seizures on the basis of historical data alone is usually not possible. Clues include a personal or family history of psychiatric disorder and a precipitant with strong emotional or psychological overlay. Repeatedly normal interictal EEGs (which include sleep and anterior temporal leads) in the face of frequent and medically refractory seizure episodes should suggest the diagnosis. Although violent flailing or thrashing of arms and legs, especially when movements are asynchronous or arrhythmic, and pelvic thrusting are considered "classic" signs of hysterical seizures,[8–10] similar phenomena can be seen during partial seizures of frontal lobe origin.[8, 11, 12] Preserved consciousness with sustained motor activity of the arms and legs is rare in epilepsy. Nonetheless, observation of an attack, even by an experienced observer, will accurately differentiate epileptic from psychogenic seizures no more than 50–80% of the time.[13] Thus, for many patients, a secure diagnosis of psychogenic seizures can be made only during a period of intensive inpatient monitoring using simultaneous video/EEG recordings. Careful analysis of the patient's behavior during a typical attack and correlation of the behavioral characteristics with simultaneous EEG activity permit definitive classification of such episodes most of the time.[8, 14] It must be remembered, however, that psychogenic seizures and epileptic seizures can coexist in the same patient, although one or the other usually predominates at any given time. Therefore, recording a nonepileptic attack in a patient with uncontrolled seizures does not, by itself, prove that all of the patient's seizures are psychogenic. It is essential to verify with the patient and family that the spontaneously recorded seizures determined to be psychogenic are typical of the habitual and disabling seizures experienced at home. Serum prolactin measurements may assist in classifying a seizure as psychogenic or epileptic if (1) the clinical behavior included bilateral convulsive movements that lasted more than 30 seconds; (2) the prolactin measurements are obtained within 15 minutes of the event and compared with interictal baseline levels drawn on a different day at the same time; and (3) values are established for what constitutes a significant rise.[15, 16]

Some types of *sleep disorders* can mimic epilepsy. In children, confusion arises most often with the parasomnias (somniloquy, somnambulism, night terrors, and enuresis).[17] In adults, the automatic behavior syndrome, which often accompanies excessive daytime somnolence and is the result of repeated episodes of microsleep that impair performance and vigilance, can result in periods of altered mental function, awareness of "lost time" having elapsed, detached behavior that seems out of touch with the environment, and amnesia.[18] Historical features that help distinguish the automatic behavior syndrome from complex partial seizures include absence of an aura or changes in affect, rarity of alimentary automatisms, and lack of postictal symptoms.[19]

Because of its protean manifestations, migraine can occasionally be confused with epilepsy. This is especially likely in children, in whom headache may be relatively inconspicuous with some presentations. Basilar artery migraine can manifest with episodic confusion and disorientation, lethargy, mood changes, alterations in and even loss of consciousness, vertigo, ataxia, and bilateral visual disturbances.[20-23] In children, migraine may take the form of cyclical vomiting with or without nausea, signs of vasomotor instability (flushing, pallor, mydriasis), and photophobia.[24] In atypical cases of migraine, a careful history will usually reveal recurrent association with at least mild headache and a family history suggesting migraine.

To Treat or Not to Treat?

Although there can be little doubt that drug treatment is indicated and beneficial for most patients with epilepsy, there are certain circumstances when antiepileptic drugs may be reasonably deferred or used for only a limited time. The common issues in such cases are (1) the probability of seizure recurrence; (2) the likelihood of substantial psychosocial, vocational, or physical consequences with further seizures;

and (3) whether the benefit to be derived from treatment substantially outweighs the chance of treatment-related side effects or inconvenience.

Acute Symptomatic Seizures

Acute symptomatic seizures are seizures caused by or associated with an acute medical or neurologic illness. The most common example of acute symptomatic seizures is febrile seizures in children (see Chapter 8), but other frequently encountered causes include metabolic or toxic encephalopathies (e.g., uremia, hypo- and hyperglycemic states, hepatic failure, drug withdrawal) and acute brain infections (encephalitis and meningitis). To the extent there is no underlying permanent brain damage, these seizures are usually self-limited. The primary therapeutic concerns in such patients should be identification and treatment of the underlying disorder. If antiepileptic drugs are used to suppress seizures acutely, they generally do not need to be continued after the patient has recovered. One caveat that should be remembered, however, is that the presence of a precipitating medical illness (e.g., uremia, hypoglycemia, hepatic failure, drug withdrawal) does not necessarily exclude the need to search for a pathologic condition in the brain. This is because underlying brain lesions increase the risk for acute symptomatic seizures (as well as epilepsy) in appropriate settings.[25]

The issue of treating acute symptomatic seizures that occur in the setting of stroke, head injury, neurosurgical procedures, and alcohol use is more complicated. Each of these is a significant risk factor both for acute symptomatic seizures as well as for epilepsy.[26] Although antiepileptic drugs can be effective in treating seizures acutely, they may not delay or reduce the development of later epilepsy. This has been shown most clearly for seizures after a head injury. For example, phenytoin is highly effective in suppressing seizures in the first week or so after head injury, but it is ineffective when continued prophylactically to prevent the development of posttraumatic epilepsy.[27] The association between alcohol and seizures is also complicated. Whereas acute alcohol withdrawal can trigger self-limited seizures that do not require treatment, chronic alcohol abuse is a major risk factor for epilepsy.[28] Thus, many alcoholics may, over time, have both acute symptomatic seizures and recurrent unprovoked seizures (epilepsy).[29, 30]

In our view, therefore, the approach to patients who have acute symptomatic seizures as well as a substantially increased risk for later epilepsy should be based on the need to suppress active seizures, not on the hope that epilepsy may be prevented. This approach is supported not only by clinical experience and the results of a limited number of clinical trials, but also by experimental evidence regarding the mechanisms of action of antiepileptic drugs now available. For the most part, current antiepileptic drugs are effective seizure suppressants but most do not appear to affect the development of epilepsy. That is, drugs such as carbamazepine and phenytoin are good anticonvulsants but seem to be ineffective antiepileptogenic agents.[31]

Benign Epilepsy Syndromes

Several electroclinical syndromes are now recognized that are characterized by seizure onset in childhood, absence of clinical or neuroimaging evidence of structural pathologic entities in the brain, relatively infrequent seizures, and a uniformly good prognosis for complete remission in mid- to late adolescence without long-term behavioral or cognitive problems. The most common and best characterized of these syndromes is benign focal epilepsy of childhood with central-midtemporal sharp waves.[32, 33] Other similar syndromes include benign partial epilepsy with occipital spike waves,[34] benign epilepsy with affective symptoms,[35] and benign frontal epilepsy of childhood.[36] When evaluating a child with seizures, it is important to determine if the clinical and EEG criteria fit one of these benign syndromes because not all of these children need to be treated. The sole goal of treatment in such cases is to prevent recurrence. Because many children have only one or a few seizures, treatment is generally necessary only in cases where multiple seizures have occurred or if the parents or child are especially fearful of further episodes. In addition, we often treat very young children (7 or 8 years of age or younger) or those who have had several seizures with only a short interval between them because these appear to be settings that increase the risk of multiple recurrences. It is a mistake, in our view, to treat until the EEG normalizes, because interictal abnormalities will persist, in the majority of cases, long after seizures have remitted clinically.

The Single Unprovoked Seizure

The majority of patients come to medical attention having had more than one seizure. About 30% of patients with unprovoked seizures, however, are seen by a physician having had only a single attack, virtually always a generalized tonic-clonic convulsion. For this group of patients, it is reasonable to consider whether treatment is indicated (see Chapter 9). Estimates of recurrence after a first unprovoked seizure vary widely, from 16% to 67%,[37–40] mainly because of differences in ascertainment methods and in the length of the interval between seizure and medical contact. We believe that the data of Hauser et al.[38] and Shinnar et al.[40] clearly establish low- and high-risk groups for recurrence after a single unprovoked seizure. The risk of further seizures is greatly increased by an abnormal EEG, a history of significant brain injury, and a family history of epilepsy. Conversely, patients without any of these factors have a lower risk of recurrence.

Until recently, an important issue in treatment decisions was the absence of data indicating any beneficial effect of treatment on preventing recurrences. Now, a large, multicenter, randomized study from Italy clearly shows that antiepileptic drug therapy reduces the risk of relapse following a first unprovoked generalized tonic-clonic seizure.[41] Among 397 patients ranging in age from 2 to 76 years, treated patients seen within 7 days of the first seizure had a recurrence rate of 25% at 2 years. In contrast, untreated patients had a recurrence rate of 51%. If patients with previous "uncertain spells" were excluded from the analysis, treatment benefit was still evident, although the magnitude of the effect was reduced (recurrence rate of 30% for treated patients, 42% for untreated patients).

Thus, there is now evidence to justify treatment based on the positive effect of therapy on reducing relapse rate even in a low risk patient group. We still believe, however, that treatment should not be automatic for this group of patients. Treatment decisions should still involve a discussion and analysis of the benefits to be gained from treatment versus the potential risks or adverse effects of therapy. For example, about 30% of patients treated with antiepileptic drugs develop side effects severe enough to require a change in treatment. Furthermore, when, as in children, there are particular concerns about the effects of antiepileptic drugs on brain development, learning, and behavior,[42, 43] we tend to avoid or defer treatment, especially if the consequences of further seizures are judged to be insignificant. Finally, there is no evidence that early treatment alters the long-term prognosis for extended remission.

The Diagnostic Evaluation

Because epilepsy is a group of conditions and not a single homogeneous disorder, and because seizures may be symptoms of both diverse brain disorders and an otherwise normal nervous system, it is neither possi-

Table 3-2. Important Historical Features of Epileptic Seizures

First event in the seizure (aura, initial movement)

Subsequent evolution of the seizure

Postictal manifestations (Todd's paresis)

Is there more than one seizure type?

Has there been a change in the seizure pattern?

Date and circumstances of first attack

Subsequent precipitating or triggering factors (alcohol, sleep deprivation)

Age of onset, frequency of attacks, and longest seizure-free interval

Response to previous medication (doses, blood levels, combinations)

Family history (parents, offspring, siblings)

Is there a history of neonatal seizures or febrile seizures?

Is there a history of previous brain injury?

Is there personal or family history of other neurologic, mental, or systemic disease?

---

ble nor desirable to develop inflexible guidelines for what constitutes a "standard" or "minimal" set of diagnostic tests. The role of the physician is threefold: (1) to determine if epilepsy or seizures exist and not some alternative diagnosis; (2) to define, if possible, an underlying cause; and (3) to optimize treatment.

The clinical data from the history (Table 3-2) and physical examination should allow a reasonable determination of probable diagnosis, seizure and epilepsy classification, and the likelihood of an underlying pathologic condition in the brain. Based on these considerations, diagnostic testing should be undertaken selectively. Thus, a normal child with brief lapses of attention whose symptoms can be reproduced in the office by hyperventilation is a very different patient than a middle-aged man who has developed partial seizures that seem to be getting progressively worse. Furthermore, diagnostic testing is never a substitute for clinical judgment and observation through follow-up and re-examination.

Initial Diagnostic Studies

Bearing in mind the foregoing caveats, we believe that an EEG should be done in every case as an aid to diagnosis or to assist in classifying the seizure or epilepsy syndrome. In some instances, EEG findings will aid in prognosis and in determining the need for treatment. Routine blood tests are rarely diagnostically useful in healthy children and adults but are necessary in newborns and in older patients with acute or chronic systemic disease to detect abnormal electrolyte, glucose, calcium, and magnesium values and impaired liver or kidney function. Any suspicion of meningitis or encephalitis mandates lumbar puncture. We obtain brain imaging routinely on (1) children with abnormal development; (2) children with abnormal findings on physical examination; (3) children whose seizures are likely to be manifestations of symptomatic epilepsy; and (4) any patient older than age 18 years. We do not routinely obtain imaging on children with idiopathic epilepsy, including the benign focal epilepsy syndromes. Brain magnetic resonance imaging (MRI), although more costly, is much more sensitive than computed tomography (CT) in detecting potentially epileptogenic lesions such as cortical dysplasia, hamartomas, well differentiated glial tumors, and cavernous malformations.[44-46] Both axial and coronal planes should be imaged using both T1 and T2 sequences. Gadolinium enhancement does not appear to increase the sensitivity for detecting cerebral lesions, but it may be helpful in differentiating among possible causes.[47]

If, after reviewing all the clinical and laboratory data, the clinical picture remains confusing and there is still uncertainty regarding the diagnosis of seizure or epilepsy, we advocate a period of "watchful waiting" and close follow-up. In general, we advise against use of antiepileptic drugs as a diagnostic test because of the high placebo effect (about 30% in most controlled clinical trials) and the fact that few antiepileptic drugs are specific for epilepsy. Consider, for example, the widespread use of carbamazepine and valproate in treating psychiatric disorders.

Repeating Laboratory Tests

Blood Tests

Laboratory tests should be repeated only to answer specific questions. "Routine" blood monitoring is both costly (estimated at more than $400 million a year in the United States) and ineffective in avoiding serious toxicity.[48] The assumption that hepatic failure, aplastic anemia, or other severe drug reactions can be averted by frequent blood tests is not supported by any scientific data.[49] Minor elevations in liver alanine aminotransferase and aspartate aminotransferase occur in about 25–30% of patients with epilepsy; however, these neither correlate with clinical symptoms nor predict development of hepatitis or liver failure.[50-52] Gamma-glutamyl transferase levels seem to be particularly useless as indicators of clinically significant liver dysfunction in people with epilepsy.[51] Nearly 20% of patients taking carbamazepine develop a benign leukopenia: white blood cell (WBC) counts below 4,000/ml.[52] A few patients will have WBC counts that drop transiently below 2,500/ml. The risk of developing aplastic anemia is not increased in this group, and no patients in this group have an increased rate of infections or other possible complications that might be attributed to leukopenia.[53, 54]

The entire issue of blood monitoring in patients with epilepsy has been critically reviewed by Pellock and Willmore,[49] and we endorse their views and recommendations. Especially in patients on monotherapy, we do not believe that asymptomatic patients require regular blood tests if initial screening laboratory studies were negative. On the other hand, an attempt should be made to identify patients, at the onset of therapy, who are at increased risk for adverse drug reactions. These include patients with known or suspected metabolic or biochemical disorders, a history of previous drug reactions, and medical illnesses affecting hematopoesis or liver and kidney function. Blood monitoring is also indicated in young children receiving multiple therapeutic agents that include valproate, and in patients who are unable to communicate symptoms and their health status effectively.

Similarly, routine measurement of plasma antiepileptic drug levels is not necessary in the majority of patients. Although therapeutic drug monitoring has been a major advance in helping determine compliance, in compensating for physiologic (age, pregnancy) or disease-related alterations in drug pharmacokinetics, and in avoiding undesirable drug interactions, drug levels must be interpreted in light of a patient's clinical progress. For example, therapeutic effectiveness is best judged by two measures of clinical effect: seizure frequency and the appearance of toxic side effects. All too often, however, the blood level, rather than the patient, becomes the goal of treatment: Therapy must be optimal if a drug's blood concentration is in the "therapeutic range." This oversimplified view, encountered all too often in our experience, can have undesirable consequences. First, it is not uncommon for low or "therapeutic" blood levels to be cited as evidence against a patient's complaint of side effects. Conversely, drug dosage is frequently reduced because of a "toxic" level even though there has been good seizure control and no indication of adverse reactions.

Neuroimaging

If the initial MR scan was interpreted as normal, brain imaging need not be repeated if seizures are controlled and the patient is neurologically normal. In patients with uncontrolled seizures, a MR scan is necessary even if multiple previous CT scans were interpreted as normal. We also advise obtaining a follow-up MR scan after about 12 months for patients whose first scan appeared normal but who are not doing as well as expected. Repeat MR scans are also necessary at an interval determined by the patient's clinical progress in two other situations: (1) if the first scan showed an equivocal abnormality or finding; and (2) if an experienced neuroradiologist concludes, on review, that the initial scan was not technically sufficient to exclude such epileptogenic lesions as cavernous malformations and cortical dysplasia.

Electroencephalographic Studies

Routinely obtaining follow-up EEGs every 6–12 months is useless. Any EEG performed after the first should be framed around a specific question. For example, if there is a need to detect epileptiform discharges for diagnostic or classification purposes, repeating the EEG up to three times (but not more) will increase the yield of positive studies.[55] Follow-up EEGs in children with absence seizures or infantile spasms may be more sensitive than casual observation in determining if optimal therapy has been achieved.[56-58] EEG recording may also be helpful in determining if a decline in the patient's behavior or mental function is the result of subclinical seizures, drug toxicity, or a progressive neurologic syndrome. Finally, EEG findings may be an important predictor of success when drug withdrawal is being contemplated for patients whose seizures are in remission.[59-61] It is important to recognize, however, that with rare exceptions (see above), routine EEG findings cannot be used by themselves to measure the success of treatment or to gauge a given patient's susceptibility to further seizures.

Initiating Treatment

Although details of treatment and relevant clinical pharmacologic issues are dealt with in detail in later chapters, there are several aspects of therapy that require comment here. First, drug choice should be based primarily on the patient's type(s) of seizure(s), modified as necessary by considerations of cost and dosing requirements and other factors that might affect compliance. Two large, multicenter, Veterans Administration collaborative studies have investigated the comparative efficacy and side effects of drugs used in treating partial and secondarily generalized seizures.[62, 63] Carbamazepine, phenytoin, primidone, and phenobarbital were equipotent in terms of anticonvulsant effect, but carbamazepine and phenytoin were considerably more successful overall because they produced fewer sedative and cognitive side effects and were thus associated with greater patient acceptance.[62] Valproate was as effective as carbamazepine, and presumably phenytoin, in treating secondarily generalized seizures but less effective in treating complex partial seizures.[63] Valproate can be used as effective monotherapy for the majority of patients with primary generalized seizures, and it is a particularly advantageous drug when several generalized-onset seizure types coexist. Ethosuximide is as effective as valproate in treating absence seizures, but it has little or no effect on generalized tonic-clonic or myoclonic seizures. Carbamazepine and phenytoin are nearly as effective as valproate against generalized tonic-clonic seizures, but they are ineffective against, and may even exacerbate, myoclonic and absence seizures.

Second, treatment should start with a single drug, generally at low dosage. This is especially important in elderly patients.Only phenytoin and phenobarbital can reasonably be started at maintenance dosage. Valproate, primidone, and carbamazepine should be introduced at a low dose to avoid toxicity and then increased in increments determined by individual patient tolerance and knowledge of the drug's pharmacokinetics. It is our experience that many patients will not tolerate 200 mg bid of carbamazepine, which is the manufacturer's recommended starting dose, and we more often begin with an initial dose of 100 mg bid. Primidone has serious sedative effects in the majority of naive patients, and most will not be able to tolerate more than 125 mg, or even 50 mg, per day at first.

Third, the dose should be increased as necessary to produce seizure control or until side effects appear. Some patients on monotherapy will have no side effects and will derive increased therapeutic benefit from phenytoin plasma levels of 25 µg/ml or carbamazepine levels of 13–14 µg/ml. Such "high" concentrations may be necessary to suppress seizures optimally in some patients. If the first drug is ineffective, an appropriate alternative drug should be substituted. Addition of a second drug improves seizure control without increasing side effects in only about 15% of patients.[62, 64]

Finally, it is important to identify any environmental or physiologic factors that can lower an individual's seizure threshold to precipitate

Table 3-3. Factors Increasing the Risk of Seizures

Common
 Sleep deprivation
 Alcohol withdrawal
 Dehydration
 Drugs and drug interactions
 Systemic infection
 Trauma
 Malnutrition
Occasional
 Barbiturate withdrawal
 Hyperventilation
 Flashing lights
 Diet and missed meals
 Specific "reflex" triggers

Source: Reproduced with permission from TA Pedley. The Challenge of Intractable Epilepsy. In D Chadwick (ed), New Trends in Epilepsy Management: The Role of Gabapentin. Royal Society of Medicine Symposium Series No. 198. London: Royal Society of Medicine, 1993;3.

seizures under certain circumstances. Sleep deprivation and irregular sleep habits are especially common triggers for some types of epilepsy, but other factors may be important in individual patients (Table 3-3).[65, 66]

When Initial Medical Treatment Fails

Psychosocial Considerations

Overall, at least 30% of patients with epilepsy continue to have seizures despite optimal drug therapy (WA Hauser, personal communication), and fewer than 50% of adult patients with partial and secondarily generalized seizures will remain seizure-free for more than 12 months.[62, 67] Thus, it is important for the physician to help each patient develop realistic treatment goals and expectations regarding outcome of therapy. For example, even patients who do not become seizure-free can reasonably anticipate that proper treatment will reduce the frequency and severity of attacks without producing chronic drug toxicity. Patients should also expect help with rehabilitation and social adjustment. In general, the degree to which seizures will be controlled is established within the first 1–2 years of treatment.[67]

To what extent patients with continuing seizures are viewed as intractable or refractory depends largely on individual perceptions of disability.[2] Some patients with incompletely controlled seizures suffer relatively few functional consequences and lead nearly normal lives. Others may find their lives severely compromised even by relatively infrequent attacks. Psychosocial dysfunction, as expressed by difficulty in establishing interpersonal relationships, building self-esteem, and obtaining or maintaining employment, is high among patients with chronic epilepsy and contributes significantly to the disability arising from the physical limitations and disruptions in daily activities imposed by the seizures themselves.[68] Assisting patients and their families in developing strategies for improved coping while educating friends, teachers, coworkers, and employers about the persistent stigma and myths that surround epilepsy can help reduce functional disability.

Neurologic Issues

Although treatment failure is frequently the result of intrinsic, unmod-ifiable factors associated with the epileptic condition, persistent seizures are not uncommonly the result of remediable, exogenous causes. Any patient with uncontrolled seizures should, at some point, be re-evaluated regarding diagnosis. Psychogenic seizures in particu-lar are a notorious and frequent cause of intractability. Another issue that can contribute to medical refractoriness is failure to identify med-ical illnesses and treatments that can cause or contribute to recurrent seizures, such as systemic lupus erythematosus, hypoglycemia, drug abuse, and theophylline toxicity. Other factors contributing to inef-fective treatment include using drugs in insufficient amounts or admin-istering them inappropriately, unrecognized or unanticipated drug interactions, and noncompliance.

In helping patients and their families develop realistic treatment goals, it is important to identify, as early as possible, any predictors that suggest that complete seizure control may be unrealistic. Structural brain disease, in particular, has a high association with intractable epilepsy irrespective of whether the pathologic entity is focal or diffuse,

Table 3-4. Predictors of Intractability of Epilepsy

Seizure onset at less than 2 years of age

Frequent generalized seizures

Atonic, atypical absence seizures

Failure to achieve control readily (within 2 years)

Evidence of brain damage

Low intelligence

A specific etiology for the seizures

Severe electroencephalographic abnormality

Source: Modified from EA Rodin. The Prognosis of Patients with Epilepsy. Springfield, IL: Thomas, 1968;175; and reproduced with permission from TA Pedley. The Challenge of Intractable Epilepsy. In D Chadwick (ed), New Trends in Epilepsy Management: The Role of Gabapentin. Royal Society of Medicine Symposium Series No. 198. London: Royal Society of Medicine, 1993;3.

static or progressive. A number of definable syndromes are also associated with persistent seizures, including early myoclonic encephalopathy; early infantile epileptic encephalopathy (Ohtahara's syndrome); infantile spasms (West's syndrome); Lennox-Gastaut syndrome and myoclonic-astatic epilepsy of Doose; various progressive metabolic or degenerative encephalopathies, including adrenoleukodystrophy, ceroid lipofuscinosis, storage diseases (Tay-Sachs disease, sialidoses), and the progressive myoclonus epilepsies; epilepsia partialis continua (Rasmussen's syndrome); and otherwise unspecified lesional epilepsies, including temporal lobe epilepsy. Several generic factors are also generally accepted predictors of poor response to treatment (Table 3-4).

Concurrent Medical Illness

All patients with epilepsy will have a concurrent medical illness requiring treatment at some time. Whether benign and self-limited or severe and life-threatening, comorbidity can complicate seizure management.[69, 70] Phenylpropanolamine, for example, a common nonprescription ingredient in cold, sinus, and allergy remedies, can precipitate seizures in people with epilepsy. Propoxyphene, ibuprofen, isoniazid, erythromycin, cimetidine, verapamil, and diltiazem are examples of drugs that significantly increase concentrations of some antiepileptic drugs and lead to clinical toxicity. Phenothiazines, antihistamines, and tricyclic antidepressants may lead to seizure breakthroughs and loss of control.

Diseases affecting liver function can affect the biotransformation and disposition of antiepileptic drugs. Clinically significant effects, however, usually only appear with moderate to severe hepatic dysfunction. In such cases, antiepileptic drug dosing must be based on antiepileptic drug levels and clinical response. When hypoalbuminemia is present, total drug concentrations can be misleading; unbound ("free") drug levels are frequently necessary to interpret clinical effects. Renal insufficiency causes accumulation of some drugs or their metabolites, and uremia can have profound effects on protein binding and the ratio of unbound to bound drug. Both peritoneal dialysis and hemodialysis substantially reduce levels of phenobarbital, primidone, and ethosuximide but usually have relatively little effect on plasma concentrations of phenytoin and carbamazepine. Management in such circumstances is facilitated by determining drug levels before and after dialysis and giving supplement doses of antiepileptic drugs postdialysis as necessary to maintain stable blood concentrations.

The Role of the Comprehensive Epilepsy Center

The majority of patients with epilepsy are well cared for in their communities by primary care physicians and general neurologists. Some patients, however, benefit from referral to a specialized center offering multidisciplinary diagnostic and treatment services. Indications for such referrals include (1) continued diagnostic uncertainty whether a patient's symptoms are caused by epilepsy, (2) persistent seizures that remain uncontrolled after 1–2 years of reasonable treatment, (3) psychosocial dysfunction related to epilepsy, (4) availability of investigational drugs through clinical trials, and (5) special diagnostic needs (e.g., progressive neurologic syndrome) or treatment needs (e.g., status epilepticus).

Several studies have demonstrated that treatment at a comprehensive epilepsy center results in an improved outcome for carefully selected patients in terms of better seizure control, reduced drug-related toxicities, alternative or additional diagnoses, and gains in social adjustment.[71-73] Although specific cost-based data are currently lacking, available information strongly supports the conclusion that comprehensive epilepsy centers are the most efficient, medically appropriate, and cost-effective way to manage patients with intractable seizures. Epilepsy centers are also the usual sites for surgical evaluations and epilepsy surgery. Finally, much epilepsy-related research, both basic and clinical, is conducted at these centers.

Indications for referral and guidelines providing basic definitions of the scope and quality of services that should be provided at a comprehensive epilepsy center have been developed by the National Association of Epilepsy Centers.[74]

References

1. Pedley TA. Differential diagnosis of episodic symptoms. Epilepsia 1983;24(Suppl 1):S31.
2. Pedley TA. The Challenge of Intractable Epilepsy. In D Chadwick (ed), New Trends in Epilepsy Management: The Role of Gabapentin. Royal Society of Medicine Symposium Series No. 198. London: Royal Society of Medicine, 1993;3.
3. Kapoor WN, Karpf M, Wieand S, et al. A prospective evaluation and follow-up of patients with syncope. N Engl J Med 1983;309:197.
4. Sra JS, Mohammad RJ, Boaz A et al. Comparison of cardiac pacing with drug therapy in the treatment of neurocardiogenic (vasovagal) syncope with bradycardia or asystole. N Engl J Med 1993;328:1085.
5. Gastaut H. Electro-encephalographic study of syncope—its differentiation from epilepsy. Lancet 1957;2:1018.
6. Egli M, O'Kane M, Mothersill I, et al. Monitoring at the Swiss Epilepsy Center. In J Gotman, JR Ives, P Gloor (eds), Long-term Monitoring in Epilepsy (EEG Suppl. No. 37). Amsterdam: Elsevier, 1985;371.
7. Rowan AJ, Siegel M, Rosenbaum DH. Daytime intensive monitoring: comparison with prolonged intensive and ambulatory monitoring. Neurology 1987;37:481.
8. Desai BT, Porter RJ, Penry JK. A study of 42 attacks in six patients with intensive monitoring. Arch Neurol 1982;39:202.
9. Gulick TA, Spinks IP, King DW. Pseudoseizures: ictal phenomena. Neurology 1982;32:24.
10. Saygi S, Katz A, Marks DA, Spencer S. Frontal lobe partial seizures and psychogenic seizures: comparison of clinical and ictal characteristics. Neurology 1992;43:1274.
11. Waterman K, Purves SJ, Strauss E, Wada JA. An epileptic syndrome caused by mesial frontal lobe foci. Neurology 1987;37:577.
12. Williamson PD, Spencer DD, Spencer SS, et al. Complex partial seizures of frontal lobe origin. Ann Neurol 1985;18:497.
13. King DW, Gallagher BB, Murvin AJ, et al. Pseudoseizures: diagnostic evaluation. Neurology 1982;32:18.
14. Luther JS, McNamara JO, Carwile S, et al. Pseudoepileptic seizures: methods and video analysis to aid diagnosis. Ann Neurol 1982;12:458.

15. Pritchard PB, Wannamaker BB, Sagel J, Daniel CM. Serum prolactin and cortisol levels in evaluation of pseudoepileptic seizures. Ann Neurol 1985;18:87.
16. Sperling MR, Pritchard PB, Engel J Jr, et al. Prolactin in partial epilepsy: an indication of limbic seizures. Ann Neurol 1986;20:716.
17. Guilleminault C, Anders TF. Sleep Disorders in Children. In I Schulman (ed), Advances in Pediatrics (Vol. 29). Chicago: Year Book, 1976;151.
18. Guilleminault C, Billiard M, Montplaisir J, Dement WC. Altered states of consciousness in disorders of daytime sleepiness. J Neurol Sci 1975;26:377.
19. Tharp BR. Narcolepsy and Epilepsy. In C Guilleminault , WC Bement, P Passouant (eds), Narcolepsy. New York: Spectrum, 1976;262.
20. Bickerstaff ER. Basilar artery migraine. Lancet 1961;1:15.
21. Gascon G, Barlow C. Juvenile migraine presenting as an acute confusional state. Pediatrics 1970;45:628.
22. Lapkin ML, Golden GS. Basilar artery migraine. Am J Dis Child 1978;132:278.
23. Sturzenegger MH, Meienberg O. Basilar artery migraine: a follow-up study in 82 cases. Headache 1985;25:408.
24. Holguin J, Fenichel G. Migraine. J Pediatr 1967;70:290.
25. Hauser WA, Annegers JF. Risk Factors for Epilepsy. In VE Anderson, WA Hauser, IE Leppik et al. (eds), Genetic Strategies in Epilepsy Research. Amsterdam: Elsevier, 1991;45.
26. Hauser WA, Hesdorffer DC. Epilepsy—Frequency, Causes and Consequences. New York: Demos, 1990;53.
27. Temkin NR, Dikmen SS, Wilensky AJ, et al. A randomized, double blind study of phenytoin for the prevention of post-traumatic seizures. N Engl J Med 1990;323:497.
28. Ng SKC, Hauser WA, Brust JCM, Susser M. Alcohol consumption and withdrawal in new-onset seizures. N Engl J Med 1988;319:666.
29. Koppel BS, Daras M, Tuchman AJ, et al. The relation between alcohol and seizures in a city hospital population. J Epilepsy 1992;5:31.
30. Simon RD. Alcohol and seizures. N Engl J Med 1988;319:715.
31. Silver JM, Shin C, McNamara JO. Antiepileptogenic effects of conventional anti-convulsants in the kindling model of epilepsy. Ann Neurol 1991;29:356.
32. Lerman P, Kivity S. Benign focal epilepsy of childhood: a follow up study of 100 recovered patients. Arch Neurol 1975;32:261.
33. Lombroso CT. Sylvian seizures and mid-temporal spike foci in children. Arch Neurol 1967;17:52.
34. Gastaut H. A new type of epilepsy: benign partial epilepsy of childhood with occipital spike-waves. Clin Electroencephalogr 1982;13:13.
35. Dalla-Bernardina B, Bureau M, Dravet C, et al. Epilepsie bénigne de l'enfant avec crises à séméiologie affective. Rev EEG Neurophysiol 1980;10:8.
36. Beaumanoir A, Nahory A. Les epilepsies bénignes partielles: Il cas d'épilepsie partielle frontale à l'évolution favorable. Rev EEG Neurophysiol 1983;13:207.
37. Hart YM, Sander JWAS, Johnson AL, Shorvon SD. National general practice study of epilepsy: recurrence after a first seizure. Lancet 1990;336:1271.

38. Hauser WA, Rich SS, Annegers JF, Anderson VE. Seizure recurrence after a first unprovoked seizure: an extended follow-up. Neurology 1990; 40:1163.
39. Hopkins A, Garman A, Clarke C. The first seizure in adult life: value of clinical features, electroencephalography, and computerized tomographic scanning in prediction of seizure recurrence. Lancet 1988;1:721.
40. Shinnar S, Berg AT, Moshe SL, et al. The risk of seizure recurrence following a first unprovoked seizure. Pediatrics 1990;85:1076.
41. First Seizure Trial Group. Randomized clinical trial on the efficacy of antiepileptic drugs in reducing the risk of relapse after a first unprovoked tonic-clonic seizure. Neurology 1993;43:478.
42. Farwell JR, Lee YJ, Hirtz DR, et al. Phenobarbital for febrile seizures—effects on intelligence and on seizure recurrence. N Engl J Med 1990;322:364.
43. Serrano EE, Kunis DM, Ransom BR. Effects of chronic phenobarbital exposure on cultured mouse spinal cord neurons. Ann Neurol 1988;24:429.
44. Laster DW, Penry JK, Moody DM, et al. Chronic seizure disorders: contribution of MR imaging when CT is normal. AJNR Am J Neuroradiol 1985;6:177.
45. Latack JT, Abou-Khalil BW, Siegel GF, et al. Patients with partial seizures: evaluation by MR, CT and PET imaging. Radiology 1986;159:159.
46. Theodore WH, Dorwart R, Holmes M, et al. Neuroimaging in refractory partial seizures: comparison of PET, CT and MRI. Neurology 1986;36:750.
47. Cascino GD, Hirschorn KA, Jack CR, Sharbrough FW. Gadolinium-DPTA-enhanced magnetic resonance imaging in intractable partial epilepsy. Neurology 1989;39:1115.
48. Camfield P, Camfield C, Dooley J, et al. Routine screening of blood and urine for severe reactions to anticonvulsant drugs in asymptomatic patients is of doubtful value. Can Med Assoc J 1989;140:1303.
49. Pellock JM, Willmore LJ. A rational guide to routine blood monitoring in patients receiving antiepileptic drugs. Neurology 1991;41:961.
50. Dreifuss FE, Langer, DH, Moline KA, Maxwell JE. Valproic acid hepatic fatalities. II. US experience since 1984. Neurology 1989;39:201.
51. Krause KH. Side effects of antiepileptic drugs in long term treatment. Klin Wochenschr 1988;66:601.
52. Leppik IE, Jacobs MP, Loewenson, RB, Beskar AM. Detection of adverse events by routine laboratory testing. [Abstract.] Epilepsia 1990;31:640.
53. Hart RG, Easton JD. Carbamazepine and hematological monitoring. Ann Neurol 1982;11:309.
54. Pellock JM. Carbamazepine side effects in children and adults. Epilepsia 1987;28(Suppl 3):S64.
55. Salinsky M, Kanter R, Dasheiff RM. Effectiveness of multiple EEGs in supporting the diagnosis of epilepsy: an operational curve. Epilepsia 1987;28:331.
56. Browne TR, Penry JK, Porter RJ, Dreifuss FE. Responsiveness before, during and after spike-wave paroxysms. Neurology 1974;24:659.
57. Kellaway P, Hrachovy RA, Frost JD, Zion T. Precise characterization and quantification of infantile spasms. Ann Neurol 1979;6:214.

58. Penry JK, Porter RJ, Dreifuss FE. Simultaneous recording of absence seizures with video tape and electroencephalography. A study of 374 seizures in 48 patients. Brain 1975;98:4272.
59. Callaghan N, Garrett A, Goggin T. Withdrawal of anticonvulsant drugs in patients free of seizures for two years. N Engl J Med 1988;318:942.
60. Overweg J, Binnie CD, Oosting J, Rowan AJ. Clinical and EEG prediction of seizure recurrence following anti-epileptic drug withdrawal. Epilepsy Res 1987;1:272.
61. Shinnar S, Vining EFG, Mellits ED, et al. Discontinuing anti-epileptic medication in children with epilepsy after two years without seizures. N Engl J Med 1985;313:976.
62. Mattson RH, Cramer JA, Collins JF, et al. Comparison of carbamazepine, phenobarbital, phenytoin and primidone in partial and secondarily generalized tonic-clonic seizures. N Engl J Med 1985;313:145.
63. Mattson RH, Cramer JA, Collins JF. Comparison of valproate with carbamazepine for the treatment of complex partial seizures and secondarily generalized tonic-clonic seizures in adults. N Engl J Med 1992;327:765.
64. Shorvon SD, Reynolds EH. Unnecessary polypharmacy for epilepsy. Br Med J 1977;1:1635.
65. Aird RB. The importance of seizure-inducing factors in the control of refractory forms of epilepsy. Epilepsia 1983;224:567.
66. Bennett DR, Mattson RH, Ziter FA, et al. Sleep deprivation: neurologic and EEG effects. Aerospace Med 1964;35:888.
67. Elwes RDC, Johnson AL, Shorvon SD, Reynolds EH. The prognosis for seizure control in newly diagnosed epilepsy. N Engl J Med 1984;311:944.
68. Scambler G, Hopkins A. Being epileptic: coming to terms with stigma. Soc Health Illness 1986;8:26.
69. Scheuer ML. Medical Patients with Epilepsy. In SR Resor Jr, H Kutt (eds), The Medical Treatment of Epilepsy. New York: Marcel Dekker, 1992;557.
70. Scheuer ML. Medical Aspects of Managing Seizures and Epilepsy. In TA Pedley, BS Meldrum (eds), Recent Advances in Epilepsy (Vol. 5). Edinburgh: Churchill Livingstone. 1992;127.
71. O'Neill BP, Ladon B, Harris LM, et al. A comprehensive interdisciplinary approach to the care of the institutionalized epileptic. Epilepsia 1977;18:243.
72. Porter RJ, Penry JK, Lacy JR. Diagnostic and therapeutic re-evaluation of patients with intractable epilepsy. Neurology 1977;27:1006.
73. Sutula TP, Sackellares JC, Miller JQ, Dreifuss FE. Intensive monitoring in refractory epilepsy. Neurology 1981;31:243.
74. National Association of Epilepsy Centers. Recommended guidelines for diagnosis and treatment in specialized epilepsy centers. Epilepsia 1990;31(Suppl 1):S1.

4

Clinical Pharmacology and Pharmacokinetics of Antiepileptic Drugs

Thomas R. Browne

The basic processes of clinical pharmacology are absorption, distribution, biotransformation, excretion, and drug interactions. An understanding of these processes is essential for optimum administration of antiepileptic drugs.

Absorption

It is a basic principle of physical chemistry that "like dissolves like." Water is a polar compound and dissolves other polar compounds, such as weak acids and weak bases containing ionized groups. Water solubility is an essential quality for a drug to be dissolved in the gastrointestinal (GI) tract for absorption. Cell membranes and the blood–brain barrier are composed of lipids, and nonpolar molecules are most readily dissolved in (and therefore cross) these structures. These observations highlight a problem for central nervous system (CNS) drugs, which must be water-soluble for absorption and lipid-soluble for distribution into the CNS.

"Prompt" Versus Sustained-Release Preparations

"Prompt" preparations are rapidly dissolved and rapidly absorbed from the GI tract. This results in relatively rapid and high peak serum concentration values and relatively low trough serum concentration values. Sustained-release preparations release the drug into solution at a relatively slow rate. Standard sustained-release preparations (e.g., phenytoin [Dilantin], divalproex [Depakote]) attain lower peak concentration values at a later time and higher trough values at a given time than prompt preparations. Some newer preparations, such as the experimental carbamazepine Tegretol OROS system, release drug at a fixed rate over time with very little fluctuation in steady-state serum concentration. The potential advantages of sustained-release preparations are (1) reduction of toxicity associated with peak serum concentration of the drug; (2) reduction in the risk of breakthrough seizures at the time of trough serum concentration; and (3) longer intervals between doses, with improved convenience and compliance. The potential disadvantage of sustained-release preparations is less complete absorption if not all of the drug is released before the tablet leaves the area(s) of the GI tract where absorption takes place (usually in the proximal small intestine).

Generic Substitution

Antiepileptic drugs present special problems for generic substitution because (1) they tend to be lipid-soluble (and water-insoluble) compounds, as lipid solubility permits them to cross the blood–brain barrier; (2) they have narrow therapeutic ranges; and (3) some have nonlinear pharmacokinetics, which amplifies differences in the steady-state serum concentration created by differences in bioavailability of preparations. These considerations are particularly applicable to carbamazepine and phenytoin.

The American Academy of Neurology appointed a subcommittee to report on the topic of generic substitution of antiepileptic drugs.[1,2] This report covers the complex pharmacologic, regulatory, and economic aspects of this issue. The clinically relevant portion of their conclusions is quoted below:

> Generic substitution may provide significant benefits because of lower cost, and in general the price competition may be a positive development. However, certain medications have inherent limitations that

make generic substitution problematic. In these cases, the following guidelines should be followed. Uncontrolled generic substitution should not be allowed for antiepileptic medications, especially phenytoin and carbamazepine. Once a patient is carefully titrated and optimally controlled on one specific formulation, the formulation should not be changed. Each generic formulation of those drugs should be clearly labeled and identified as to the manufacturer. Switching between different formulations should be disallowed, except with the informed consent of the physician and the patient.

Oral Suspensions

Oral suspension preparations contain drug dispersed as fine particles. Such preparations have two advantages. First, they permit swallowing of amounts of a drug that could not be swallowed if contained in a single pill or tablet. This accounts for the more frequent use of oral suspensions in pediatric practice. Second, suspensions of poorly soluble (in water) drugs such as phenytoin may permit more complete absorption of the drug.

Intramuscular Route

Intramuscular administration of antiepileptic drugs is complicated by the observation that antiepileptic drugs are poorly water-soluble compounds injected to an aqueous medium (muscle). Dissolution of drug and absorption from muscle are therefore relatively slow.

Peak serum phenytoin concentrations occur approximately 24 hours after a single intramuscular injection and are significantly less than the peak concentrations produced by the same dose given by rapid intravenous infusion. Peak phenobarbital and diazepam concentrations are reached in 1–12 hours and 45–60 minutes, respectively, after intramuscular injection. Peak serum concentrations of diazepam after intramuscular injection are substantially less than the peak concentrations produced by the same dose given as an intravenous bolus. Antiepileptic drugs should not be given via the intramuscular route in status epilepticus and in other emergencies because of the slowness of absorption and the relatively low peak serum concentrations produced by this route.

In most situations, maintenance doses of antiepileptic drugs should not be given via the intramuscular route because of the slowness and variability of absorption and because of the danger of overmedication and undermedication when switching to and from other routes of administration. See Browne (1983) for a discussion of intramuscular administration of antiepileptic drugs.[3]

Distribution

Volume of Distribution

Volume of distribution is a mathematic concept that relates the concentration of drug in serum to the remaining portions of the body. The larger the volume of distribution, the greater the tissue concentration of drug in the body. Volume of distribution is proportional to a drug's lipid solubility and increases with increasing values of lipid solubility.[4]

Route of Administration

After administration of an antiepileptic drug by the oral or intramuscular route, there is a rise and then a fall in the serum concentration of the drug. The rates of the rise and fall of the drug's serum concentration depend on the rate of the drug's absorption, distribution, and elimination. After intravenous administration of a drug, there is a high initial peak drug serum concentration followed by a rapid fall in serum concentration, corresponding to the distribution of the drug into various compartments. There is then a second phase in which serum concentration declines more slowly, corresponding to the elimination of the drug by the process of biotransformation and excretion. Phenytoin and diazepam demonstrate this type of "biphasic" fall in serum concentration after intravenous administration. When a loading dose of intravenous drug is administered, it is necessary to give a dose large enough to maintain a therapeutic serum concentration after the rapid fall in serum concentration during the distribution phase (see next section).

Distribution to the Active Site

Antiepileptic drugs act on neurons or glial cells of the CNS. To enter these cells, the drug molecules must pass the blood–brain barrier and the cell membrane. The rate of penetration of the blood–brain barrier by an antiepileptic drug depends on lipid solubility and cerebral blood flow. The concentration of phenytoin and phenobarbital in the brain parenchyma and cerebrospinal fluid (CSF) may not reach peak levels in humans until an hour or more after an intravenous injection.[5] However, studies in both animals and humans indicate that the concentration of phenytoin in the brain parenchyma remains greater than the serum concentration of unbound phenytoin once peak brain concentrations have been reached, presumably because of binding by tissue protein and phospholipids. Diazepam enters the brain parenchyma very rapidly, and the brain concentration of diazepam closely parallels the serum concentration.[6] Thus, the brain concentration of diazepam peaks soon after an intravenous injection but falls rapidly in association with the rapidly falling serum concentration. These observations provide a basis for the therapeutic strategy of treating status epilepticus with a single dose of intravenous diazepam (to stop the seizures quickly) followed immediately by a loading dose of phenytoin to provide long-term antiepileptic activity.[7]

Protein Binding

On entering the bloodstream, antiepileptic drugs are bound, to differing degrees, by plasma proteins, principally albumin. The extent of protein binding by various antiepileptic drugs is listed in Table 4-1. Protein binding has several important clinical implications.[8] First, the serum drug concentration determinations performed by most laboratories measure the total drug serum concentrations, not the free (non–protein-bound) serum concentration. Second, only the free drug can enter active sites from the plasma, and there is evidence that the concentration of free antiepileptic drug in the serum correlates better with efficacy and toxicity than does the total drug concentration. Third, the percentage of free drug in the serum is inversely proportional to the albumin concentration. Patients with low plasma albumin concentrations have a higher percentage (but not higher concentration) of free antiepileptic drug and a greater probability of developing antiepileptic drug toxicity for a given total drug serum concentration than do patients with a high plasma albumin concentration. Fourth, other drugs given in addition to an antiepileptic drug may displace the antiepileptic drug from its protein-binding sites (see Drug Interactions).

Table 4-1. Pharmacologic Data on Antiepileptic Drugs

Drug	Elimination Half-life in Adults (hrs)	Elimination Half-life in Children (hrs)	Time to Reach Steady State (days)	Therapeutic Range of Serum Concentration (µg/ml)	Protein Binding (%)
Carbamazepine	14–27	14–27 (children) 8–28 (neonates)	3–4	4–12	66–89
Clonazepam	20–40	20–40	—	0.005–0.070	47
Ethosuximide	20–60	20–60	7–10	40–100	0
Phenobarbital	46–136	37–73 (children) 61–173 (neonates)	14–21	10–40	40–60
Phenytoin	24–36[a]	5–14 (children) 10–60 (neonates) 10–140 (prematures)	7–28	10–20	69–96
Primidone	6–18	5–11	4–7	5–12[b]	0
Valproic acid	6–15	8–15	1–2	40–150	80–95

[a]At serum concentrations of 10–20 µg/ml.
[b]May be higher in patients taking primidone alone.

Reduced protein binding (increased *free fraction*) of a drug does *not* result in a change in the concentration of free drug.[8] Free drug concentration is determined only by the dosing rate and the ability of clearing organs to biotransform or excrete the free drug. If dosing rate and free drug clearance remain constant, total concentration of the drug will fall and the free fraction will increase when protein binding decreases; however, free concentration, and therefore clinical activity, will remain unchanged.

Transcellular Fluids: Cerebrospinal Fluid, Saliva, and Tears

CSF may be viewed as a plasma ultrafiltrate with a low protein concentration (and hence little protein binding). The concentrations of phenytoin, phenobarbital, primidone, carbamazepine, and ethosuximide in CSF are essentially identical to the concentrations of free drug in the serum.[9] Similar considerations apply to saliva and tears.

Biotransformation and Excretion

Basic Principles

Most antiepileptic drugs are inactivated and eliminated as a result of biotransformation by the hepatic microsomal mixed function oxidase system (cytochrome P-450 system), which transforms antiepileptic drugs into oxidized metabolites. These metabolites are usually less effective antiepileptic drugs than the parent drug, but biotransformation to active metabolites also occurs (see next section). The oxidized metabolites are usually more polar than the parent drug and more easily excreted by the kidney.

Usual Routes of Biotransformation and Excretion

Phenytoin, phenobarbital, and ethosuximide first undergo an oxidation reaction and are then excreted partly as oxidized metabolite and partly as conjugated oxidized metabolite. The initial oxidation step renders these drugs inactive as antiepileptic drugs. Primidone is oxidized to two active metabolites, phenobarbital and phenylethylmalonamide. Carbamazepine may undergo oxidation to form carbamazepine-10,11-

epoxide or carbamazepine-10,11-dihydroxide. Carbamazepine may also undergo loss of the carbamide group to form iminostilbene. Carbamazepine-10,11-dihydroxide has antiepileptic activity. Valproic acid is eliminated by direct conjugation of the parent drug and by oxidation of the parent drug. The major metabolic pathway of clonazepam is reduction of the nitro group to form an inactive 7-amino derivative.

Acetazolamide, bromide, and dimethadione are eliminated almost entirely by direct renal excretion. Phenobarbital, primidone, and ethosuximide are partly eliminated by direct renal excretion but principally as biotransformed metabolites.

Effects of Age

The rates of biotransformation of drugs may change with age. Many drugs are slowly metabolized by neonates because of their immature hepatic microsomes. Hydroxylation of phenytoin and conjugation of phenobarbital proceed more slowly in neonates than in children and adults.[3, 10] On the other hand, children metabolize phenytoin and phenobarbital more rapidly than adults and require higher doses of phenytoin and phenobarbital (in milligrams per kilograms) to achieve a given serum concentration.[3, 9, 10] Biotransformation rates may change (decrease) very abruptly at puberty.[10]

At the other end of the age spectrum, there is evidence that the elimination half-lives of phenytoin, phenobarbital, and diazepam are longer in elderly persons than in young adults.[3] These changes appear to be chiefly the result of slower metabolism.[3, 11]

Renal excretion also changes with age. Neonates have a lower renal clearance of drugs than older infants and children.[10] The glomerular filtration rate and renal excretion of intact drug declines predictably in old age, with a mean 35% reduction in elderly persons compared with young adults.[11]

Clinical Pharmacokinetics

Pharmacokinetics is the quantitative study of the combined processes of drug absorption, distribution, biotransformation, and excretion to produce mathematical models that will predict the concentration of a drug in various parts of the body as a function of dosage, route of administration, and time after administration. Drug metabolism by enzymes is the principal determinant of the pharmacokinetic properties of most antiepileptic drugs.

Rate of Enzymatic Drug Metabolism and Types of Enzyme Kinetics

The rate of metabolism of a drug by an enzyme system (V) can be expressed by the Michaelis-Menten equation:

$$V = \frac{V_{max} \times C}{K_m + C} \tag{1}$$

where V_{max} is the maximum velocity of the enzyme system, K_m is the Michaelis constant of the enzyme system, and C is drug serum concentration.

Three types of enzyme kinetics are encountered commonly in clinical practice: (1) with linear (first-order) kinetics, C is small in relation to K_m, the term $V_{max}/(K_m + C)$ does not vary with serum concentration, and V varies linearly with C; (2) with nonlinear (concentration-dependent) kinetics, the term $V_{max}/(K_m + C)$ varies inversely with C, and V varies in a nonlinear fashion with C; (3) with time-dependent kinetics, V_{max}, K_m, or both change with time with resulting changes in V.

Linear (First-Order) Kinetics

With linear kinetics, C is small in relation to K_m, the term $V_{max}/(K_m + C)$ does not vary with C, and V varies linearly with drug serum concentration (equation 1). Phenobarbital is a prototype drug with linear kinetics. Drugs with linear kinetics exhibit a number of properties outlined below.

1. Steady-state serum concentration varies linearly with dosing rate (Figure 4-1).

2. Serum concentration at one dosing rate directly predicts serum concentration at a second dosing rate (see Figure 4-1).

3. Drug clearance (equal to $V_{max}/[K_m + C]$), and elimination half-life (equal to $0.693 \times$ volume of distribution/clearance) do not vary with serum concentration.

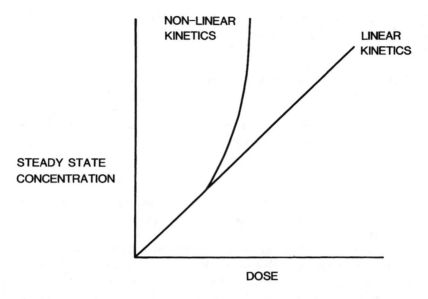

Figure 4-1. *Relationship between dosing rate and steady-state serum concentration for drugs with linear kinetics and for drugs with nonlinear kinetics.*

4.   Drug serum concentration will rise or fall exponentially over time with an increase or decrease in dosing rate (Figures 4-2 and 4-3).

Figure 4-2 shows the fundamental pharmacokinetic relationships predicted by the linear kinetic model. When administration of a drug is stopped, the concentration of the drug in the serum decreases exponentially. After one elimination half-life, the concentration of the drug has decreased by 50%; after five elimination half-lives, the concentration of the drug has decreased by more than 95%.

Conversely, when a constant intravenous infusion of a drug is begun, the concentration of the drug in the serum will accumulate at a rate that is the reciprocal of its rate of elimination. After one elimination half-life, the concentration of drug in the serum is 50% of the steady-state concentration. After five elimination half-lives, the serum concentration is essentially at its steady-state value. At this point, the rate of infusion is equal to the rate of elimination of the drug from the body.

Most drugs are not given as constant intravenous infusions but as fixed doses at fixed intervals. Figure 4-3 shows the rise in serum con-

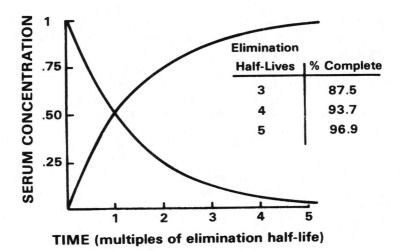

Figure 4-2. *Fundamental relationships predicted by linear kinetics. Inset table indicates the percentages of completion of elimination or buildup to steady-state concentration after multiples of the drug's elimination half-life. (Reprinted with permission from TR Browne. Pharmacologic Principles of Antiepileptic Drug Administration. In TR Browne, RG Feldman [eds], Epilepsy: Diagnosis and Management. Boston: Little, Brown, 1983.)*

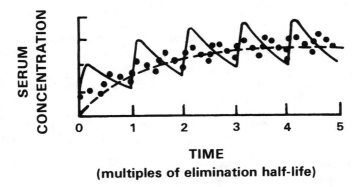

Figure 4-3. *Predicted kinetic patterns when the same dose per unit of time of a drug is given by constant intravenous infusion (dashed line), at intervals equal to the elimination half-life (solid line), and at intervals equal to one-half the elimination half-life (dotted line). (Reprinted with permission from TR Browne. Pharmacologic Principles of Antiepileptic Drug Administration. In TR Browne, RG Feldman [eds], Epilepsy: Diagnosis and Management. Boston: Little, Brown, 1983.)*

centration when the same dose per unit time of a drug is given by constant infusion, at intervals equal to the elimination half-life, and at intervals equal to one-half the elimination half-life. The time required to reach steady-state and the mean serum drug concentration are the same for all three schedules; all that varies is the range of fluctuations of serum concentration between doses. The relationships shown in Figure 4-3 apply to intravenously administered drugs and to orally administered drugs that have rapid absorption and distribution relative to elimination.

Table 4-1 lists the elimination half-lives and the time required to reach steady-state serum concentration with chronic oral administration of the most commonly prescribed antiepileptic drugs. It will be seen that the time required to reach steady-state serum concentration is approximately five times the elimination half-life for phenobarbital and several other drugs.

Nonlinear (Concentration-Dependent) Kinetics

With nonlinear (concentration-dependent) kinetics, C is relatively large in comparison with K_m, the term $V_{max}/(K_m + C)$ varies inversely with C, and V varies in a nonlinear fashion with C (equation 1). Phenytoin is a prototype drug with nonlinear kinetics. Drugs with nonlinear kinetics exhibit a number of properties outlined below.

1.   Steady-state serum concentration varies in a nonlinear fashion with the dosing rate (i.e., serum concentration increases faster than the dosing rate when the dosing rate is increased, and serum concentration decreases faster than the dosing rate when the dosing rate is decreased) (see Figures 4-1 and 4-4).

2.   Serum concentration at one dosing rate does not predict accurately serum concentration at a second dosing rate (see Figure 4-1).

3.   Drug clearance (equal to $V_{max}/[K_m + C]$) varies inversely with serum concentration, and drug elimination half-life (equal to $0.693 \times$ volume of distribution/clearance) varies directly with serum concentration.

4.   The time required to reach a steady-state serum concentration will vary directly with the dosing rate and may greatly exceed five times the elimination half-life at usual therapeutic serum concentrations (see Figure 4-4).

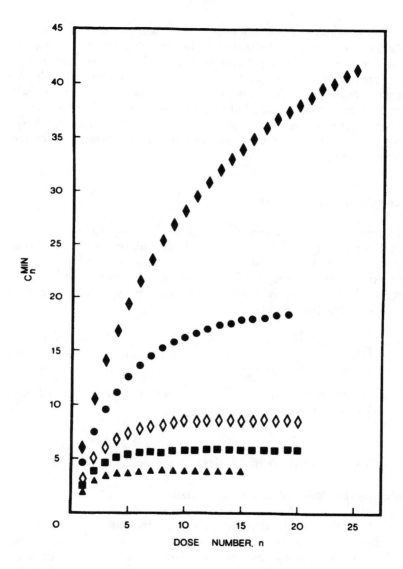

Figure 4-4. *Plot of minimum phenytoin serum concentration after the nth dose, versus the dose number, n. Symbols and dose rates (D/r, g/day) are:* ◆ = 0.50, ● = 0.40, ◇ = 0.30, ■ = 0.25, ▲ = 0.20. *(Reprinted with permission from JG Wagner. Time to reach steady state and prediction of steady-state concentration for drugs obeying Michaelis-Menten elimination kinetics. J Pharmacokinet Biopharm 1978;6:209.)*

As drug serum concentration rises, drug clearance decreases because of substrate saturation (see property No. 3 above). This results in a further rise in drug serum concentration and a further decrease in drug clearance. This self-propagating cycle can require a long period of time to go to completion. For example, phenytoin has an elimination half-life of approximately 1 day but may require up to 28 days to arrive at a steady-state serum concentration after a reduction in dosage. For a more detailed review of nonlinear pharmacokinetics see Browne and Chang (1989).[12]

Time-Dependent Kinetics

With time-dependent kinetics, $V_{max}/(K_m + C)$ changes with time, with resulting changes in V (equation 1). The common change in V is an increase (enzyme induction). Carbamazepine is a prototype drug with time-dependent kinetics exhibiting enzyme induction over the first 2 weeks of administration.[13] Drugs with time-dependent kinetics exhibit the properties outlined below.

1. Drug clearance (equal to $V_{max}/[K_m + C]$) and drug elimination half-life (equal to 0.693 × volume of distribution/clearance) will vary over time as values of V_{max} and K_m vary.

2. Drug serum concentration at a constant dosing rate will vary over time as values of V_{max} and K_m vary.

Practical Applications of Clinical Pharmacology

Therapeutic Range of Serum Concentration

The lower limit of the therapeutic range of serum concentration of antiepileptic drugs is usually defined as the serum concentration below which a majority of patients fail to have a significant reduction in seizure frequency. The upper limit of the therapeutic range of the serum concentration is usually defined as the serum concentration above which a majority of patients develop disturbing signs or symptoms of intoxication. Published therapeutic ranges of serum concentration of antiepileptic drugs thus represent values indicative of the majority of patients, but not all patients. Some patients may have

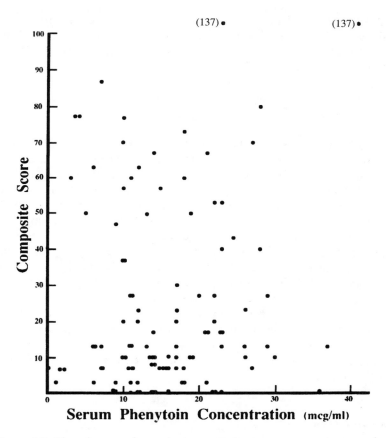

Figure 4-5. *Plot of serum phenytoin concentration versus composite score for overall response (efficacy and toxicity) to drug (0 = no seizures and no side effects; 1–20 = good response; 21–49 = acceptable but less than optimal response; 50+ = unacceptable seizure frequency, toxicity, or both). (Reprinted with permission from GE Schumacher, JT Barr, TR Browne, et al. Test performance characteristics of the serum phenytoin concentration (SPC): the relationship between SPC and patient response. Ther Drug Monit 1991;13:318.)*

good therapeutic responses with drug serum concentrations below the lower limit of the therapeutic range (Figure 4-5). Some patients may exhibit considerable intoxication with serum concentrations that are within the therapeutic range. Other patients may require serum concentrations above the therapeutic range for seizure control and show no signs or symptoms of intoxication with such concentrations (see Figure 4-5). The therapeutic ranges of serum concentration of antiepileptic drugs are listed in Table 4-1. See Schumacher et al. (1991) for further details.[14]

Dosing Interval

Antiepileptic drugs should be administered using an interval between doses that is as long as practical. Drug regimens requiring more frequent administration than once per day are not followed as well by outpatients as are regimens requiring once-daily administration. Because of the toxicity associated with high peak serum concentrations of antiepileptic drugs, the choice of dosage interval must represent a compromise that maximizes the duration of effective serum concentration and minimizes the toxicity associated with peak serum concentrations. In practice, antiepileptic drugs that have half-life elimination of 24 hours or longer usually need to be given only once daily to maintain a therapeutic serum concentration. The daily dose is usually best given at bedtime to avoid the sedative effects associated with peak levels of antiepileptic drugs. Drugs with elimination half-lives of less than 24 hours usually are given at intervals of approximately one half-life to reduce peak to trough variations in serum concentration.

Loading Dose

As noted above, the time required to attain a steady-state serum concentration is five times the drug's elimination half-life or longer. To attain steady-state serum concentration immediately, it is necessary to give a loading dose of the drug.

The loading dose of a drug is defined as:

$$LD = C \text{ (mg/L)} \times VD \text{ (liter/kg)} \qquad (2)$$

where *LD* is the loading dose, *C* is desired drug serum concentration, and *VD* is drug volume of distribution. For example, a loading dose of 14 mg/kg of phenytoin will produce a serum concentration of 20 mg/liter given phenytoin's volume of distribution of 0.7 liter/kg.

Drug Interactions

Antiepileptic drugs are frequently administered in combination. This creates the possibility of pharmacodynamic and pharmacokinetic drug interactions.

Pharmacodynamic Drug Interactions

Pharmacodynamic drug interactions are those involving the effects of two or more drugs at a common receptor site. Such effects may be agonistic or antagonistic and may be more or less than the mathematic sum of the effects of the drugs given singly.

Pharmacokinetic Drug Interactions

Pharmacokinetic drug interactions are those resulting from alterations in absorption, distribution, biotransformation, or excretion of a drug as a consequence of coadministration of one or more additional drugs. Three forms of clinically important pharmacokinetic drug interactions have been found for antiepileptic drugs: (1) induction of biotransformation of a coadministered drug, (2) inhibition of biotransformation of a coadministered drug, and (3) displacement from protein-binding sites by coadministration of drugs.[15] Pharmacokinetic drug interactions may be bidirectional (i.e., the pharmacokinetics of both drugs are affected by the presence of the other drug), and one drug may have more than one type of pharmacokinetic drug interaction with the other drug. The topic of antiepileptic drug interactions has been reviewed in depth by Pitlick et al. (1989).[16]

Pharmacokinetic drug interactions between antiepileptic drugs likely to be encountered in clinical practice are listed in Table 4-2. Note that there are also reports of less common drug interactions among antiepileptic drugs and that certain nonantiepileptic drugs (e.g., cimetidine and erythromycin) can have clinically significant drug interactions with antiepileptic drugs. Whenever an additional drug of any type is to be added to a patient's antiepileptic drug regimen, it is prudent to consult a listing of possible drug interactions such as that of Hanson and Horn (1992).[17]

Acknowledgment

Supported in part by the Department of Veterans Affairs.

Table 4-2. Commonly Encountered Pharmacokinetic Drug Interactions
Among Antiepileptic Drugs

Original Drug	Added Drug	Effect of Added Drug on Serum Concentration of Original Drug
Carbamazepine	Phenobarbital	Decrease
	Phenytoin	Decrease
	Primidone	Decrease
Phenobarbital	Valproic acid	Increase
Phenytoin	Carbamazepine	Increase
	Valproic acid	Decrease in total, no change in free concentration
Primidone	Carbamazepine	Increased concentration of derived phenobarbital
	Phenytoin	Increased concentration
Valproic acid	Carbamazepine	Decrease
	Phenobarbital	Decrease
	Primidone	Decrease

References

1. Report of the Therapeutics and Technology Assessment Subcommittee of the American Academy of Neurology. Assessment: generic substitution for antiepileptic medication. Neurology 1990;40:1641.
2. Nuwer MR, Browne TR, Dodson WE, et al. Views and reviews: generic substitution for antiepileptic drugs. Neurology 1990;40:1647.
3. Browne TR. Pharmacologic Principles of Antiepileptic Drug Administration. In TR Browne, RG Feldman (eds), Epilepsy: Diagnosis and Management. Boston: Little, Brown, 1983.
4. Arendt RM, Greenblatt DJ, DeJong RH. In vivo correlates of benzodiazepine cerebrospinal fluid uptake, pharmacodynamic action and peripheral uptake. J Pharmacol Exp Ther 1983;227:98.
5. Wilder BJ, Ramsay RE, Willmore LJ, et al. Efficacy of intravenous phenytoin in the treatment of status epilepticus: kinetics of central nervous system penetration. Ann Neurol 1977;1:511.
6. Ramsay RE, Hammond EJ, Perchalski RJ, et al. Brain uptake of phenytoin, phenobarbital, and diazepam. Ann Neurol 1979;36:355.
7. Browne TR, Mikati M. Status Epilepticus. In AH Ropper (ed), Neurological and Neurosurgical Intensive Care. Rockville, MD: Aspen, 1993.

8. Greenblatt DJ, Sellers EM, Koch-Weser J. Importance of protein binding for the interpretation of serum or plasma drug concentrations. J Clin Pharmacol 1982;22:259.
9. Browne TR. Clinical pharmacology of antiepileptic drugs. Drug Ther Rev 1979;2:469.
10. Pippenger CE. Absorption, Distribution, Protein Binding, Biotransformation, and Excretion of Antiepileptic Drugs. In PL Morselli, JK Penry, CE Pippenger (eds), Antiepileptic Drug Therapy in Pediatrics. New York: Raven, 1982.
11. Greenblatt DJ, Sellers EM, Shader RI. Drug therapy: drug disposition in old age. N Engl J Med 1982;306:1081.
12. Browne TR, Chang T. Phenytoin: Biotransformation. In RH Levy, FE Dreifuss, RH Mattson et al. (eds), Antiepileptic Drugs. New York: Raven, 1989.
13. Mikati MA, Browne TR, Collins J, et al. Time course of carbamazepine autoinduction. Neurology 1989;39:592.
14. Schumacher GE, Barr JT, Browne TR, et al. Test performance characteristics of the serum phenytoin concentration (SPC): the relationship between SPC and patient response. Ther Drug Monit 1991;13:318.
15. Browne TR, Greenblatt DJ, Schumacher GE, et al. Comparison of Methods for Determination of Pharmacokinetic Drug Interactions and Proposals for New Methods. In WH Pitlick, HJ Kupferberg, RH Levy, et al. (eds), Antiepileptic Drug Interactions. New York: Demos, 1989.
16. Pitlick WH, Kupferberg HJ, Levy RH, et al. Antiepileptic Drug Interactions. New York: Demos, 1989.
17. Hanson PD, Horn JR. Drug Interactions and Updates. Vancouver, WA: Applied Therapeutics, 1992.

5

Role of Electroencephalography in Epilepsy

Sudhansu Chokroverty

Introduction

Epilepsy is a clinical diagnosis. Therefore, a careful history must be obtained from patients, relatives, witnesses, and the medical or paramedical personnel in the hospital. This history must include ictal, preictal, postictal, and interictal periods; family and drug histories; as well as any history of significant medical or surgical illnesses that may have been responsible for triggering the seizures. The history is then followed by physical examination to evaluate the patient for any evidence of neurologic or other medical disorders. A history of recurrent true seizures is strongly suggestive of epilepsy. In a minority of patients, when an adequate history cannot be obtained or the history is equivocal, the diagnosis remains in doubt. In such cases as well as in strongly suspected cases, an electroencephalogram (EEG) is the single most important diagnostic laboratory test. To be of practical value, an EEG must be obtained according to the guidelines recommended by the American Electroencephalographic Society[1] and must include activation procedures (sleep, hyperventilation, and photic stimulation). In this chapter, the EEG findings of epilepsy and the role of EEG monitoring in the diagnosis, differential diagnosis, prognosis, and management decisions in patients with epilepsy are discussed.

The Electroencephalographic Signs of Epilepsy

Certain characteristic EEG waveforms are correlated with a high percentage of patients with clinical seizures and therefore can be considered of potentially epileptogenic significance. These epileptiform patterns generally consist of the following: spikes, sharp waves, spike and waves, and sharp and slow wave complexes.[2-5] In addition, an evolving pattern of focal rhythmic activities[6-8] (rhythmic theta or delta waves), especially in neonatal seizures, has been correlated with the behavioral pattern of clinical seizures and therefore can be considered of epileptiform significance. Temporal intermittent rhythmic delta activity (TIRDA) has recently been thought to be highly correlated with partial complex seizure.[9, 10]

A spike is defined as a waveform of brief duration (lasting 20–70 msec) that suddenly comes out of the background rhythm with a field of distribution and often is followed by an after-going slow wave.[11] A true epileptiform spike is generally biphasic or triphasic in appearance and has a sharp ascending limb followed by a slow descending limb in contrast to a sharp-appearing augmented background rhythm that generally is monophasic and has uniform ascending and descending limbs (Figure 5-1). The amplitude of a true epileptiform spike is at least 30% higher than the background activity. In addition, the duration of the epileptiform spike is generally different from the duration of the general background rhythm, and often there is disturbance of the background rhythm in the neighboring region.[2, 4, 5] Usually, the spikes are surface-negative but rarely may be surface-positive.

A sharp wave fulfills all the criteria described for a spike, except the duration is 70–200 msec.[11] Spike and wave and sharp and slow wave complexes have all the characteristics of spikes or sharp waves and are always followed by slow waves, which may be transient or repeat for several seconds or longer and in some patients may repeat in a rhythmic manner (e.g., 3-Hz spike and waves in absence seizures).[11]

To make a positive diagnosis of epilepsy, the EEG must show any or all of the above discriminating EEG features that fulfill the characteristics of epileptiform spikes or sharp waves and be accompanied by the behavioral correlates simultaneously during EEG recording in the laboratory. It is generally rare to observe the occurrence of the clinical seizure during an EEG recording in the laboratory; therefore, even in the presence of the characteristic EEG signs of epilepsy, a definitive statement about the diagnosis of epilepsy in a particular patient cannot be made. The findings are potentially epileptogenic in nature and must be correlated with the clinical history.

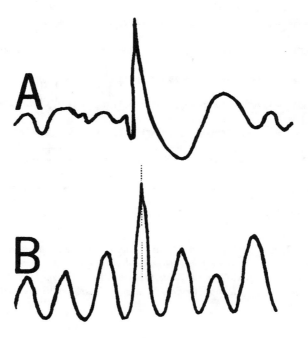

Figure 5-1. *Diagram of an epileptic spike (A) and an augmented background sharp rhythm (B). (Reprinted with permission from C Ajmone-Marsan. Electroencephalographic studies in seizure disorders: additional considerations. J Clin Neurophysiol 1984;1:143.)*

To bring out the ictal or interictal epileptiform patterns, the EEG study must routinely include activation procedures, such as sleep, hyperventilation, and photic stimulation. Also, in suspected partial complex seizures, special basal temporal electrodes (e.g., nasopharyngeal, T1, T2, sphenoidal electrodes) should be used.

To differentiate between true seizures and pseudoseizures, ictal EEG abnormalities (characteristic EEG epileptiform discharges combined with the patient's usual clinical spells) must be documented. For this purpose, simultaneous video-EEG monitoring in a special unit is often necessary. Perfectly normal ictal and postictal EEG findings in the presence of an alleged usual clinical spell suggests that the so-called ictal attacks are pseudoseizures. The incidence of pseudoseizures in epilepsy monitoring units may be up to 30%.[12] It must be remembered, however, that many epileptics (60–70%) have both true and pseudoseizures.

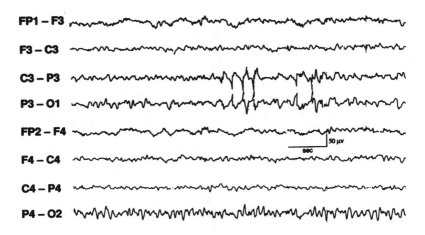

Figure 5-2. *Electrode pops at P3 electrode. (Reprinted with permission from T Walczak, S Chokroverty. Electroencephalography, Electromyography and Electrooculography: General Principles and Basic Technology. In S Chokroverty [ed], Sleep Disorders Medicine. Boston: Butterworth-Heinemann, 1994;95.)*

Differentiating Features Between True Epileptiform and Nonepileptiform Patterns

There are several EEG findings that may mimic epileptiform patterns but that are not of epileptogenic significance. It is important to identify these patterns in order to determine whether the patient has real epilepsy. These EEG findings may include the following[2, 4, 13–17]:

1. A variety of **sharp artifacts** (e.g., electrode pops, intravenous drip artifacts, electrocardiographic artifacts, muscle artifacts related to eye movement or muscle contraction). These sharp artifacts are easy to identify from their distribution and morphologic appearance. If necessary, electrocardiographic artifacts can be identified by the findings on a one-lead electrocardiogram. Electrode pops are limited to one channel (Figure 5-2), and the artifacts will be eliminated after the electrode problems are corrected. Muscle artifacts should be eliminated by having the patient relax rather than by reducing the high-frequency filter settings.

2. **Sharp transients** (e.g., positive occipital sharp transients [POSTs][18] [Figure 5-3; see also Figure 5-5]; mu rhythms[19] [Figure 5-4]; posterior

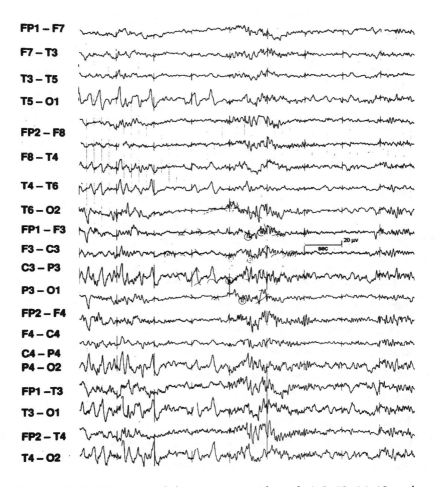

Figure 5-3. *Positive occipital sharp transients (channels 4, 8, 12, 16, 18, and 20 from the top) during stage II sleep.*

slow waves of youth; posterior slow-wave transients associated with eye blinks;[20, 21] lambda waves;[22] vertex sharp waves [Figure 5-5]; K complexes; sharp-appearing spindles [Figure 5-6]; hypnagogic or hypnopompic hypersynchrony [HH], which resemble spike and wave complexes [Figure 5-7]; harmonics of normal rhythms, which resemble spikes or sharp waves; photic driving responses, which resemble spike

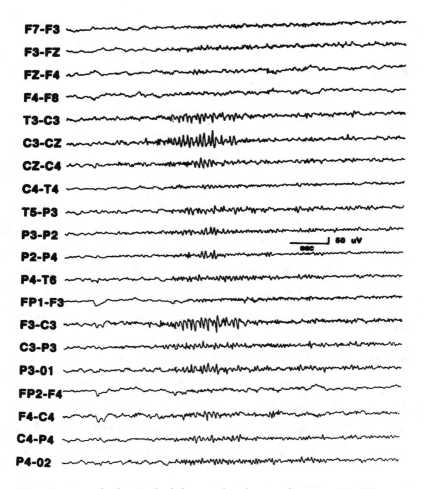

Figure 5-4. *Mu rhythm in the left central and parietal regions (C3, P3). There is phase reversal of a 10-Hz comblike rhythm at C3 and P3.*

and waves [Figure 5-8]; augmentation of an ongoing background rhythm that assumes a sharp or spike-like appearance [see Figure 5-1]). Sharp transients are sometimes seen during sleep and wakefulness in normal individuals.[15, 23] The sharp transients listed above can be differentiated by paying close attention to their distribution and morphology, to any accompanying slow waves or other disturbances of the

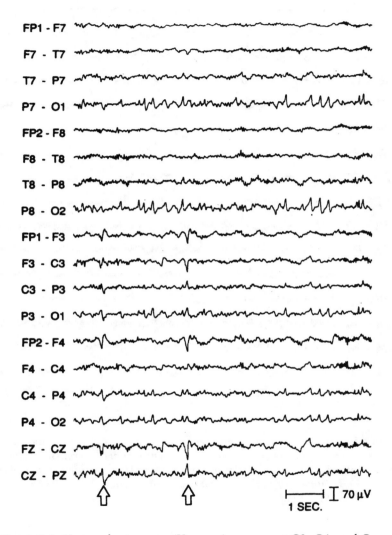

Figure 5-5. *Vertex sharp waves (V waves) are seen at C3, C4, and Cz electrodes (arrows) with spread of activities to the neighboring electrodes. Note also positive occipital sharp transients in channels 4 and 8 from the top. (Reprinted with permission from S Noachter, E Wyllie. EEG Atlas of Epileptiform Abnormalities. In E Wyllie [ed], The Treatment of Epilepsy: Principles and Practice. Philadelphia: Lea & Febiger, 1993;298.)*

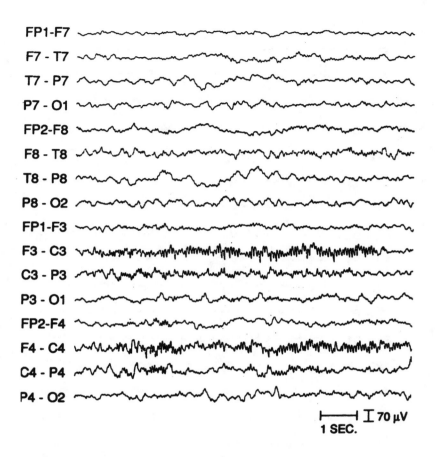

Figure 5-6. *Sharp appearing sleep spindles at C3 and C4 electrodes during stage 2 non–random eye movement sleep. (Reprinted with permission from S Noachter, E Wyllie. EEG Atlas of Epileptiform Abnormalities. In E Wyllie [ed], The Treatment of Epilepsy: Principles and Practice. Philadelphia: Lea & Febiger, 1993;298.)*

neighboring background activities, and to the state of the patient's alertness. For example, vertex sharp waves, sharp-appearing K complexes and spindles, POSTs, and HH are state-dependent and have a characteristic distribution. Some are age-dependent, such as HH and posterior slow waves of youth. Lambda waves resemble POSTs but are seen during scanning of some visual patterns. The differentiating features of

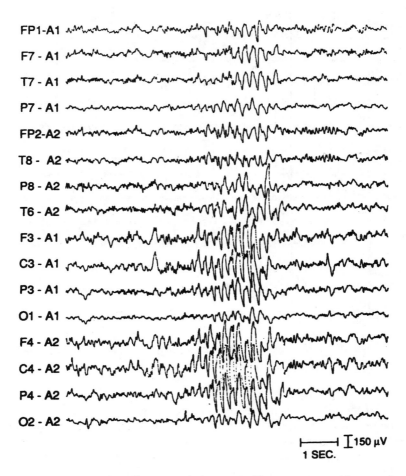

Figure 5-7. *Hypnagogic hypersynchrony resembling paroxysmal bursts of sharp waves. (Reprinted with permission from S Noachter, E Wyllie. EEG Atlas of Epileptiform Abnormalities. In E Wyllie [ed], The Treatment of Epilepsy: Principles and Practice. Philadelphia: Lea & Febiger, 1993;298.)*

true spikes and sharp waves of epileptiform significance and augmented background rhythm have already been described above. Mu rhythms may be described as an amplified and halved beta rhythm, have a comb-like appearance, are seen in the central regions (C3 and C4 of the International Nomenclature), and are attenuated by clenching of the hands, usually contralaterally.

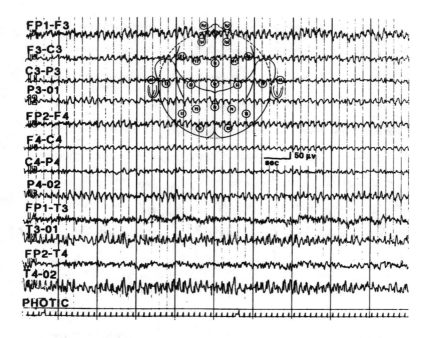

Figure 5-8. *Photic driving responses seen diffusely at 7 Hz resembling spike and wave bursts.*

3. Certain sharp transients of doubtful significance that are thought to be normal variants.[2, 4, 16, 17, 24–26] These may include the following 14- and 6-Hz positive spikes[27, 28] (Figure 5-9), small sharp spikes or benign epileptiform transients of sleep (BETSs)[29, 30] (Figure 5-10), 6-Hz spike and waves (phantom spike and waves)[31] (Figure 5-11), Wicket spikes[32] (Figure 5-12), and psychomotor variant (rhythmic midtemporal) discharge (Figure 5-13). Each of the above has a characteristic pattern; the recognition of this pattern is important for the diagnosis and differential diagnosis of true epileptiform discharges.

Fourteen- and 6-Hz positive spikes or cetenoids are seen in children and adolescents during sleep in the posterior temporal regions. BETSs are of low amplitude, have a wide distribution, are best seen in the referential montages, and may be unilateral or bilateral. Six-Hz spikes and waves show an attenuated spike component (low-amplitude spike), which may be seen in the anterior temporal, frontal, or posterior temporal distribution. Wicket spikes are generally seen

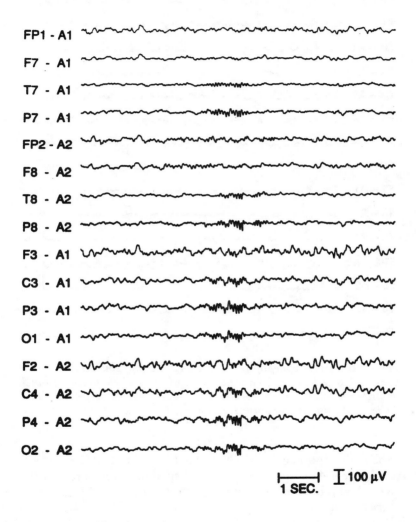

Figure 5-9. *Fourteen- and 6-Hz positive spikes seen bilaterally in the posterior regions. (Reprinted with permission from S Noachter, E Wyllie. EEG Atlas of Epileptiform Abnormalities. In E Wyllie [ed], The Treatment of Epilepsy: Principles and Practice. Philadelphia: Lea & Febiger, 1993;298.)*

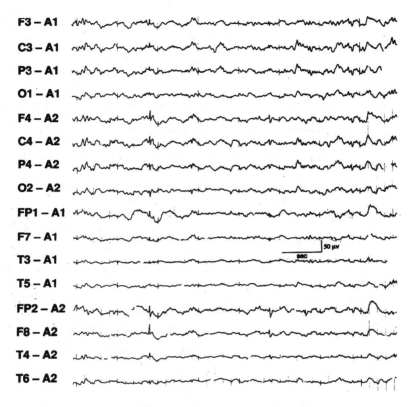

Figure 5-10. *Benign epileptiform transients of sleep or small sharp spikes in channels 5–8 and 13–16 from the top. (Reprinted with permission from S Chokroverty. Sleep and Epilepsy. In S Chokroverty [ed], Sleep Disorders Medicine. Boston: Butterworth-Heinemann, 1994;429.)*

in the midtemporal area (see Figure 5-12) and resemble mu rhythms (see Figure 5-4). Often one or several spike-like waves repeat themselves. A psychomotor variant pattern (see Figure 5-13) has a characteristic flat- or square-topped appearance and is seen during stages I–II of non–rapid eye movement (NREM) sleep, maximally in the midtemporal regions.

4. Patterns that may mimic epileptiform discharges but that have no epileptogenic significance.[2, 24, 33] These patterns include triphasic waves[34, 35] (Figure 5-14); periodic or pseudoperiodic lateralized epilep-

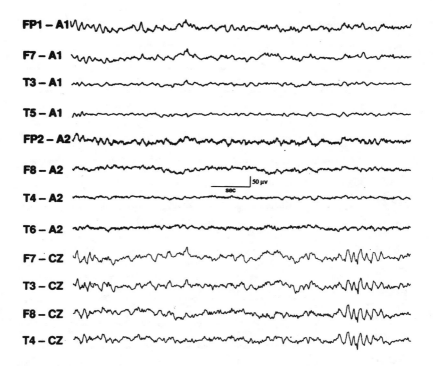

Figure 5-11. *Six-Hz spike and wave pattern seen in the last four channels. (Reprinted with permission from T Walczak, S Chokroverty. Electroencephalography, Electromyography and Electrooculography: General Principles and Basic Technology. In S Chokroverty [ed], Sleep Disorders Medicine. Boston: Butterworth-Heinemann, 1994;95.)*

tiform discharges (PLEDs)[36] (Figure 5-15); periodic complexes[37] (Figure 5-16); subclinical rhythmic epileptiform discharges of adults[38] (Figure 5-17); burst-suppression patterns[37] (Figure 5-18); and occipital needle spikes in infants or children with retrolental fibroplasia, choreoretinitis, or other visual problems.[37, 39]

Triphasic waves (see Figure 5-14) have a characteristic morphology and distribution. As its name suggests, the waves have a triphasic appearance with an initial positive component. These waves are seen synchronously and symmetrically with frontal dominance of the amplitude. The waves show an anteroposterior phase shift. Triphasic waves were originally described as being specific for hepatic

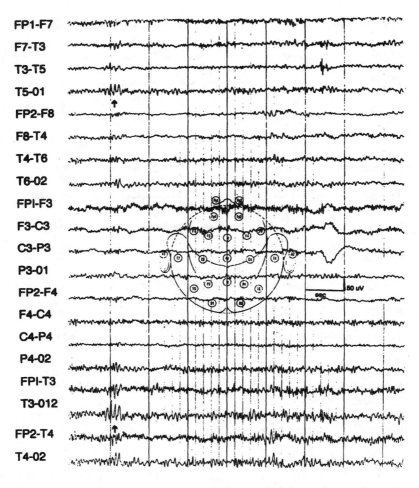

Figure 5-12. *Several spike-like waves (Wicket spikes) repeating rhythmically at T3–T5 (arrows) as well as in T4 with reduced amplitude in an adult without any history of seizure.*

encephalopathy but later were found to be in other metabolic, toxic, and even some anoxic encephalopathies. There is some resemblance to the epileptiform spikes. In fact, in their original description, these waves were termed *blunt spike waves*,[34] but they are not potentially epileptogenic in nature.

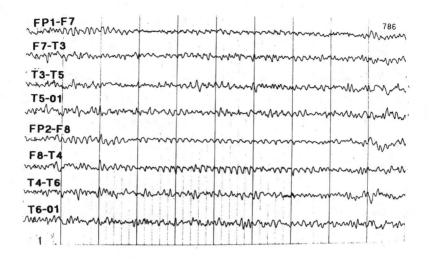

Figure 5-13. *Psychomotor variant pattern of 5- to 6-Hz square-topped or notched waves at F8–T4 during stage I non–random eye movement sleep.*

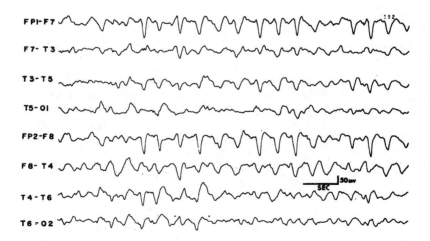

Figure 5-14. *Triphasic waves seen synchronously with dominance of the amplitude frontally. (Reprinted with permission from S Chokroverty, ME Bruetman, V Berger, MG Reyes. Progressive dialytic encephalopathy. J Neurol Neurosurg Psychiatry 1976;39:411.)*

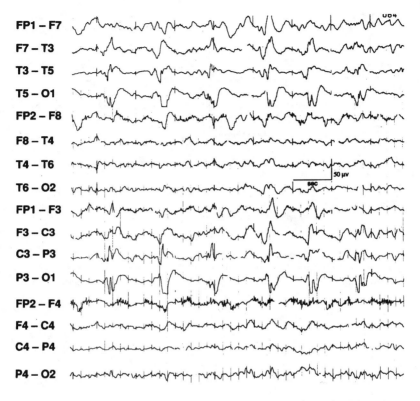

Figure 5-15. *Periodic lateralized epileptiform discharges in the left hemisphere originating predominantly from the parietal and posterior temporal regions (P3, T5) at a rate of approximately 0.8/second in a 72-year-old woman with history of confusion and falling episodes. (Reprinted with permission from T Walczak, S Chokroverty. Electroencephalography, Electromyography and Electrooculography: General Principles and Basic Technology. In S Chokroverty [ed], Sleep Disorders Medicine. Boston: Butterworth-Heinemann, 1994;95.)*

PLEDs (see Figure 5-15) were described by Chatrian et al.[36] as periodic or pseudoperiodic lateralized discharges consisting of complexes of sharp and slow waves, spike and slow waves, or bursts of rhythmic slow waves with sharp appearance and seen unilaterally. Most commonly, PLEDs are found in acute cerebral lesions such as infarction but have been described in many other conditions. Patients with PLEDs

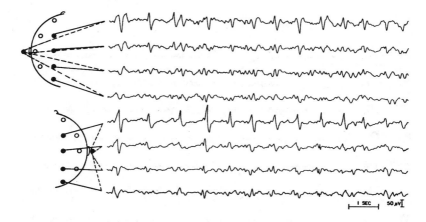

Figure 5-16. *Periodic complexes (frontally dominant bilateral sharp waves at a rate of about 1 Hz) in a patient with Jakob-Creutzfeldt disease. (Reprinted with permission from BJ Fisch. Spehlmann's EEG Primer. New York: Elsevier, 1991.)*

often have an altered state of alertness and, many times, contralateral clonic movements of their bodies. These discharges are not thought to be part of the EEG findings of chronic epilepsy, but sometimes these findings closely resemble the EEG findings of focal status epilepticus. Sometimes, PLEDs may be seen independently on both sides, in which case they are termed *BIPLEDs.*

In addition to PLEDs, there are other periodic complexes,[33, 37] such as complexes of sharp waves or spikes (see Figure 5-16) or multiple sharp waves and spikes with or without a mixture of slow waves seen in a periodic fashion. These complexes may be seen in a variety of disorders such as in Jakob-Creutzfeldt disease, herpes simplex encephalitis, and subacute sclerosing panencephalitis (SSPE). The periodic complexes seen in Jakob-Creutzfeldt disease (see Figure 5-16) occur approximately at a rate of one per second, whereas in SSPE, the discharges are much slower, usually one every 3–4 seconds. These do not signify chronic epileptogenicity. Periodic complexes in herpes simplex encephalitis are usually unilateral but sometimes may be seen bilaterally.

A burst-suppression pattern (see Figure 5-18) is characterized by bursts of complexes that consist of a mixture of sharp waves, spikes or slow waves, and other faster rhythms, followed by marked atten-

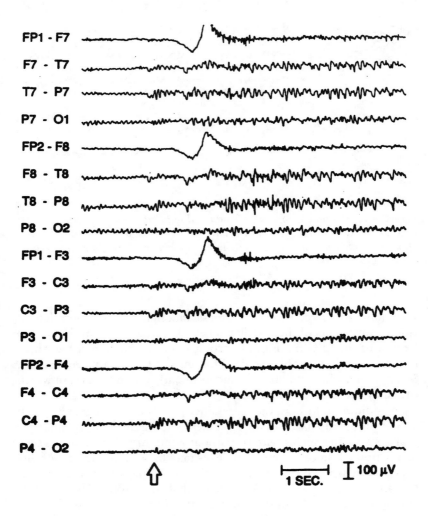

Figure 5-17. *Subclinical rhythmic electrographic discharges of adults resembling ictal epileptiform discharges but without any clinical association. Arrow indicates the onset of the discharges. (Reprinted with permission from S Noachter, E Wyllie. EEG Atlas of Epileptiform Abnormalities. In E Wyllie [ed], The Treatment of Epilepsy: Principles and Practice. Philadelphia: Lea & Febiger, 1993:298.)*

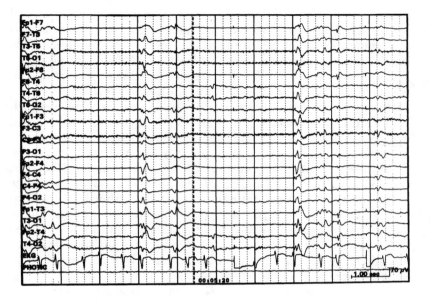

Figure 5-18. *Burst-suppression pattern. Note bursts of a mixture of slow and sharp waves or spikes interspersed with periods of marked attenuation of activities seen synchronously and symmetrically.*

uation of the activities that give rise to the characteristic pattern of burst-suppression. The pattern occurs irregularly rather than periodically, signifies severe cortical anoxia, and is seen characteristically in anoxic encephalopathy. A similar pattern has also been noted in comatose patients after barbiturate overdose or other severe metabolic or toxic encephalopathy that causes diffuse cerebral anoxia and in some patients after prolonged synchronous and symmetric epileptiform discharges. A burst-suppression pattern does not signify chronic epileptogenicity.

Ictal and Interictal Patterns

Characteristic ictal patterns that occur during EEG monitoring may suggest a particular type of epilepsy. EEG monitoring may thus help in classifying the types of epilepsy and the epileptic syndromes (see Chapter 2), which is important in initiating pharmacotherapy. EEG monitoring may help differentiate between primary generalized and partial seizures with or without secondary generalization, which is important because the treatment is different in these conditions. EEG monitoring may also help identify different varieties of interictal and ictal epileptiform discharges that are associated with specific epileptic syndromes,[13–15, 37] such as Lennox-Gastaut syndrome[40, 41] (Figure 5-19), infantile spasms[42] (Figure 5-20), benign rolandic epilepsy (sylvian seizure) with centrotemporal spikes[43] (Figure 5-21), childhood benign seizure with occipital spikes (Figure 5-22), and juvenile myoclonic epilepsy of Janz (Figure 5-23). Treatment is different in these different epileptic syndromes. For example, infantile spasms respond to corticotropin and prednisone. Lennox-Gastaut syndrome is difficult to treat, but some patients improve with valproic acid or clonazepam. Juvenile myoclonic epilepsy responds to valproic acid. Sylvian seizures have good prognosis and often remit by 15–20 years of age. Those having clinical seizures respond to the standard first-line antiepileptic drugs. Recognizing the patterns of the above epileptic syndromes is therefore important.

The EEG findings in Lennox-Gastaut syndrome[40, 41] (see Figure 5-19) are characterized interictally by slow spike and wave discharges at a rate of 1.5–2.5 Hz that are seen synchronously and symmetrically on a diffuse slow background rhythm. Tonic seizure is the most common clinical presentation in Lennox-Gastaut syndrome.[41] Tonic seizures often occur during sleep at night, and the EEG shows sudden paroxysms of 10- to 25-Hz fast rhythms followed by sharp and slow wave complexes. Ictal EEG patterns during atonic, akinetic, clonic, or tonic-clonic presentations in Lennox-Gastaut syndrome may include prolonged bursts of generalized spike and wave rhythms, paroxysmal generalized fast rhythms, or generalized bursts of sharp waves followed by marked attenuation of EEG activity (Figure 5-24). Sometimes electrodecremental responses are seen.

Infantile spasms show the characteristic hypsarrhythmic EEG patterns[42] (see Figure 5-20) of multifocal high-amplitude slow waves and sharp waves or spikes seen bilaterally. During sleep, the EEG may assume an appearance of suppression-burst–like patterns. During a clinical ictus with spasms, the EEG may show a generalized electrodecremental pattern (Figure 5-25). A variety of ictal patterns have been noted during infantile spasms[42, 44, 45]: an electrodecremental pattern (see Figure 5-25) as described by Bickford and Klass,[44] high-amplitude diffuse bilateral spikes or polyspikes (see

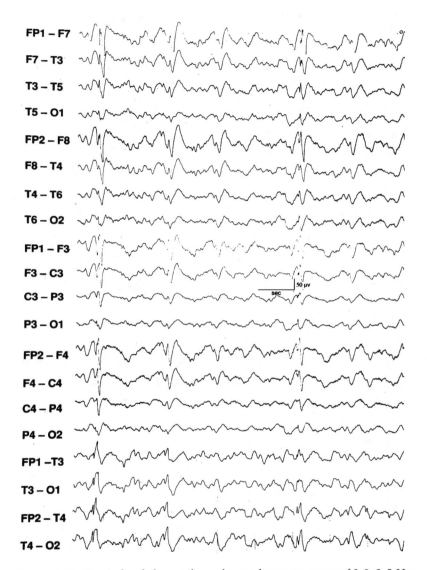

Figure 5-19. *Generalized slow spike and wave bursts at a rate of 2.0–2.5 Hz in the interictal period in a patient with Lennox-Gastaut syndrome. (Reprinted with permission from S Chokroverty. Sleep and Epilepsy. In S Chokroverty [ed], Sleep Disorders Medicine. Boston: Butterworth-Heinemann, 1994;429.)*

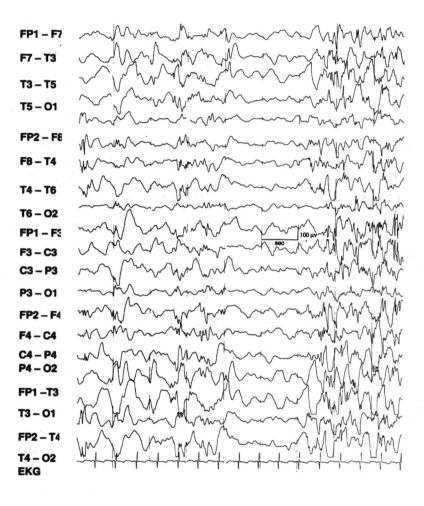

Figure 5-20. *Electroencephalogram showing multifocal high amplitude slow waves and sharp waves or spikes (hypsarrhythmic pattern) in a 9-month-old girl with infantile spasms. (Reprinted with permission from S Chokroverty. Sleep and Epilepsy. In S Chokroverty [ed], Sleep Disorders Medicine. Boston: Butterworth-Heinemann, 1994.)*

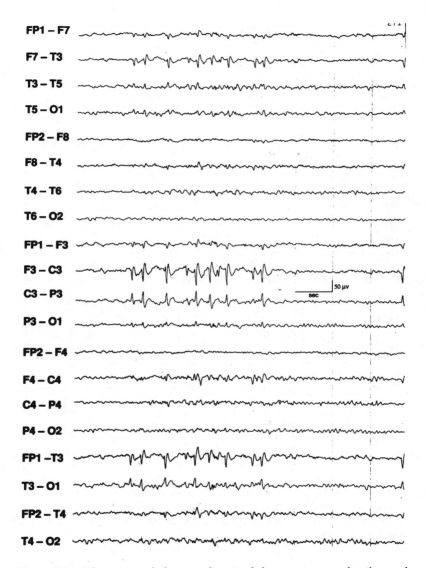

Figure 5-21. *Electroencephalogram showing left centrotemporal spikes and sharp waves in a patient with benign rolandic epilepsy (sylvian seizures). (Reprinted with permission from S Chokroverty. Electroencephalography, Electromyography and Electrooculography: General Principles and Basic Technology. In S Chokroverty [ed], Sleep Disorders Medicine. Boston: Butterworth-Heinemann, 1994;95.)*

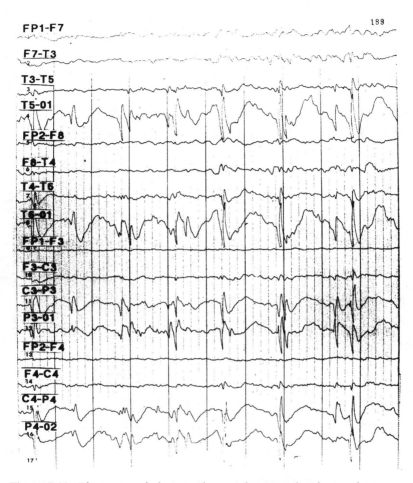

Figure 5-22. *Electroencephalogram showing bioccipital spikes or sharp waves accompanied by after-going slow waves in a patient with benign childhood seizure with occipital spikes. Note an error in channel 8: T6–01 should read T6–02.*

Figure 5-20), burst-suppression patterns, generalized anteriorly dominant high-amplitude sharp and slow wave complexes, or slow waves with or without interspersed background attenuation.

Rolandic epilepsy is characterized by centrotemporal spikes (see Figure 5-21). Juvenile myoclonic epilepsy shows multiple spike and wave

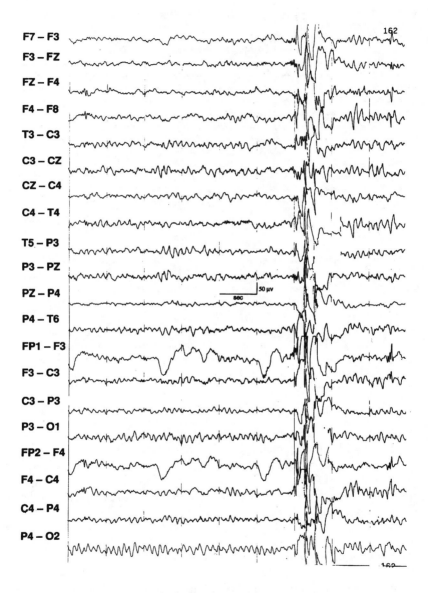

Figure 5-23. *Interictal generalized multiple spike and wave discharges in the electroencephalogram seen synchronously.*

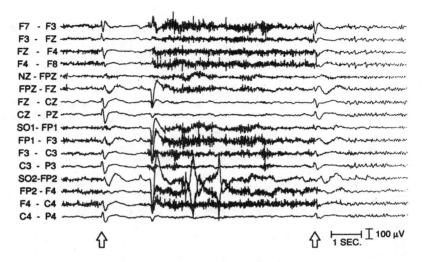

Figure 5-24. *An electroencephalogram showing an ictal pattern in a patient with Lennox-Gastaut syndrome during an attack of atonic seizures. Left-hand arrow indicates the onset of the ictus, characterized clinically by limp head nodding, tonic stiffening, and elevation of both arms, and electro-graphically by a burst of generalized sharp wave followed by attenuation of electroencephalographic rhythm. After cessation of muscle activity, a second similar ictus (right hand arrow) was noted. (Reprinted with permission from S Noachter, E Wyllie. EEG Atlas of Epileptiform Abnormalities. In E Wyllie [ed], The Treatment of Epilepsy: Principles and Practice. Philadelphia: Lea & Febiger, 1993;298.)*

discharges transiently seen synchronously and symmetrically (see Figure 5-23) and accompanied by clinical myoclonic jerks.[46]

An electrographic seizure pattern is potentially epileptogenic and is defined as an EEG pattern showing epileptiform discharges accompanied by a clinical seizure. In the absence of a clinical seizure, such discharges are termed a *subclinical electrographic seizure.*

Partial Complex Seizure of Temporal Lobe Origin

Interictal EEG findings of partial complex seizures of temporal lobe origin[47] may show focal temporal, particularly anterior and midtemporal (Figure 5-26), sharp waves or spikes accompanied by

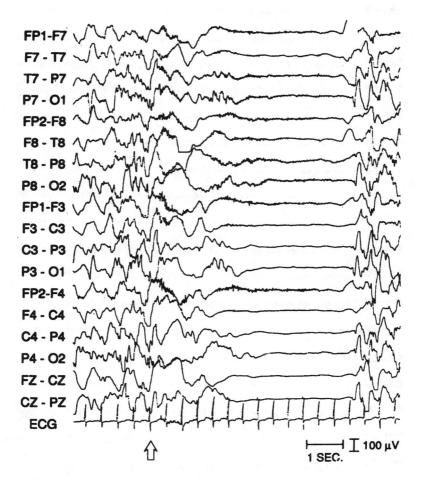

Figure 5-25. *An electroencephalogram showing a generalized electrodecremental pattern during a spasm (onset at the arrow) in an 8-month-old baby with infantile spasms. (Reprinted with permission from S Noachter, E Wyllie. EEG Atlas of Epileptiform Abnormalities. In E Wyllie [ed], The Treatment of Epilepsy: Principles and Practice. Philadelphia: Lea & Febiger, 1993;298.)*

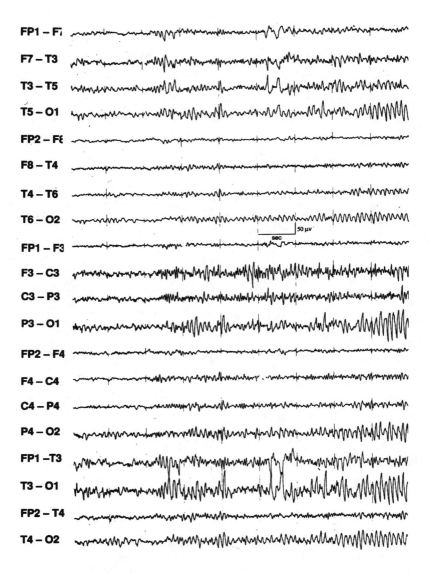

Figure 5-26. *Focal left midtemporal (T3) interictal spikes in a patient with partial complex seizure. Also note breach rhythm at C3, which may have the appearance of multiple spikes.*

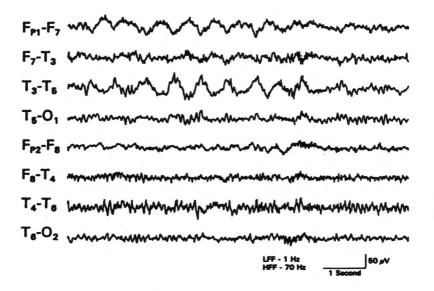

Figure 5-27. *Left temporal intermittent rhythmic delta activity during wakefulness in a 30-year-old woman with partial complex seizure. (Reprinted with permission from MM Normand, ZK Wszolek, DW Klass. Temporal intermittent rhythmic delta activity in electroencephalograms. J Clin Neurophysiol 1995;12:280.)*

after-going slow waves, or they may show TIRDA (Figure 5-27). The ictus may begin with sudden attenuation[48, 49] of the background rhythm or attenuation of the focal temporal spikes or sharp waves followed by rapidly evolving rhythmic discharges (e.g., rhythmic waves in the alpha, theta, or delta frequencies) with or without spikes or sharp waves[47, 50, 51] (Figure 5-28) and accompanied by behavioral correlates of a clinical seizure. The discharges may rapidly involve the entire ipsilateral hemisphere (see Figure 5-28) or may spread to involve the contralateral hemisphere, giving rise to a secondary bilateral synchrony. The postictal EEG may show diffuse slowing of the background rhythm with more marked focal slowing, focal spikes or sharp waves, or focal attenuation of the background rhythm.

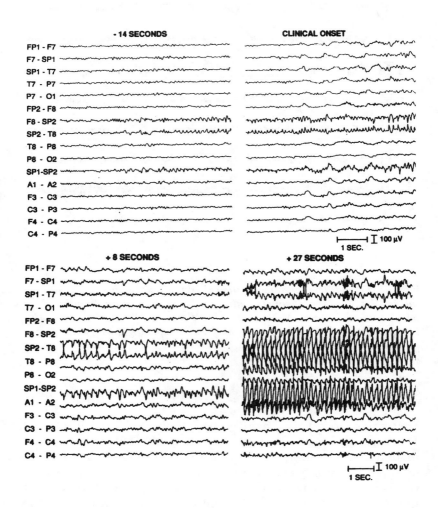

Figure 5-28. *A patient with a complex partial seizure showing a sudden burst of rhythmic spikes maximally at the right sphenoidal (SP2) electrode 14 seconds before the clinical onset of staring, unresponsiveness, and automatisms, followed by the spread of epileptiform discharges. (Reprinted with permission from S Noachter, E Wyllie. EEG Atlas of Epileptiform Abnormalities. In E Wyllie [ed], The Treatment of Epilepsy: Principles and Practice. Philadelphia: Lea & Febiger, 1993;298.)*

Simple Partial Seizure

Ictal EEG patterns in simple partial seizures are similar to those seen in patients with partial complex seizures of temporal origin except for the site of the abnormalities.[47] However, ictal patterns may not be detected in surface EEG monitoring in many patients with simple partial seizures because of a very localized focus or a distant location.[52, 53]

Partial Complex Seizures of Extratemporal Origin

The interictal patterns (Figure 5-29) and ictal patterns (Figure 5-30) of partial complex seizures of extratemporal origin[14, 15, 57] are similar to those seen in partial complex seizures of temporal origin except for the location. It is, however, difficult to detect seizures of extratemporal (frontal) origin because the ictal discharges often begin with fast rhythms and then are mixed with muscle artifacts resulting from clinical jerking of the body.

Absence Spells

The ictal pattern in the primary generalized epilepsy of the absence type[14, 15, 54] is similar to the interictal pattern (Figure 5-31), showing symmetric and synchronous frontally dominant 3-Hz spike and wave discharges.[14, 15] Generally, when the duration exceeds 3 seconds, there is a clinical seizure, with impairment of awareness, and a vacant and staring appearance. Occasionally, there may be clonic movements of the eyelids.[54]

Primary Generalized Tonic-Clonic Seizure

The ictal pattern is different in the tonic and in the clonic phases (Figure 5-32).[14, 15, 54] The clinical tonic seizure is accompanied by EEG attenuation of the background rhythm followed by the appearance of paroxysmal fast rhythms around 10 Hz (so-called epileptic recruiting rhythms). As the patient enters the clonic phase, the EEG shows a mixture of fast rhythms and slow waves that give rise to spike wave paroxysms that initially may be in the range of 4–6 Hz and then gradually slow down and stop before the postictal phase. The postictal EEG is characterized by diffuse slow waves or background attenuation, with

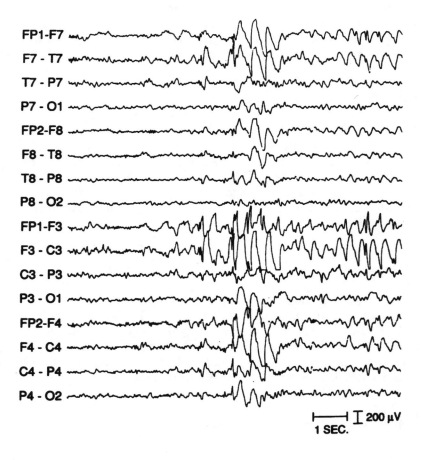

Figure 5-29. *Interictal electroencephalogram in a patient with partial complex seizure of extratemporal origin (frontal lobe seizure) showing sharp and slow wave complexes maximally in the left frontal region with intermittent secondary bilateral synchrony. (Reprinted with permission from S Noachter, E Wyllie. EEG Atlas of Epileptiform Abnormalities. In E Wyllie [ed], The Treatment of Epilepsy: Principles and Practice. Philadelphia: Lea & Febiger, 1993;298.)*

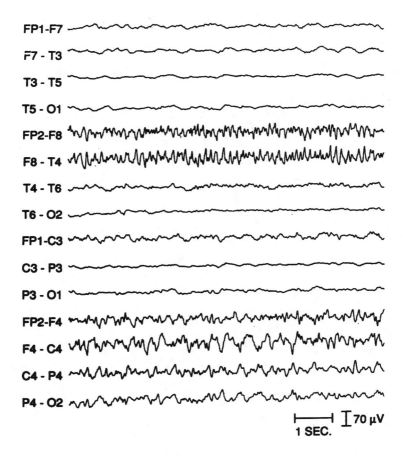

Figure 5-30. *Subclinical electrographic seizure in a patient with frontal lobe seizure showing an electroencephalographic seizure pattern 50 seconds after the onset in the right frontal region. (Reprinted with permission from S Noachter, E Wyllie. EEG Atlas of Epileptiform Abnormalities. In E Wyllie [ed], The Treatment of Epilepsy: Principles and Practice. Philadelphia: Lea & Febiger, 1993;298.)*

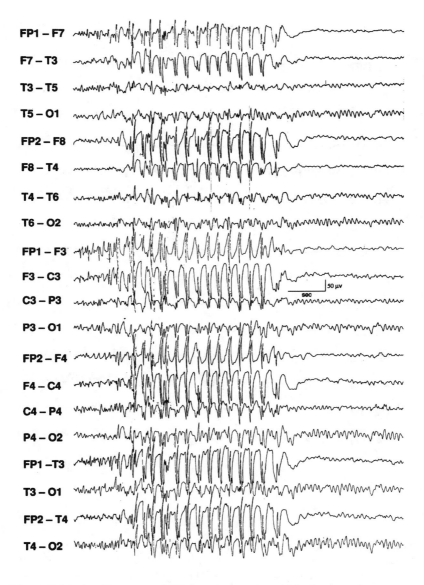

Figure 5-31. *An electroencephalogram in a patient with absence seizure showing frontally dominant generalized 3-Hz spike and wave discharges seen synchronously and symmetrically.*

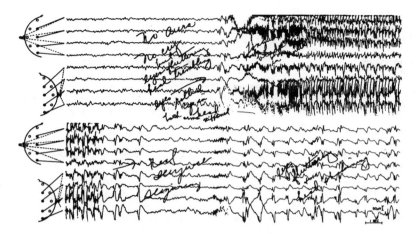

Figure 5-32. *Ictal pattern in an 18-year-old girl with generalized tonic-clonic seizure. Note that the tonic phase of the ictus begins with intermittent generalized spikes and movement artifacts followed by rhythmic repetitive spikes of increasing amplitude and decreasing frequency. The technician's notes are in the upper left hand side of the tracing. Ten seconds later at the onset of the clonic phase, the electroencephalogram shows slow waves intermixed with spikes giving rise to high amplitude generalized spike and wave complexes. The technician's clinical note on the electroencephalographic tracing now reads, "Real seizure, seizuring. Eyes fluttering and head shaking." (Reprinted with permission from BJ Fisch. Spehlmann's EEG Primer. New York: Elsevier, 1991.)*

gradual recovery to the preictal normal background rhythm after several hours or 1 to 2 days. The interictal EEG may show generalized synchronous and symmetric 4- to 6-Hz spike and wave discharges or multiple spike and waves (Figure 5-33).

Role of Electroencephalography in the Differential Diagnosis Between Epileptic and Nonepileptic Conditions

True epileptic attacks, which are characterized by episodic loss of awareness or consciousness with or without partial or generalized body movements, may mimic closely some other clinical conditions, making differentiation a difficult task. In this situation, the EEG findings may

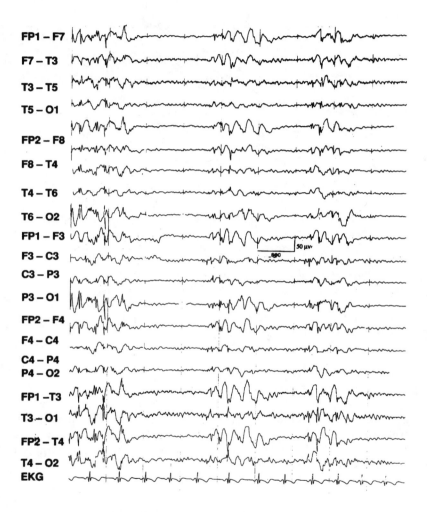

Figure 5-33. *Interictal electroencephalogram in a patient with primarily generalized tonic-clonic seizures showing 4- to 5-Hz generalized spike and wave and multiple spike wave discharges in synchronous and symmetrical fashions with frontal dominance of amplitude. (Reprinted with permission from S Chokroverty. Sleep and Epilepsy. In S Chokroverty [ed], Sleep Disorders Medicine. Boston: Butterworth-Heinemann, 1994;429.)*

make a significant contribution toward a diagnosis. A careful history and physical examination, however, constitute the most important first step in the diagnosis. Some conditions that mimic true epilepsy are syncope, cardiac arrhythmias, transient ischemic attacks, transient global amnesia, migraine with visual symptoms, pseudoseizures (hysterical or other psychogenic seizures), parasomnias (e.g., night terror and sleep walking, nightmare, bruxism, REM-behavior disorder, confusional arousals), narcoleptic sleep attacks, breath-holding spells, hyperventilation syndrome, apnea in infants, panic attacks, certain movement disorders (e.g., paroxysmal choreoathetosis, dystonia, myoclonus), and acute confusional states in the elderly (see also Chapter 3). It is beyond the scope of this chapter to discuss the characteristic clinical and the differential diagnostic features of all of these conditions. It is, however, possible to diagnose many of these conditions on the basis of the history and physical findings. Many patients will require laboratory testing. Important tests in such situations are EEG, including ambulatory cassette EEG recording and long-term video-EEG monitoring if necessary; polysomonographic recording; and electrocardiographic examination.

Limitations of Electroencephalography in Diagnosing Epilepsy

Limitations of the EEG in diagnosing epilepsy include the following:

1. Normal EEG findings do not exclude a diagnosis of epilepsy; there may be several reasons for this.[2, 4, 13, 16] Epilepsy is a paroxsymal event; therefore, during the short recording (e.g., 20–30 minutes), paroxsymal epileptiform discharges are not necessarily seen. Hence, on repeating the EEG, there is a better chance of getting positive interictal EEG findings. The initial EEG recording may show normal results in 50% of true epileptics. Even after three or four EEGs, 8–10% may show normal EEG findings.[55–57] The yield after three or four EEG recordings obtained after activation procedures (sleep, sleep deprivation, hyperventilation, photic stimulation) does not increase. Increasing the duration of recording to several hours or days (i.e., long-term monitoring), however, increases the chance of obtaining a positive EEG result.

The second reason for obtaining a normal EEG recording even in a patient with true epilepsy is that the discharging focus may be in a deep location or buried in a sulcus and therefore inaccessible to surface EEG recording.[2, 13] Furthermore, the discharges may have been attenuated considerably or may have changed morphologically by the time the discharges arrive at the surface.[2, 13]

2. True interictal epileptiform activity does not necessarily indicate the patient has epilepsy. In two important series,[58-60] 1–2% of normal individuals had true interictal epileptiform abnormalities in EEG findings.

3. The siblings of patients with absence seizures may show transient bursts of typical 3-Hz spike and wave discharges in EEG recordings but without any clinical evidence of absence spells.

4. There is no clear relationship between EEG epileptiform discharges, the clinical improvement in the epileptic attacks, and the serum levels of antiepileptic drugs (AEDs) except in absence spells (petit mal). Kellaway and others[2, 61] have clearly shown through automated spike counting a significant decrease in the number of spikes associated with clinical improvement in petit mal epilepsy. With some AEDs (for example, carbamazepine), the EEG epileptiform discharges may increase, and the background activities may show deterioration (slowing) in the presence of clear improvement in the clinical spells.[62, 63]

5. Extracranial (surface EEG) recordings in some cases of partial complex seizure may falsely localize or lateralize the epileptic foci as documented by the depth recording during presurgical evaluation.[64]

6. On rare occasions, even ictal EEG recordings may not be diagnostic.[47, 54] This is true in patients with simple partial seizures with motor manifestations. Some patients with partial complex seizures with only psychic manifestations have ictal scalp EEG findings. In many patients during a generalized ictus, the muscle and the movement artifacts may obscure the EEG evidence of epilepsy, whereas in other cases, subtle ictal EEG findings, such as an electrodecremental response followed by rhythmic fast discharges, may be missed or mistaken for artifacts.

7. Certain EEG patterns that resemble epileptiform patterns have no specific epileptiform significance (see paragraphs 3 and 4 under Differentiating Features Between True Epileptiform and Nonepileptiform Patterns).

8. Many sharp artifacts may resemble EEG signs of epilepsy (see paragraph 1 under Differentiating Features Between True Epileptiform and Nonepileptiform Patterns).

9. Some sleep or awake EEG waves may be normal variants (see paragraph 2 under Differentiating Features Between True Epileptiform and Nonepileptiform Patterns) and mimic epileptiform discharges but are not of potentially epileptogenic significance.

Factors for the Maximal Yield of Interictal Discharges in Electroencephalography

Factors for the maximal yield of interictal discharges in the EEG[2, 4, 13, 16, 17, 55, 56, 65] may be summarized as follows:

1. The maximal yield of interictal epileptiform activity (IEA) usually occurs by the third or fourth EEG.

2. A high yield of IEA is seen within the first 24 hours or 1 week after a seizure.

3. A higher yield is observed in children than in adults.

4. The longer the duration of EEG recording, the higher the yield.

5. Sleep and sleep deprivation (24 hours or partial deprivation) guarantee a higher yield.

6. Activation procedures such as hyperventilation and photic stimulation are associated with a higher yield.

7. A higher yield is often seen in patients with generalized epilepsy.

8. A higher yield occurs if EEG monitoring is 24 hours or longer.

9. In some epileptics, the time of EEG recording (nocturnal versus diurnal) determines the yield. Epileptiform discharges frequently show both circadian and ultradian patterns. For example, epileptiform discharges commonly increase during sleep (circadian pattern) and show cyclic changes with the NREM-REM cycle (ultradian), with increments during NREM and decrements during REM sleep. Other changes that may be noted during sleep: Generalized discharges may become fragmented and irregular (e.g., 3-Hz spike and waves), and secondarily generalized discharges may become lateralized during REM sleep because of a tonic inhibition of the interhemispheric transfer of impulse traffic across the corpus callosum.

10. A higher yield is noted if the anticonvulsants are temporarily withdrawn; this should be performed only during presurgical evaluation for the purpose of localization of the foci, otherwise status epilepticus may be precipitated, or the EEG may show nonspecific paroxysmal discharges of spike and wave during the postwithdrawal phase.

11. A higher yield is frequently observed after EEG recording using additional or special (e.g., nasopharyngeal, T1 and T2, sphenoidal, zygomatic) electrodes.

12. An algorithm for EEG recording in patients suspected of epilepsy is as follows:[65]

    a. Record a routine EEG during sleep (natural or induced), hyperventilation, and photic stimulation, and look for IEA.

    b. If the patient's EEG findings are negative for IEA, record an EEG with sleep deprivation (partial [at least 4 hours] or total [24 hours]).

    c. If the patient's EEG findings are negative for IEA after three or four EEGs, record a prolonged (4–6 hours) daytime EEG with induced sleep.

    d. If the patient's EEG findings with induced sleep are negative for IEA, perform an overnight polysomnographic (PSG) study, preferably a video-PSG for electroclinical correlation. If computer facilities exist for reformatting, change the paper speed to 30 mm/second instead of the usual sleep recording speed of 10 mm/second. If computer facilities are not available, record the PSG at 30 mm/second, particularly during suspicious behavioral episodes. Use an appropriately devised seizure montage with the full complement of electrodes or special electrode placements (e.g., T1 and T2).

    e. If the patient's EEG findings are negative for IEA after steps a–d, perform an ambulatory cassette EEG recording.

    f. If the patient's EEG findings are negative for IEA after steps a–e, perform long-term video-EEG monitoring for 24–72 hours or longer if necessary.

g. Finally, in some patients, invasive EEG monitoring using subdural grid or depth electrodes may be necessary for localizing and lateralizing a focus.

Prognosis

EEG monitoring may be helpful in evaluating the reasons for a patient's
behavioral deterioration.[2, 13] Focal or diffuse slow waves in the EEG
accompanied by spikes or sharp waves may be secondary to repeated
seizures. Excessive slow waves in the EEG may indicate overmedication
(antiepileptic drug side effects). A progressive slow wave may indicate
a focal structural lesion; however, postictal focal EEG abnormalities
should be excluded first in such cases.

Role of Electroencephalography in the Management Decisions

EEG monitoring plays an important role[2, 13] in the following situations:
(1) in determining the type of pharmacotherapy in epilepsy, (2) in assessing the effects of AEDs on the clinical outcome, (3) in documenting the
undesirable side effects of AEDs on EEG recordings, (4) in assessing the
possibility of recurrence after withdrawal of AEDs, and (5) in presur-
gically evaluating patients with medically refractory seizures.

The type of AED to be used in a particular patient depends on the
type of the epilepsy and the epileptic syndrome as outlined in the International Classification. This is an electroclinical determination. The
EEG recording shows a characteristic pattern in partial seizures with
or without secondary generalization, in primary generalized seizure,
and in various epileptic syndromes as discussed previously.

The value of EEG monitoring in predicting the chances of recurrence
of seizures after AED withdrawal in patients who remain seizure-free
2–4 years remains controversial (see Chapters 15 and 19). It is agreed
by the majority of investigators, however, that EEG monitoring in conjunction with other features is an important predictor of whether AEDs
can be withdrawn without a recurrence of seizures.

In cases of status epilepticus where the patient remains comatose
because of prolonged or repeated seizures, intravenous AEDs, or anesthetic agents, EEG monitoring remains the only laboratory test for
monitoring the progress of the epileptiform discharges.

Presurgical Evaluation

EEG monitoring may be helpful in localizing the epileptiform focus during presurgical evaluation for partial complex seizures (see also Chapter 16).[2, 13] Presurgical evaluation involves intensive EEG monitoring that may require both noninvasive and invasive long-term recording. The initial step should be prolonged noninvasive video-EEG inpatient monitoring in a dedicated unit.

The indications for long-term monitoring in epilepsy are (1) to identify the type of seizure, (2) to differentiate epileptic from nonepileptic events, (3) to quantitate the seizure control (long-term monitoring can help assess quantitatively the degree of seizure control, which can then be correlated with the efficacy of anticonvulsants or other forms of treatment), (4) to preoperatively identify the site of the seizure onset in patients with poorly controlled partial seizure who were candidates for neurosurgery, (5) to assess the effects of antiepileptic drugs, (6) to identify circadian variations of seizures, and (7) to differentiate sleep disorders from true epilepsy.

Special electrodes, such as sphenoidal electrodes, nasopharyngeal electrodes, and T1 and T2 basal temporal electrodes, should be used. The use of these electrodes increases the likelihood of demonstrating epileptic seizure discharges in partial complex seizures. Also, the use of multiple, closely spaced electrodes over a region suspected to be potentially epileptogenic on the basis of a standard EEG may increase the chances of detecting epileptiform discharges.[66] If the focus is in the anterior temporal region and unilateral or dominantly unilateral or independently bilateral, if the patient is free from diffuse cerebral dysfunction (e.g., marked mental deterioration) and language dysfunction, and if the patient is an adolescent or a young adult, anterior temporal lobectomy may improve the patient's intractable seizures.[2, 13] If the lesions are extratemporal and multiple, the prognosis is not so favorable.

In a complicated case, if the focus cannot be delineated by standard EEG monitoring or prolonged video-EEG monitoring, an invasive technique of recording EEG must be used.[2, 13, 66–68] These techniques may include depth electrographic recording or EEG recordings obtained after placement of subdural or epidural grids or strips over the cortical convexity. Several investigators found the subdural method of recording useful in locating the site and the extent of the focal epileptiform discharges.[66–68] Depth electrodes should not be left in place for more than 4 weeks, and subdural grid electrodes should not be used for more than 2 weeks because of potential complications, such as infections, hemorrhage, and current leakage.

References

1. Lesser RP. American Electroencephalographic Society Guidelines in EEG and Evoked Potentials. J Clin Neurophysiol 1986;3:1.
2. Engel J Jr. A practical guide for routine EEG studies in epilepsy. J Clin Neurophysiol 1984;1:109.
3. Maulsby RL. Some guidelines for assessment of spike and sharp waves in EEG tracings. Am J EEG Technol 1971;11:3.
4. Pedley TA. Interictal epileptiform discharges: discriminating characteristics and clinical considerations. Am J EEG Technol 1980;20:101.
5. Ajmone-Marsan C. Electroencephalographic studies in seizure disorders: additional considerations. J Clin Neurophysiol 1984;1:143.
6. Sharbrough FW. Scalp-recorded ictal patterns in focal epilepsy. J Clin Neurophysiol 1993;10:262.
7. Klass DW. Electroencephalographic manifestations of complex partial seizures. Adv Neurol 1975;11:113.
8. Blume WT, Young GB, Lemieux JF. EEG morphology of partial epileptic seizures. Electroencephalogr Clin Neurophysiol 1984;57:295.
9. Reiher J, Beaudry M, Leduc CP. Temporal intermittent rhythmic delta activity (TIRDA) and the diagnosis of complex partial epilepsy: sensitivity, specificity and predictive value. Can J Neurol Sci 1989;16:398.
10. Normand MM, Wszolek ZK, Klass DW. Temporal intermittent rhythmic delta activity in electroencephalograms. J Clin Neurophysiol 1995;12:280.
11. Chatrian GE, Bergamini L, Dondey M, et al. A Glossary of Terms Most Commonly Used by Clinical Electroencephalographers. In The International Federation of Societies for Electroencephalography and Clinical Neurophysiology. Recommendations for the Practice of Clinical Neurophysiology. Amsterdam: Elsevier, 1983;11.
12. Pedley TA. The Challenge of Intractable Epilepsy. In D Chadwick (ed), New Trends in Epilepsy Management: The Role of Gabapentin. Royal Society of Medicine Symposium Series No. 198. London: Royal Society of Medicine, 1993;3.
13. Engel J Jr. Seizures and Epilepsy. Philadelphia: FA Davis, 1989;340.
14. Daly DD, Pedley TA. Current Practice of Clinical Electroencephalography. New York: Raven, 1990.
15. Niedermeyer E, Lopes Da Silva F. Electroencephalography: Basic Principles, Clinical Applications and Related Fields (3rd ed). Baltimore: Urban & Schwarzenberg, 1993.
16. Drury I, Beydoun A. Pitfalls of EEG interpretation in epilepsy. Neurol Clin 1993;11:857.
17. Sato S, Rose DF. The electroencephalogram in the evaluation of the patient with epilepsy. Neurol Clin 1986;4:509.

18. Vignaendra V, Matthews RL, Chatrian GE. Positive occipital sharp transients of sleep: relationships to nocturnal sleep cycle in man. Electroencephalogr Clin Neurophysiol 1974;37:239.
19. Kazelka JW, Pedley TA. Beta and mu rhythms. J Clin Neurophysiol 1990;7:191.
20. Westmoreland BF, Sharbrough FW. Posterior slow wave transients associated with eye blinks in children. Am J EEG Technol 1973;15:14.
21. Belsh JM, Chokroverty S, Barabas G. Posterior rhythmic slow activity in EEG after eye closure. Electroencephalogr Clin Neurophysiol 1983;56:562.
22. Barlow JS, Ciganek L. Lambda responses in relation to visual evoked responses in man. Electroencephalogr Clin Neurophysiol 1969;26:183.
23. Kellaway P. An Orderly Approach to Visual Analysis: Characteristics of the Normal EEG of Adults and Children. In DD Daly, TA Pedley (eds), Current Practice of Clinical Electroencephalography (2nd ed). New York: Raven, 1990;139.
24. Westmoreland BF. Benign EEG Variants and Patterns of Uncertain Clinical Significance. In DD Daly, TA Pedley (eds), Current Practice of Clinical Electroencephalography (2nd ed). New York: Raven, 1990;243.
25. Pedley TA. EEG Patterns that Mimic Epileptiform Discharges But Have No Association with Seizures. In CE Henry (ed), Current Clinical Neurophysiology. Update on EEG and Evoked Potentials. New York: Elsevier, 1980;307.
26. Klass DW, Westmoreland BF. Nonepileptogenic epileptiform electroencephalographic activity. Ann Neurol 1985;18:627.
27. Gibbs FA, Gibbs EL. Fourteen and six per second positive spikes. Electroencephalogr Clin Neurophysiol 1963;15:553.
28. Eeg-Olofsson O. The development of the electroencephalogram in normal children from the age of 1 through 15 years: 14 and 6 positive spike phenomenon. Neuropaediatrie 1971;2:405.
29. Reiher J, Klass DW. Two common EEG patterns of doubtful clinical significance. Med Clin North Am 1968;52:933.
30. White JC, Langston JW, Pedley TA. Benign epileptiform transients of sleep: clarification of the small sharp spike controversy. Neurology 1977;27:1061.
31. Thomas JE, Klass DW. Six-per-second spike-and-wave pattern in the electroencephalogram: a reappraisal of its clinical significance. Neurology 1968;18:587.
32. Reiher J, Lebel M. Wicket spikes: clinical correlates of a previously undescribed EEG pattern. Can J Neurol Sci 1977;4:39.
33. Zifkin BG, Cracco RQ. An Orderly Approach to the Abnormal EEG. In DD Daly, TA Pedley (eds), Current Practice of Clinical Electroencephalography (2nd ed). New York: Raven, 1990;253.
34. Bickford RG, Butt AR. Hepatic coma: the electro-encephalographic pattern. J Clin Invest 1955;34:790.
35. Fisch BJ, Klass DW. The diagnostic specificity of triphasic wave patterns. Electroencephalogr Clin Neurophysiol 1988;70:1.
36. Chatrian GE, Shaw CM, Leftman H. The significance of periodic lateralized epileptiform discharges in EEG: an electrographic, clinical and pathological study. Electroencephalogr Clin Neurophysiol 1964;17:177.

37. Fisch BJ. Spehlmann's EEG Primer. New York: Elsevier, 1991.
38. Westmoreland BF, Klass DW. A distinctive rhythmic EEG discharge of adults. Electroencephalogr Clin Neurophysiol 1981;51:186.
39. Stillerman ML, Gibbs EL, Perlstein MA. Electroencephalographic changes in strabismus. Am J Ophthalmol 1952;35:54.
40. Gastaut H, Roger J, Soulayrol R, et al. Childhood epileptic encephalopathy with diffuse spike-waves (otherwise known as "petit mal variant") or Lennox syndrome. Epilepsia 1966;7:139.
41. Blume WT. Lennox-Gastaut Syndrome. In H Luders, RP Lesser (eds), Epilepsy: Electroclinical Syndrome. New York: Springer-Verlag, 1987;73.
42. Westmoreland BF, Gomez MR. Infantile Spasms (West syndrome). In H Luders, RP Lesser (eds), Epilepsy: Electroclinical Syndrome. New York: Springer-Verlag, 1987;49.
43. Luders H, Lesser RP, Dinner DS, Morris HH. Benign Focal Epilepsy of Childhood. In H Luders, RP Lesser (eds), Epilepsy: Electroclinical Syndrome. New York: Springer-Verlag, 1987;303.
44. Bickford RG, Klass DW. Scalp and depth electrographic studies of electro-decremental seizures. Electroencephalogr Clin Neurophysiol 1960;12:263.
45. Kellaway P, Hrachovy RA, Frost JD, Zion T. Precise characterization and quantification of infantile spasms. Ann Neurol 1979;6:214.
46. Dinner DS, Luders H, Morris HH, Lesser RP. Juvenile Myoclonic Epilepsy. In H Luders, RP Lesser (eds), Epilepsy: Electroclinical Syndrome. New York: Springer-Verlag, 1987;131.
47. Sharbrough FW. Scalp-recorded ictal patterns in focal epilepsy. J Clin Neurophysiol 1993;10:262.
48. Ralston BL, Paptheodorou CA. The mechanism of transition of interictal spiking foci into ictal seizure discharges. Part II: observations in man. Electroencephalogr Clin Neurophysiol 1960;12:297.
49. Geiger LR, Harner RN. EEG patterns at the time of focal seizure onset. Arch Neurol 1978;35:276.
50. Klass DW, Espinosa RE, Fischer-Williams M. Analysis of concurrent electroencephalographic and clinical events occurring sequentially during partial seizures. Electroencephalogr Clin Neurophysiol 1973;34:728.
51. Blume WT, Young GB, Lemieux JF. EEG morphology of partial epileptic seizures. Electroencephalogr Clin Neurophysiol 1984;57:295.
52. Devinsky O, Kelley K, Porter RJ, Theodore WH. Clinical and electroencephalographic features of simple partial seizures. Neurology 1988;38:1347.
53. Devinsky O, Sato S, Kufta CV, et al. Electroencephalographic studies of simple partial seizures with subdural electrode recordings. Neurology 1989;39:527.
54. Drury I, Henry TR. Ictal patterns in generalized epilepsy. J Clin Neurophysiol 1993;10:268.
55. Salinsky M, Kanter R, Dasheiff RM. Effectiveness of multiple EEGs in supporting the diagnosis of epilepsy: an operational curve. Epilepsia 1987;28:331.

56. So NK. The Electroencephalogram. In PM Matthews, DL Arnold (eds), Diagnostic Tests in Neurology. New York: Churchill Livingstone, 1991;133.
57. Ajmone-Marsan C, Zivin LS. Factors related to the occurrence of typical paroxysmal abnormalities in the EEG records of epileptic patients. Epilepsia 1970;11:361.
58. Zivin L, Ajmone-Marsan C. Incidence and prognostic significance of epileptiform activity in the EEG of non-epileptic subjects. Brain 1968;91:751.
59. Petersen I, Eeg-Olofsson O, Sellden U. Paroxysmal Activity in EEG of Normal Children. In P Kellaway, I Petersen (eds), Clinical Electroencephalography of Children. New York: Grune & Stratton, 1968;167.
60. Eeg-Olofsson O, Petersen I, Sellden U. The development of the electroencephalogram in normal children from the age of one through fifteen years. Neuropaediatrie 1971;4:375.
61. Kellaway P, Saltzberg B, Frost JD Jr, Crawley JW. Relationship between clinical state, ictal and interictal EEG discharges, and serum drug levels: generalized epilepsy/ethosuximide. Neurology 1979;29:559.
62. Snead OC, Hosey LC. Exacerbation of seizures in children by carbamazepine. N Engl J Med 1985;313:916.
63. Sachdeo R, Chokroverty S. Increasing epileptiform activities in EEG in presence of decreasing clinical seizures after carbamazepine. Epilepsia 1985;26:522.
64. Spencer SS. Depth electroencephalography in selection of refractory epilepsy for surgery. Ann Neurol 1981;9:207.
65. Chokroverty S. Sleep and Epilepsy. In S Chokroverty (ed), Sleep Disorders Medicine. Boston: Butterworth-Heinemann, 1994;429.
66. Lesser RP, Luders H, Dinner DS, et al. EEG in epilepsy. Barrow Neurological Institute 1987;3:42.
67. Wyler AR, Ojemann GA, Lettick E, et al. Subdural strip electrodes for localizing epileptogenic foci. J Neurosurg 1984;60:1195.
68. Lueders H, Hahn J, Lesser RP, et al. Localization of Epileptogenic Spike Foci: Comparative Study of Closely Spaced Scalp Electrodes, Nasopharyngeal, Sphenoidal, Subdural and Depth Electrodes. In H Akimoto, H Kazamatsuri, M Seino, et al. (eds), Advances in Epileptology: XIIIth Epilepsy International Symposium. New York: Raven, 1982;185.

6

Treatment of Primary Generalized Seizures: Tonic-Clonic and Absence Seizures

Roger J. Porter

Introduction

Generalized tonic-clonic seizures and absence seizures are quite different entities, but they are often treated with the same medications, notably valproate. The common classification of these two seizure types comes from the notion that both attacks can be considered primarily generalized—that is, either may arise without evidence of a local onset. It is unlikely that this concept will stand the test of time, but current dogma places these two epileptic events together on this basis. One concept that separates the two is the process of secondary generalization, which is discussed under Which Drugs to Use. Appropriate treatment of these seizures depends on the correct diagnosis. For this reason, the seizure type is described in detail before therapeutic options are considered.

Generalized Tonic-Clonic Seizures

Diagnosis

Generalized tonic-clonic seizures do not involve random flailing of the body and limbs, but are surprisingly stereotyped, although isolated fragments do occur. The fragments may be the result of partially effective antiepileptic drug treatment, and either tonic or clonic motions may be separately observed.[1] When the typical attack occurs, it usually follows the pattern described by Gastaut and Broughton.[2] The tonic phase lasts approximately 10–20 seconds and is characterized by the onset of brief bilateral flexion followed by extension of the arms and legs. The tonic phase usually does not end abruptly, but forms a continuum with the clonic phase that follows. As the rigid tonicity is increasingly interrupted by decreased tone, a fine tremor gradually appears as the muscular relaxations completely interrupt the tonic contractions, and the clonic phase begins. Clonic jerks are brief, violent flexor spasms of the entire body; they typically last about 30 seconds and end with slowing and finally cessation of the jerking. The patient is usually comatose or stuporous at the end of the attack.

In addition to the above sequence of events, autonomic changes are prominent. The heart rate and blood pressure may double, and bladder pressure may increase up to sixfold. Pupillary mydriasis and glandular hypersecretion of the skin and salivary glands occur. Cyanosis is correlated with the accompanying apnea.[2]

The electroencephalographic (EEG) accompaniments of generalized tonic-clonic seizures are dramatic but often obscured by muscle artifact. The initial EEG change is usually desynchronization that lasts 1–3 seconds, followed by 10 seconds of 10-Hz spikes. Because the clonic phase predominates, the spikes are mixed with slow waves and finally become a polyspike and wave pattern. The EEG is flat, or nearly flat, after a severe generalized tonic-clonic seizure but gradually recovers to normal rhythms.[1]

Generalized tonic-clonic seizures may represent the maximum expression of epilepsy in adult human beings. Support for this notion is based on the observation of the large number of seizure types that may progress directly to this seizure type. In fact, most generalized tonic-clonic seizures occur secondarily to a less dramatic seizure type. Patients often have a history of partial seizures that progress to generalized tonic-clonic seizures. When these generalized attacks occur in patients with partial epilepsy, most—if not all—of the attacks are secondarily induced. Similar observations have been made in generalized seizures other than tonic-clonic seizures. For example, the progression of absence seizures to generalized tonic-clonic seizures has been documented clinically and electrographically,[3–5] and the progression of clonic seizures to generalized tonic-clonic seizures has been noted.[5, 6] Clearly, in patients with generalized tonic-clonic seizures, the nature of any other seizure type must be established. Appropriate therapy can then be instituted for the fundamental seizure type, as well as for the tonic-clonic seizures.[1]

The stereotypical nature of generalized tonic-clonic seizures makes them relatively easy to distinguish by the patient's medical history. Other seizure types are more subtle and often more heterogeneous. When taking the patient's medical history, first establish whether or not generalized tonic-clonic seizures (e.g., psychogenic attacks) are present, then search for a history of other seizure types.[1]

Treatment

Whom to Treat

The decision to treat generalized tonic-clonic seizures revolves around the question of how many seizures the patient has had and whether patients who have had only a single seizure should be treated. This is a controversial subject. Much of the controversy surrounds the likelihood of seizure recurrence after the first attack. Hauser and colleagues[7, 8] suggested that the 3-year recurrence rate may be as low as 27%, whereas Elwes et al.[9] found a recurrence rate of 71%, and Hopkins et al.[10] a rate of 52%. The lower rate may be the result of a higher percentage of treated patients and of a less rapid entry into the study after the first event.[11] A study of generalized tonic-clonic seizures conducted in Italy found that patients given phenytoin, phenobarbital, carbamazepine, or valproic acid after a first seizure were less likely (18% versus 38%) to have a second attack in the subsequent 2 years than patients who were untreated.[12] It is not uncommon for a patient to have a single, unprovoked generalized tonic-clonic seizure, and most clinicians—barring evidence that repetitive seizures might occur—would choose not to treat the patient. This approach is not necessarily the case with other seizure types.[1]

The reasons usually given for not treating a single generalized tonic-clonic attack are that a significant percentage of patients will never have another seizure and that many have only toxicity to gain from the medication.[1] Hachinski[13] summarizes the current, rational approach to patients with single seizures by noting that those who have structural or electroencephalographic evidence of lesions should be approached less conservatively than those who have negative investigations. In addition, the occupation and attitude of the patient must be considered. Finally, the certainty of the diagnosis plays some role. Hachinski[13] notes that "it is usually only after a second seizure that both physicians and patients are prepared for their respective roles in anticonvulsant treatment." This view, however, may be altered by future studies and is not universally supported. Hopkins et al.,[10] for example, believe that early treatment not only suppresses attacks in the short term, but also the long-term tendency to recurrence.

Which Drugs to Use

The therapy of generalized tonic-clonic seizures is often thought to depend on the nature of the onset of the attack—that is, secondarily generalized attacks may respond to different medications than those arising primarily. In the latter, there is no antecedent seizure leading directly to the generalized tonic-clonic attack.

What remains unknown is whether treating the antecedent seizure type instead of the generalized tonic-clonic seizure itself is an acceptable medical approach. We know, for example, that phenytoin or carbamazepine is effective in the treatment of partial seizures and that secondarily generalized seizures occurring in patients with partial seizures respond quite well to these same medications. The unanswered question is whether the medication, by decreasing the number and severity of partial seizures, makes secondary spread less likely or whether it has a primary effect on the generalized tonic-clonic attacks themselves. For generalized tonic-clonic seizures accompanying absence seizures, the issue is even more difficult. Valproate is highly effective against absence seizures and apparently against the associated generalized tonic-clonic seizures as well. Ethosuximide, however, which is also effective against absence seizures, has been thought by some to exacerbate other seizure types, but there is no conclusive evidence that it exacerbates generalized tonic-clonic seizures. In fact, the effect of the drugs in decreasing absence seizure frequency may also lead to a decrease in secondary generalization of the seizures.

These observations aside, current dogma suggests that the treatment of generalized tonic-clonic seizures occurring secondarily to partial seizures is similar to that of partial seizures themselves. Carbamazepine and phenytoin are the current drugs of choice. Although the efficacy of valproate against secondarily generalized tonic-clonic seizures appears to be equal to that of carbamazepine,[14] many epileptologists believe that valproate is less effective than carbamazepine or phenytoin for such attacks. However, valproate is effective against primary generalized tonic-clonic seizures, whether they occur in isolation or in combination with other generalized seizures such as absence or myoclonia.[15, 16] The role of the newer antiepileptic drugs in the treatment of generalized tonic-clonic seizures may be substantial, especially for patients refractory to or intolerant of current medications (see the paragraph below). Even though the majority of clinical trials were conducted with patients who had secondarily generalized tonic-clonic seizures, these drugs are likely to prove effective against primarily generalized attacks as well.

Phenytoin and Carbamazepine

Generalized tonic-clonic seizures respond to a variety of medications, including carbamazepine, hydantoins, barbiturates, valproate, and the newer medications. The drugs of choice for secondarily generalized tonic-clonic attacks are carbamazepine and phenytoin. In choosing a drug, the physician should weigh factors other than efficacy. Phenytoin and carbamazepine are almost equally efficacious but differ in their potential toxicity. Neither phenytoin nor carbamazepine has sedative effects.

Phenytoin has several advantages. It is an old, safe compound, and most physicians are familiar with its use. Serious side effects are rare and almost always reversible. The parenteral formulation is useful, although intramuscular administration is not recommended. Methods for determining the plasma phenytoin level are commonly available.

The starting dose of phenytoin in adults is typically 300 mg/day; divided daily doses may be necessary if the generic compound is used. The optimum dose in an individual patient is determined by the effectiveness of the drug, with guidance from the drug level. The drug can be increased at approximately weekly intervals, although special care should be taken at higher doses to avoid toxicity related to saturation kinetics. The maximal dose is the maximal tolerated dose, but is typically between 300 and 400 mg/day—e.g., 350 mg/day.

The disadvantages of phenytoin use include hirsutism; gingival hyperplasia; coarsening of the features; and a teratogenic potential, including the fetal hydantoin syndrome. Dose-related toxicity is occasionally a problem because of the drug's nonlinear kinetics. Phenytoin, discovered in the late 1930s, was marketed before controlled clinical trials were required; therefore, evidence of its effectiveness against partial seizures and generalized tonic-clonic seizures is mainly anecdotal.[1]

Carbamazepine has some advantages. It is easily tolerated by most patients and does not cause hirsutism or gingival hyperplasia. In one study,[17] it outperformed phenytoin in the evaluation of behavioral toxicity, and the drug may have a positive psychotropic effect. In a different study of normal volunteers, phenytoin and carbamazepine impaired memory and performance equally.[18] Carbamazepine should be started slowly. In adults, 100 mg twice daily is appropriate, increasing the dose as necessary every few days, typically up to 800–1,000 mg/day; some patients require up to 1,600 mg/day for maximal seizure control. The drug is best given in divided doses because of its short half-life.

The disadvantages of carbamazepine use include the risk of blood dyscrasias, which is an overrated fear, and a short half-life, which may necessitate a dosing schedule of several times a day.[1] There is evidence that carbamazepine may be as teratogenetic as other antiepileptic compounds.[19]

Barbiturates are occasionally useful but have the serious disadvantage of sedating the patient, even at plasma levels within the "therapeutic range." Benzodiazepines are usually ineffective for the long-term control of generalized tonic-clonic seizures. Valproate is discussed in the section on ethosuximide and valproate.

The appropriate use of these standard drugs depends on their therapeutic plasma levels (Table 6-1). The pharmacokinetic principles for achieving these levels are discussed in Chapter 4.

Absence Seizures

Diagnosis

Absence seizures were among the first seizure types to be adequately described. Their high frequency in children, modern techniques of intensive monitoring, and a large population of patients with absence seizures gathered by Dreifuss at the University of Virginia[1] made it possible to conduct the early descriptive studies.[20] Absence seizures begin in childhood or early adolescence. The patient is unresponsive throughout the attack. Although unresponsiveness is the rule, motionlessness occurs in less than 10% of absence attacks. In fact, many other phenomena may accompany such attacks.[20] Absence seizures are generally

Table 6-1. Therapeutic Levels of Standard Antiepileptic Drugs

Drug	Effective Level (mg/liter)	High Effective Level* (mg/liter)	Toxic Level (mg/liter)
Carbamazepine	6–15	12	8
Phenytoin	10–20	18	15
Phenobarbital	10–30	25	20
Primidone	5–15	12	10
Valproic acid	50–100	80	100
Ethosuximide	50–100	80	100

*Minimum levels that should be reached (particularly during monotherapy) in patients with refractory seizures before deciding the drug has failed to help. Higher levels are often possible with monotherapy. Levels are trough levels drawn before the morning medication.

brief, usually lasting less than 10 seconds and rarely longer than 45 seconds. The attacks are not associated with auras; postictal abnormalities; hallucinations; formed speech; or other symptoms characteristic of partial seizures, generalized tonic-clonic seizures, or infantile spasms. In a video analysis of 374 recorded absence seizures, the attacks were characterized by some combination of the features given in Table 6-2. Automatisms are common in absence seizures. Any seizure lasting longer than 7 seconds has a 50% or greater chance of having associated automatisms; a seizure lasting longer than 18 seconds has a 95% chance of associated automatisms.[20] The automatisms commonly occurring in absence seizures are much the same as those in complex partial seizures, although they are usually somewhat less complicated or prolonged. Lip smacking, chewing, and fumbling of the fingers are commonly observed in absence seizures; less common are swallowing, lip licking, grimacing, yawning, scratching, rubbing, shuffling the legs, walking, and stepping in place.[1]

An important study of 926 videotaped absence seizures by Holmes et al.[21] differentiated between typical and atypical absence attacks. The patients with atypical attacks had a much higher likelihood of having developmental delay or retardation, other types of seizures (other than partial seizures), and EEGs with interictal abnormalities. The differences between the seizures of each group are also noteworthy. Typical absence seizures were more likely to be characterized by automatisms and eye blinking, whereas atypical absence seizures were typified by more prominent increases or decreases in muscle tone. Atypical absence

Table 6-2. Features of Absence Seizures

Feature	Percentage of Seizures*
Automatisms	63
Mild clonic motion (usually eyelids)	46
Decreased postural tone (usually head nodding)	23
Increased postural tone (usually arching of the back)	5
Autonomic phenomena	?

*Many patients had more than one feature.
Source: Reprinted with permission from JK Penry, RJ Porter, FE Dreifuss. Simultaneous recording of absence seizures with video tape and electroencephalography: a study of 374 seizures in 48 patients. Brain 1975;98:427.

seizures were significantly longer than typical absence seizures. The onset and cessation of the seizures were abrupt in each type and were not useful in distinguishing between the two groups. Finally, the authors concluded that typical and atypical absence attacks are not discrete entities but form a continuum.

Treatment

Whom to Treat

The majority of patients with absence seizures require medication to abolish their attacks. The interruption of consciousness interferes with normal daily functioning and necessitates the use of antiepileptic drugs. The response to antiabsence medication can be quantified. Absence seizures are characteristically associated with generalized, high-voltage spike and wave discharges in the EEG that occur at 2.5–3.5 Hz. A large number of behavioral measures have shown that performance is decreased during the spike and wave discharge.[22] The generalized spike and wave abnormality, therefore, unlike most electrographic abnormalities, correlates directly with the seizure itself, and obviously the number of generalized spike and wave paroxysms will give an excellent estimate of the seizure frequency. A decrement in consciousness occurs even if the paroxysm lasts less than 2–3 seconds. Antiabsence therapy therefore should be aimed at eliminating not only the clinical seizures, but also as many generalized spike and wave discharges as possible. Many brief absence attacks may go unnoticed clinically, and the EEG is the best way of identifying them. Prolonged EEG recording before and after medication changes is helpful for assessing the effectiveness of therapy.

Which Drugs to Use

Ethosuximide and valproate are the primary drugs for treating absence seizures. Ethosuximide, a relatively nontoxic and nonsedative drug, has been the drug of choice for the treatment of absence attacks since its introduction in 1960. Valproate is preferred if the patient has generalized tonic-clonic seizures in addition to absence attacks. Although the liver toxicity and teratogenicity of valproate have received much publicity, these side effects are uncommon, and the drug is use by hundreds of thousands of patients with no difficulty.

Other drugs are effective but more toxic than ethosuximide and valproate. Nitrazepam and clonazepam, both benzodiazepines, are quite effective but cause problems of tolerance and adverse effects on behavior. Trimethadione has a series of different side effects. Acetazolamide is effective for a few months, but the development of tolerance is common. Phensuximide and methsuximide, two other succinimides, are less useful than ethosuximide in most patients.

Ethosuximide and Valproate

As with all antiepileptic drugs, ethosuximide should be used vigorously and fully before being abandoned as ineffective for absence seizures. Plasma ethosuximide levels in the range of 60–100 µg/ml should be achieved. In resistant patients, even higher levels, occasionally as high as 150 µg/ml, may be needed.[23] Ethosuximide has a long half-life, but spacing of the daily dosage is necessary to avoid the side effects of nausea, vomiting, headache, and anorexia. Initial drowsiness rarely persists. The side effects necessitate a regimen that achieves gradual buildup of the drug. Although a dose of 1,500–2,000 mg daily may be required to achieve seizure control, it may be necessary to start with a dose of 250–500 mg daily to avoid gastrointestinal upset. The drug is typically given in divided doses because of its potential for causing nausea, even though the half-life of the drug is relatively long. The dose can be increased every few days. The gastrointestinal side effects can often be alleviated by temporary dose reduction. Bone marrow depression is an exceedingly rare idiosyncratic side effect of ethosuximide, but it can be fatal.

Valproate is perhaps the most widely used antiepileptic drug for absence seizures, in part because of its effectiveness against a broad spectrum of seizure types, including the generalized tonic-clonic attacks that sometimes accompany absence seizures. Valproate is highly effective against absence seizures[24] and decreases the generalized spike and wave paroxysms that accompany them.[25] With the use of 12-hour telemetered EEGs to measure the frequency of generalized spike and wave discharges, valproate was compared with ethosuximide in a double-blind, response-conditional crossover study of absence seizures in 45 patients.[26] Valproate was found to be as effective as ethosuximide.

Patients who meet the diagnostic criteria for absence seizures and who do not respond to ethosuximide should be considered for treatment with valproate. The drug should be started in relatively low doses, with gradual buildup to a therapeutic level. Valproate shares with ethosuximide a tendency to irritate the gastrointestinal tract. This tendency can usually be overcome with slowly increasing doses and considerable patience. The dose of valproate necessary for seizure control is often more than 30 mg/kg. In some patients, doses of 60 mg/kg are required to reach reasonable plasma valproate levels and maximal efficacy. The therapeutic level (before the morning dose) ranges from 60 µg/ml to 100 µg/ml, but in resistant cases every effort should be made to exceed 80 µg/ml before abandoning the drug. Furthermore, many patients tolerate levels considerably higher than 100 µg/ml.[27] Valproate has a short half-life, and as higher doses are approached, it should be recognized that a dosing regimen of four times a day will allow the maximal daily dose with minimal side effects. In less severely affected patients, less frequent administration is satisfactory.[28, 29]

Certain side effects are unique to valproate. Weight gain is a problem in a few patients, presumably from increased appetite. Although hair loss is temporary and reversible on dose reduction or discontinuation of the drug, it may be dramatic in a few affected patients. A fine tremor occurs at higher doses. Reversible amenorrhea has been noted. A decrease in the platelet count has been reported, but bleeding is not well documented enough to cause concern. Drug interactions are a problem, especially with phenobarbital. The teratogenicity of valproate is discussed in Chapter 11.

The most important idiosyncratic side effect of valproate is acute hepatotoxicity. There is virtually no evidence that this side effect is dose-related. The hepatotoxicity may begin insidiously and may not be accompanied by specific laboratory abnormalities. Even the aspartate aminotransferase (AST) level may not rise dramatically and is a limited predictor of eventual outcome. It is, nevertheless, the best biochemical indicator available and should be monitored for the first few months of therapy. Although the AST level may return to normal in some patients if the drug is stopped, the clinical course in others appears to be inexorable. The initial clinical signs of hepatotoxicity may be nausea, sleepiness, vomiting, and jaundice.

Although acute hepatotoxicity is rare, the following specific recommendations for the use of valproate[30, 31] recognize that it is more common in very young children and in patients receiving multiple drug therapy:

1.   Avoid administering valproate as part of anticonvulsant polytherapy in children younger than 3 years of age unless monotherapy has failed or the potential benefits of polypharmacy merit the risks.

2.   Avoid administering valproate to patients with pre-existing liver disease or a family history of childhood hepatic disease.

3.   Administer valproate in as low a dose as possible consistent with seizure control.

4.   Avoid the concurrent administration of valproate and salicylates, and avoid fasting in children with intercurrent illnesses.

5.   Observe the patient clinically for vomiting, headache, edema, jaundice, or seizure breakthrough, especially after a febrile illness. If any of these symptoms develop, discontinue valproate therapy until a definitive diagnosis is established.

Multiple Drug Therapy

Although many patients are well controlled on a single medication and although one of the goals of the physician should be to simplify the regimen as much as possible (e.g., aiming for monotherapy), some patients require more than one drug. The advantages of limiting medication to a single drug are many[1]:

1.   Adverse drug interactions are much less likely; they obviously do not even occur with monotherapy.

2.   Side effects in general may be fewer, although this issue is complex.

3.   Compliance by the patient may be better; however, compliance problems may also relate to inadequate attention by the physician to this issue.

4. Cost may be lower; it may also be higher if more expensive drugs are chosen.

5. Seizure control is better in some patients, but improvement in seizure control may not relate to a fundamental alteration in the propensity to have seizures. Rather, it may relate to increased compliance because of few adverse side effects.

In spite of these advantages, some patients, usually with severe epilepsy, respond better to a multidrug regimen. If a patient does poorly on a single drug, the physician should consider two simultaneous drugs as a reasonable alternative.

Summary

Both generalized tonic-clonic seizures and absence seizures are often treated with valproate. The epileptic events themselves, however, are entirely different and require completely different therapeutic strategies. A full knowledge of the form and variety of the epileptic syndromes associated with these seizure types will permit the physician to choose the appropriate therapy.

References

1. Theodore WH, Porter RJ. Epilepsy: 100 Elementary Principles, London: Saunders, 1995.
2. Gastaut H, Broughton R. Epileptic Seizures: Clinical and Electrographic Features, Diagnosis and Treatment. Springfield, IL: Thomas, 1972;286.
3. Oller-Daurella L. The confusional states (absence status). Acta Neurol Belg 1974;74:265.
4. Niedermeyer E. Immediate transition from a petit mal absence into a grand mal seizure: Case report. Eur Neurol 1976;14:11.
5. Theodore WH, Porter RJ, Albert P, et al. The secondary generalized tonic-clonic seizure: a video-tape analysis. Neurology 1994;44:1403.
6. Porter RJ, Sato S. Secondary Generalization of Epileptic Seizures. In H Akimoto, H Kazamatsuri, M Seino, AA Ward Jr. (eds), Advances in Epileptology; XIIIth Epilepsy International Symposium. New York: Raven, 1982;47.
7. Hauser WA, Anderson VE, Loewenson RB, McRoberts SM. Seizure recurrence after a first unprovoked seizure. N Engl J Med 1982;307:522.
8. Hauser WA. Should people be treated after a first seizure? Arch Neurol 1986:43:1287.
9. Elwes RDC, Chesterman P, Reynolds EH. Prognosis after a first untreated tonic-clonic seizure. Lancet 1985;2:752.

10. Hopkins A, Garman A, Clarke C. The first seizure in adult life. Lancet 1988;1:721.
11. Elwes RDC, Reynolds EH. Should people be treated after a first seizure? Arch Neurol 1988;45;490.
12. First Seizure Trial Group. Randomized clinical trial on the efficacy of antiepileptic drugs in reducing the risk of relapse after a first unprovoked tonic-clonic seizure. Neurology 1993;43:478.
13. Hachinski V. Management of a first seizure. Arch Neurol 1986;43:1290.
14. Mattson RH, Cramer JA, Collins JF, et al. A comparison of valproate with carbamazepine for the treatment of complex partial seizures and secondary generalized seizures in adults. N Engl J Med 1992;327:765.
15. Collaborative Study Group: Bourgeois B, Beaumanoir A, Blajev B, de la Cruz N, et al. Monotherapy with valproate in primary generalized epilepsies. Epilepsia 1987;28(Suppl 2):S8.
16. Chadwick DW. Valproate monotherapy in the management of generalized and partial seizures. Epilepsia 1987;28(Suppl 2):S12.
17. Smith DB, Mattson RH, Cramer JA, et al. Results of a nationwide Veterans Administration cooperative study comparing the efficacy and toxicity of carbamazepine, phenobarbital, phenytoin, and primidone. Epilepsia 1987;28(Suppl 3):S50.
18. Meador KJ, Loring DW, Abney OL, et al. Effects of carbamazepine and phenytoin on EEG and memory in healthy adults. Epilepsia 1993;34:153.
19. Jones KL, Lacro RV, Johnson KA, Adams I. Pattern of malformations in the children of women treated with carbamazepine during pregnancy. N Engl J Med 1989;320:1661.
20. Penry JK, Porter RJ, Dreifuss FE. Simultaneous recording of absence seizures with video tape and electroencephalography: a study of 374 seizures in 48 patients. Brain 1975;98:427.
21. Holmes GL, McKeever M, Adamson M. Absence seizures in children: clinical and electroencephalographic features. Ann Neurol 1987;21:268.
22. Penry JD. Behavioral Correlates of Generalized Spike-Wave Discharge in the Electroencephalogram. In MAB Brazier (ed), Epilepsy: Its Phenomena In Man. New York: Academic, 1973;171.
23. Sherwin AL. Ethosuximide. Relation of Plasma Concentration to Seizure Control. In DM Woodbury, JK Penry, CE Pippenger (eds), Antiepileptic Drugs (2nd ed). New York: Raven, 1982;637.
24. Simon D, Penry JK. Sodium di-N-propylacetate (DPA) in the treatment of epilepsy A review. Epilepsia 1975;16:549.
25. Penry JK, Porter RJ, Sato S, et al. Effect of Sodium Valproate on Generalized Spike-Wave Paroxysms in the Electroencephalogram. In NJ Legg (ed), Clinical and Pharmacological Aspects of Sodium Valproate (Epilim) in the Treatment of Epilepsy. Tunbridge Wells, England: MCS Consultants, 1976;158.
26. Sato S, White BG, Penry JK, et al. Valproic acid versus ethosuximide in the treatment of absence seizures. Neurology 1982;2:157.
27. Hurst DL. Expanded therapeutic range of valproate. Pediatr Neurol 1987;3:342.
28. Wilder BJ, Karas BJ, Hammond EJ, Perchalski RJ. Twice daily dosing of valproate with divalproex. Clin Pharmacol Ther 1983;34:501.

29. Gjerloff I, Arentsen J, Alving J, Secher BG. Monodose versus three daily doses of sodium valproate: a controlled trial. Acta Neurol Scand 1984;69:120.
30. Dreifuss FE, Santilli N, Langer DH, et al. Valproic acid hepatic fatalities: a retrospective review. Neurology 1987;37:379.
31. Dreifuss FE, Langer DH. Hepatic considerations in the use of antiepileptic drugs. Epilepsia 1987;28(Suppl 2):S23.

Appendix: New Medications

Four new medications have been introduced in most countries in the past 5 years: felbamate, gabapentin, lamotrigine, and vigabatrin. All but vigabatrin are available in the United States. The drugs were primarily studied in adults with complex partial seizures, but their use in treating patients with secondarily generalized tonic-clonic seizures has also been demonstrated for some. Effectiveness against all generalized tonic-clonic seizures appears evident. A comprehensive overview is available.[1] For the limited purposes of this chapter, suffice it to say that any one of these drugs may prove effective for treating patients with generalized tonic-clonic seizures and that the usual reasons for choosing one of them (instead of, for example, phenytoin, carbamazepine, or valproate) is on the basis of adverse effects rather than efficacy. Three of the four (lamotrigine excluded) are sufficiently nonpotent that the dose is often measured in grams per day. A summary of relevant pharmacology of these drugs is included in Chapters 18 and 19. A few sentences on each of these four medications follow:

Felbamate was exceedingly promising, but idiosyncratic toxicity to bone marrow and to the liver have limited its use. The drug is often well tolerated, and anecdotal reports of patients who respond only to felbamate abound. Drug interactions may be a problem.

Gabapentin is very potent but has pharmacologic advantages. It is not metabolized and has no drug interactions. The drug has a short half-life and must usually be administered multiple times per day.

Lamotrigine is more potent than the others discussed here; doses range from 200 mg/day to 700 mg/day. Drug interactions must be considered, especially with valproate.

Vigabatrin is an inhibitor of gamma-aminobutyric acid transaminase and therefore has the advantage of a new, specific mechanism of action. It is not yet available in the United States, but the European experience is vast. Although the half-life is short, the pharmacodynamic effect may be prolonged. Toxicity includes psychiatric disturbances such as psychosis, which is seen in a small percentage of patients.

7

Practical Approach to Management of Simple and Complex Partial Seizures

Peter W. Kaplan and Ronald P. Lesser

Definition

Focal epileptic seizures arise from a localized region in one cerebral hemisphere, and their clinical expression derives from the cortical areas involved in the discharge. The International Classification of Epileptic Seizures[1] categorizes these events into two groups: those that affect consciousness (complex) and those that do not (simple). Simple partial seizures produce motor, sensory, autonomic, and psychic symptoms without impairment of consciousness. Complex partial seizures involve impairment of consciousness or vigilance and typically include stereotyped, semipurposeful movements or automatisms, loss of awareness, and a variable period of confusion.

Seizure Spread

Both simple and complex partial seizures may spread within one hemisphere or involve both hemispheres. Secondarily generalized seizures occur when seizure activity spreads to both hemispheres with loss of consciousness. During the course of ictal spread, a patient may progress through several clinical stages, passing, for example, from simple partial seizures to complex partial seizures and then to secondarily generalized tonic-clonic seizures. The greater the impairment of consciousness, the greater the impact on educational, social, and professional activities. Seizure type and frequency therefore determine the treatment and decisions regarding antiepileptic drug (AED) treatment.

Diagnosis

Paroxysmal disturbances of movement, sensation, behavior, and consciousness may be due to a variety of causes aside from seizures[2-5] (Table 7-1). The overall management of epileptic seizures is predicated on the accurate categorization of such an event as an epileptic seizure. Although making a diagnosis of seizures may appear to be a straightforward process, it is frequently problematic. When there is a clear, spontaneous description of urinary incontinence, tongue biting, postictal confusion, and drowsiness, the diagnosis is usually unambiguous. Often, however, the patient and witnesses to the event are unable to say whether automatisms were present, what the duration of the event was, or whether there were focal or generalized convulsive movements (often witnesses appear after the event has occurred). Frequently, a patient is seen by a physician without a witness and may have difficulty relating significant features of the episode, thus leaving the diagnosis in doubt. Much art in deduction and careful and perceptive questioning, along with the availability of sufficient facts, are required to establish a diagnosis of an epileptic seizure[5] and thus to differentiate it from other paroxysmal organic disturbances, let alone psychogenic seizures.[6, 7]

Seizure Classification

The diagnosis of an epileptic seizure should be further extended to involve classification into seizure type, since treatment and prognosis may vary according to categorization.[7] For example, the onset of focal seizures involving the tongue and face in a 12-year-old boy accompanied by an electroencephalographic (EEG) recording of cen-

Table 7-1. Frequent Causes of Nonepileptic Spells

Hypovolemic or hypotensive syncope

Transient ischemic attacks

Migraine

Cardiac dysrhythmias and drop attacks

Vasovagal syncope

Hypoglycemia

Vestibular or inner ear disease

Delirium and encephalopathy

Alcohol or drug-related syndromes

Menopausal "hot flashes"

Hyperventilation episodes

Transient global amnesia

Psychogenic seizures

Conversions disorder

Somatization disorder

Depression

Factitious disorder

Panic attacks

Pheochromocytoma

Intermittent movement disorders

---

trotemporal spikes leads to the diagnosis of the electroclinical syndrome of rolandic epilepsy. This self-limited, generally benign disorder responds well to certain AEDs and may be differentiated from less benign focal epilepsies. Furthermore, AED therapy may often be discontinued in early adulthood with the regression of the seizure disorder. Conversely, multifocal epileptiform discharges on EEG findings associated with complex partial seizures that follow a multifocal cerebral insult (e.g., severe head trauma, encephalitis) may be more resistant to treatment and necessitate lifelong AED therapy. Seizure types, then, help delineate an epilepsy syndrome; delineation of an epilepsy syndrome carries with it knowledge of prognosis and guidance in management.

Etiology

Because seizures are a clinical expression of several factors that produce a lowered seizure threshold, it is also essential to identify features other than seizure type and EEG pattern. Several epilepsies are genetic in nature, and inquiry into a family history of seizures and age of onset may identify a familial tendency. Rarely, other genetic disorders in which seizures appear as secondary phenomena may be revealed. Acquired causes of seizure disorders may be uncovered with questions about gestational prematurity, concurrent viral infection during pregnancy, perinatal trauma or infection, and infantile or childhood trauma. In this way, for example, benign febrile seizures with little risk for later epilepsy may be differentiated from more serious disorders of infancy and childhood. In adolescence and adulthood, acquired causes of seizures may also be uncovered; seizures may be precipitated by therapeutic drugs such as theophylline; "recreational" drugs such as cocaine, amphetamines, and phencyclidine; or by withdrawal from benzodiazepines, barbiturates, and alcohol. Information about genetic, environmental, emotional, toxic, and medicinal factors is valuable in the optimal management of a seizure disorder.

Physical Examination

Physical and neurologic examinations are essential in any patient with seizures. Although the examination findings are often normal, certain disorders have clinical manifestations of diagnostic importance. Cutaneous abnormalities may be seen with tuberous sclerosis, von Recklinghausen's disease, or Sturge-Weber syndrome—all of which may be associated with seizures. Stigmata of collagen vascular diseases or systemic disorders (e.g., hepatic, renal, endocrine disorders) may be found. Focal neurologic deficits may be noted, correlating with previous trauma or stroke, or may suggest previously unsuspected disease (e.g., intracranial neoplasia). Often, however, no particular syndrome of focal neurologic deficit is uncovered, and, with normal studies, a focal seizure disorder may be described as cryptogenic.

Investigations

Serum electrolytes, liver function tests, computed tomographic (CT) or magnetic resonance imaging (MRI) scans, and psychometric testing may reveal other disorders or more fully delineate recognized abnormalities. Congenital systemic or metabolic disorders may be delineated with a battery of specialized tests often routinely applied in disorders of infancy. Acquired metabolic disorders may be revealed by abnormal serum electrolyte levels, liver function, and the results of other specific tests. Computed tomographic and MRI scans of the head may reveal evidence of abnormal cerebral development, calcification caused by infection or neoplasia, evidence of injury or trauma, the presence of a vascular malformation, and, significantly, the absence of abnormality. Positron emission tomography and single-photon emission computed tomography may have a secondary role in the evaluation of seizure disorders.[8, 9]

Electroencephalography

The EEG has long been an essential test in the diagnosis, classification, and management of seizure disorders.[10–13] Outpatient, daytime EEG recordings with patients awake and asleep, with hyperventilation, and with intermittent photic stimulation may reveal epileptic abnormalities occurring, for example, only during sleep, or these procedures may induce epileptic discharges and help to substantiate a diagnosis of epilepsy. Furthermore, such patterns help to classify the disorder as a focal or generalized disturbance. Localization of a focus to one hemisphere may then be isolated further to a particular lobe or lobes. When several routine EEGs are normal and should the patient's paroxysmal events persist despite therapy, more prolonged inpatient EEG-video monitoring may help clarify whether these events are epileptic or not.

Treatment

General Issues

There are frequent misperceptions regarding seizures, their cause, and consequence. It therefore is essential to explain to the patient and family members the nature of the disorder and to allay unwarranted feelings of inadequacy, guilt, and stigma. The patient should be fully encouraged to adapt to the disability and to assume, as much as possible, a normal lifestyle. General advice should be given with regard to regularizing the time and duration of sleep, moderating the use of alcohol and drugs with a central stimulant effect, and adhering to the AED intake regimen. School children should be encouraged to participate normally in sports and scholastic activities, although sports such as swimming and climbing should be engaged in with proper precautions. Adults are usually able to maintain employment, although, again, occupations involving heights, dangerous machinery, driving, or working near or in water require precautions. Also, people with disorders that interfere with driving ability are subject to appropriate regulations of their right to drive; this includes many (although not all) patients with epilepsy. It is difficult to evaluate all the risks of daily living, but evaluation, discussion, and a "game plan" for all of these issues are important. Patients with poorly controlled convulsive seizures, mental retardation, or severe disability may need to remain under supervised home care or institutionalization. Care centers for patients with severe epilepsy may be found in most communities.

Modification of lifestyle and behavior may decrease the triggering of epileptic seizures. Regularization of meals and sleep time and the avoidance of sleep deprivation and of stress may improve control. Use of amphetamines and other stimulants, alcohol intake, and fever are other factors that can lower the seizure threshold in some patients.

Antiepileptic Drug Treatment

The Decision to Initiate Antiepileptic Drug Therapy

Decisions about whether and when to initiate AED therapy involve the certainty of diagnosis; the frequency of seizures; the type of seizures; and the degree to which a patient's social, scholastic, and professional life may be adversely affected by them. Not only the diagnosis of seizures and epilepsy but also the prolonged intake of AEDs may have a major impact on the psychological and physical aspects of daily living. Quite aside from the impact of having a seizure disorder, patients may need to take medications with unpleasant side effects for prolonged periods of time. Clearly, if a patient has frequent tonic-clonic seizures, the decision to initiate treatment is not difficult. Conversely, in a patient with daily activities requiring a high level of intellectual activity but who suffers from simple partial seizures (posing little danger to the patient), one might question the use of AEDs that could control seizures but impair cognition.

A diagnosis of seizures and epilepsy must be firm. Clearly defining features typical of partial seizures by witnessing an event or by capturing a seizure or epileptiform activity on an EEG ensure a high probability of diagnosis, although misdiagnoses do occur, especially in patients with pseudoseizures. Patients with epilepsy should be treated. Patients with infrequent, poorly described spells with clinical features suggestive of fainting, hypoglycemia, panic attacks, or psychogenic seizures,[5-7] to name a few, do not warrant AED therapy, and often require additional assessment, for example, with EEG monitoring. There is much controversy surrounding the use of AEDs after a single seizure.[14, 15] The decision to treat is often complex, and many facets of a patient's social, general medical, and epileptic condition need to be considered (see Chapter 9). Studies suggest that if the event occurs with acute toxic or metabolic imbalance, alcohol withdrawal, or drug withdrawal, therapy is not indicated. If the EEG shows a clear focus, the probability of subsequent seizures may be increased. This is also the case if a seizure occurs in the setting of a progressive structural abnormality such as a malignancy or with an arteriovenous malformation; in such instances AEDs may be warranted. Homebound patients may be at less of a health risk if they have another seizure than those who drive. Patients in some occupations may be at greater risk of experiencing job-related difficulties after a seizure than others. Usually after two events, the probability of further seizures is increased, and AED therapy is indicated. It is essential to discuss all these issues freely with the patient, incorporating contributory factors in the consensus to treat with AEDs. The options available; the nature and side effects of AEDs; and restrictions on driving, swimming, and working at heights or with dangerous machinery should be addressed. The discussion also should include the duration and manner of treatment, further investigations such as imaging studies, when AED levels need to be monitored, alternatives in treatment, and the importance of compliance with any instituted therapy. A patient and family members will retain only some of this information after one visit, and much essential information will be forgotten. Explanations must often be repeated on follow-up visits as new questions arise. A sympathetic and careful approach is needed, if possible incorporating a nurse-practitioner, in order to build a relationship that fosters optimal treatment.

Considerations in Choosing an Antiepileptic Drug

The choice of AED for the treatment of simple or complex partial seizures is partly determined by their focal onset rather than by a particular underlying cause, whether the seizures arise from cerebral infarction, from congenital abnormalities such as arteriovenous malformations, or from acquired insult such as head trauma. Once the decision has been reached to initiate drug therapy, several factors must be taken into consideration.[16–19]

Drug Effectiveness

The choice of an AED is largely determined by the probability of seizure control and the profile of side effects.[16–19] This profile determines whether a drug is referred to as "a drug of first choice" (first-line AED) or "a drug of second choice" (second-line AED drug). Phenytoin and carbamazepine (CBZ) are drugs of first choice for simple partial, complex partial, and secondarily generalized seizures. Although its use is becoming more widespread, sodium valproate remains a drug of second choice. Primidone and phenobarbital, long used in focal seizure disorders, are now less popular because of their higher incidence of unpleasant side effects. The newer benzodiazepines such as clorazepate and clobazam are also second-line choices.

Frequency of Medication Intake

It is convenient to take a medication only once or twice during the day. For example, a child and parents wanting to minimize the awkwardness of taking tablets during school time may opt for a twice-daily regimen so that pills can be taken before and after school. Patients with poor memories or difficulties with compliance may find it convenient to take a single daily dose at a fixed time of day, linking medication intake with an invariant daily activity such as breakfast, dinner, or some other habitual activity. Conversely, patients with poorly controlled seizures, good compliance, and self-motivation who may experience side effects when AEDs are taken at higher dosages once or twice a day may prefer or need first-line AEDs taken at a lower dosage three or more times daily.

Side Effects

The profile of AED side effects may play an important role in the choice of medication. For example, for young women, the less severe side effects of CBZ, which does not produce coarsening of the facies, hirsutism, and gum hyperplasia (as phenytoin sometimes does), can offset the inconvenience of having to take the AED three times daily. Patients with painful neuropathies and particular psychiatric disorders in addition to epileptic seizures can benefit from the therapeutic effects of CBZ. Conversely, patients with low white blood cell and platelet counts or with a low serum sodium level might need to avoid CBZ, which has a high incidence of causing these problems. Some patients may experience gastrointestinal distress or visual difficulties with CBZ and may therefore prefer phenytoin. Finally, the sedative effects of primidone or phenobarbital may be unacceptable in patients requiring maximal alertness.

Valproate can produce hyperammonemia in young or elderly patients who are taking one or more AEDs. Severe hepatic reactions to valproate occur in only a small number of patients, primarily those younger than 2 years of age.[20] However, increased serum ammonia, alterations in liver enzyme levels, or encephalopathy may occur in others, making it necessary to discontinue the drug. Asymptomatic patients with these changes often can continue to take valproate but should be closely monitored.

In pregnancy, all first-line AEDs can cause fetal abnormalities, but there is particular concern with valproate and, to a slightly lesser extent, with CBZ during the first trimester because of the high incidence of serious dysraphic disorders.[21] With polytherapy, the incidence of abnormalities markedly increases, as does the general incidence of AED side effects.[22]

Ability to Monitor Antiepileptic Drug Levels

In many patients, titrating the AED dosage ensures adequate seizure control.[23] Patients with poor seizure control may require careful manipulation in AED intake to achieve control. In such patients, small changes in dose may mean the difference between breakthrough seizures on the one hand and AED toxicity on the other. Although clear "landmarks" for empiric therapy can be used (breakthrough seizures representing suboptimal dosage, unacceptable side effects indicating excess intake or drug toxicity), these large swings in response can be minimized by monitoring AED blood levels.

Of necessity, AEDs that are easily monitored in a particular laboratory should be chosen. Most laboratories have the ability to measure phenytoin, phenobarbital, CBZ, primidone, and valproate levels.

Starting Antiepileptic Therapy

When starting patients on AED therapy, a single medication should be started at a low dosage to avoid side effects. This low dosage can then be raised by increasing the frequency of intake to several times a day or by increasing the dosage of the particular intake gradually over days to weeks depending on the AED selected. Dosage increments are variably tolerated by different people, but typical increases can be made every

3–7 days during initial treatment. A steady state of AED metabolism is reached after five half-lives. Typically, therefore, a steady state usually will be reached with CBZ, which has a half-life of 8–12 hours, in 40–60 hours. Phenobarbital, which has a much more prolonged half-life, takes 3–4 weeks to reach steady state. If seizures occur during the course of medication increase, a further increase in dosage or modification of the daily regimen should be made. Even if blood levels are high, AEDs may be increased if there are no clinical side effects or hematologic, renal, or hepatic impairment. If AED levels are low but the patient has no further seizures, the regimen often may be maintained as is. Once a satisfactory dosing schedule has been found, a steady-state "baseline" level can be useful. Thereafter, determinations of serum AED levels usually need be obtained only once yearly.

Monotherapy

It is now generally recognized that monotherapy is preferable to polytherapy in many patients.[11, 24–27] Most patients can be satisfactorily managed with a single AED even if this means treatment above the so-called therapeutic range,[27] if maintenance at this level occurs in the absence of unacceptable side effects. If this schema is not effective, another first-line AED should be gradually instituted as previously outlined to reach either a therapeutic blood level or satisfactory seizure control together with gradual discontinuation of the ineffective medication. This process may be repeated sequentially with each drug before considering maintaining the patient on two AEDs. Toxicity problems not infrequently arise during the increasing phase of the second AED because of additive toxic effects during polytherapy. A patient can experience side effects despite having subtherapeutic levels of both AEDs; this will require more frequent monitoring and adjustments in therapy. The same dosages and better seizure control without side effects may be obtained by altering the particular regimen. For example, if side effects occur when both medications are taken together at the same times during the day, they can be intercalated throughout the day. Altering the regimen in this way, however, increases the number of times the patient must take medication and hence can affect compliance.

Compliance can further be enhanced by using a pillbox containing the daily doses of medication to be taken or by having the patient use a digital watch with multiple alarms. A seizure calendar can be used to jot down the time medication was taken and the type and time of a particular seizure on a particular day. This stratagem allows the patient and physician to maximize communication and therapeutic effort.

Inadequate Control on One Antiepileptic Drug

A minority of patients will not achieve adequate or complete eradication of epileptic seizures after AED monotherapy for several weeks or months. There may be several reasons for such inadequate control: Compliance may be inadequate (the medication is being taken at the wrong time or wrong dose, in insufficient amounts, or not at all), the AED may be ineffective, or the patient may not have epilepsy. All of these possibilities should be considered, since each is frequently encountered in practice. Ensuring that the diagnosis of epilepsy is accurate, maintaining a careful history of AED intake, asking a companion about seizure manifestations and medication compliance, and measuring AED levels will remedy poor seizure control in some cases. A patient should preferably be restarted on monotherapy with an agent that has had an inadequate trial before considering polytherapy, provided, of course, that there is no history of allergy or serious side effects. Some patients have long and convoluted histories of AED treatment, often with a history of allergy, side effects, or ineffective treatment, all of which must be re-examined. Re-evaluation of a changing pattern of neurologic deficit or change in seizure type may uncover a progressive central nervous system lesion that necessitates other therapy.

When there is inadequate control with good compliance and when sequential monotherapy has failed, a second AED should be added and gradually increased while the patient is monitored for side effects and AED levels are measured until a steady-state situation has been reached.[28] The choice of AEDs should be rational and implemented in an organized fashion. The combinations should include, if possible, first-line therapeutic agents; should have a history of tolerable or no side effects; and usually should be selected on the basis of complementary actions. For example, valproate and phenytoin or CBZ work by different mechanisms, so the combination constitutes an effective choice. Lamotrigine or gabapentin (see the section on new antiepileptic drugs) with phenytoin, CBZ, or valproate are other good combinations.

A special problem encountered in female patients is catamenial seizures. Catamenial seizures are those that occur before, during, or after the menstrual period. Despite excellent seizure control during most of the month, some women experience breakthrough seizures regularly in association with menses. If a specific time for such breakthrough seizures can be identified, an increased dosage should be given 2–4 hours before that time, depending on the drug. The time at which the dosage is increased should be tailored to the particular needs of the patient. If seizures occur at predictable times before, during, or after menstruation, increased intake is best instituted several days before this period. If there is a general increase in seizures around the time of menstruation without a fixed relationship to menstruation or time of day, an empiric increase in dosage may be attempted 3–5 days before menstruation and continued 5–7 days after. If seizure control cannot be obtained by such increases in the first-line AED, other second-line AED adjuvants may be helpful. For example, acetazolamide, clorazepate, or clobazam may be instituted a few days before menstruation and taken for the duration of the perimenstrual period.

New Antiepileptic Drugs

After many years without new AEDs, several new drugs have become available in the United States: felbamate, gabapentin, and lamotrigine. This new generation of agents has been approved for add-on therapy for the treatment of partial seizures with or without secondary generalization.

While the exact role these newer agents play in epilepsy management is still being worked out, their most evident role is in the treatment of the approximately 30% of patients with intractable seizures.[29] These new drugs may offer patients not only improvement in the number of seizures, but also improvement in the overall quality of life, particularly if the older AEDs produced adverse effects.

All the newer AEDs have undergone controlled clinical trials examining their efficacy and safety in patients with partial seizures with or without generalized tonic-clonic seizures and have demonstrated efficacy in double-blind trials. Lamotrigine appears to have broad antiepileptic activity as add-on therapy in patients with partial seizures and Lennox-Gastaut syndrome.[30, 31] Some of the benefits of gabapentin are the relatively mild transient central nervous system side effects, the lack of interaction with other drugs, and the relatively rapid rate of dosage increase possible.[32] Although experience with felbamate has been good regarding seizure control in some of the most refractory patients,[33] the high incidence of aplastic anemia and liver problems has led to its limitation to patients in whom a possibility of dangerous AED side effects is outweighed by the danger of refractory seizures.

There are several other newer antiepileptic agents that are in trial in the United States or have not yet received approval by the Food and Drug Administration. These include vigabatrin, topiramate, tiagabine, and drugs chemically related to CBZ and phenytoin.

The use of previous AED combinations (e.g., phenytoin and CBZ) were in some cases limited by the fact that the AEDs not only acted by the same mechanism, but also produced many of the same toxic effects, with these side effects being more likely when more than one drug was given at the same time. Newer combinations of agents that include previous first-line drugs (e.g., CBZ, valproate, phenytoin) with one of the newer drugs (e.g., lamotrigine or gabapentin) may offer some advantages: The mechanisms of action may complement each other, and drug toxicity may not be additive to the same degree as in pervious AED combinations. Some combinations have the potential for either increasing the blood level of other AEDs or decreasing the dosage needed for therapeutic effect (e.g., lamotrigine when used with valproate). No single new AED would seem to have advantages with no disadvantages. New data are being accumulated regarding the use of the newer agents as monotherapy.

Problems with Polypharmacy

When AEDs are used concurrently, toxicity and side effects are more frequent, often at levels at which the individual agent would not produce symptoms. Ataxia, blurred vision, dizziness, and somnolence all can appear de novo when new agents are added or maintained. Intercurrent illness, fever, or other medication can precipitate side effects.

Duration of Therapy

Combination therapy should be continued in order to obtain maximal seizure control. Since the process of sequentially trying all monotherapies that may eventually prove ineffective requires many months, often with close supervision and occasionally with hospitalization, the decision of when to discontinue (if at all) one of the drugs is difficult (see Chapter 14) and unclear.[14, 34–37] Occasionally, seizure control improves with time, possibly requiring only one AED; seizure disorders in childhood may be less problematic in adulthood.

Decisions to withdraw AEDs must be thoroughly discussed with the patient, taking into account personal preferences, occupation, driving permits, and more general psychosocial concerns.[38] The data available to guide the clinician and a patient in decisions on whether and when to consider discontinuation of AEDs are variable depending on the population studied. After a seizure-free period of 2–3 years, the chance of seizure recurrence off AEDs varies from 20% to 70%. The most vulnerable period for seizure recurrence is during the withdrawal period. Factors mitigating against successful withdrawal of AEDs include a history of prolonged, difficult seizure control; multifocal central nervous system disease and mental retardation; and multifocal and active epileptiform foci on the EEG. Elements that portend successful AED withdrawal include few seizures over a brief period and self-limited child-hood epilepsy syndromes such as benign focal epilepsy of childhood.

After particularly difficult seizure control, two AEDs may need to be continued for several years before one agent is discontinued. Many times, discontinuation of either drug is not appropriate, but if the decision is made to taper medication, the drug apparently most likely to produce side effects or to be less effective should be discontinued first. This should be done as slowly as possible to ensure as little perturbation as possible in the remaining AED levels and in control and to reduce the likelihood of withdrawal effects. It may take months to wean a patient off phenobarbital or benzodiazepines because of problems with habituation, the possibility of barbiturate-induced or benzodiazepine-induced withdrawal seizures, and the appearance of insomnia and agitation.

Continued Intractability

Surgery has proved to be very effective in treating complex partial seizures. When seizures continue despite efforts at medical control, the surgical option should be considered. The diagnostic and therapeutic strategies for such patients are considered in Chapter 15.

References

1. Commission on Classification and Terminology of the International League Against Epilepsy. Proposal for revised clinical and electroen-cephalographic classification of epileptic seizures. Epilepsia 1981;22:489.
2. Burnstine H, Lesser RP. Focal Seizure Disorders. In RT Johnson (ed), Current Therapy in Neurologic Disease (3rd ed). Philadelphia: B.C. Decker, 1990;36.
3. Wayne HH. Syncope. Physiological considerations and an analysis of the clinical characteristics in 510 patients. Am J Med 1961;30:418.
4. Fisher CM. Syncope of obscure nature. Can J Neurol Sci 1979;6:7.
5. Kaplan PW. Spells: Syncope, Seizures and Other Episodic Disorders. In JD Stobo, DB Hellmann, PW Ladenson, et al. (eds), The Principles and Practice of Medicine (23rd ed). Stamford, CT: Appleton & Lange, 1996.
6. Lesser RP. Psychogenic Seizures. In TA Pedley, BS Meldrum (eds), Recent Advances in Epilepsy (2nd ed). New York: Churchill Livingstone 1985;273.
7. Ramani SV, Quesney LF, Olson D, Gumnit RJ. Diagnosis of hysterical seizures in epileptic patients. Am J Psychiatry 1980;137:705.
8. Gaillard WD, Bhatia S, Bookheimer SY, et al. FDG-PET and volumetric MRI in the evaluation of patients with partial epilepsy. Neurology 1995;45:123.

9. Stefan H, Bauer J, Feistel H, et al. Regional cerebral blood flow during focal seizures of temporal and frontocentral onset. Ann Neurol 1990;27:162.
10. Lesser RP, Fisher RS, Kaplan PW. The evaluation of patients with intractable complex partial seizures. Electroencephalogr Clin Neurophysiol 1989;73:381.
11. Lesser RP, Dinner DS, Luders H, Morris HH. Differential diagnosis and treatment of intractable seizures. Cleve Clin Q 1984;51:227.
12. Escueta AV, Bacsal FE, Treiman DM. Complex partial seizures on closed-circuit television and EEG: a study of 691 attacks in 79 patients. Ann Neurol 1982;11:292.
13. Kaplan PW, Lesser RP. Long-Term EEG Monitoring. In DD Daly, TA Pedley (eds), Current Practice of Clinical EEG (2nd ed). New York: Raven, 1990.
14. Fromm GH, Fisher RS, Dasheiff R, Hachinski V (Discussants). Controversies in neurology: first seizure management reconsidered. Arch Neurol 1987;44:1189.
15. First Seizure Trial (FIR.S.T.) Group. Randomized clinical trial on the efficiency of antiepileptic drugs in reducing the risk of relapse after a first unprovoked tonic-clonic seizure. Neurology 1993;43:478.
16. Kaplan PW, Loiseau P, Fisher RD, Jallon P. Epilepsy A to Z: A Glossary of Epilepsy Terminology. New York: Demos-Vermande, 1995.
17. Pisani F, Perruca E, DiPerri R. Clinically relevant antiepileptic drug interactions. J Int Med Res 1990;18:115.
18. Smith DB, Mattson RH, Cramer JA, et al. Results of a nationwide Veterans Administration Cooperative Study comparing the efficacy and toxicity of carbamazepine, phenobarbital, phenytoin and primidone. Epilepsia 1987;28(Suppl 3):S50.
19. Meador KJ, Loring DW, Allen ME, et al. Comparative cognitive effects of carbamazepine and phenytoin in healthy adults. Neurology 1991;41:1537.
20. Driefuss FE, Langer DH, Moline KA, Maxwell JE. Valproic acid hepatic fatalities. II. US experience since 1984. Neurology 1989;39:201.
21. Jones KL, Lacro RV, Johnson KA, Adams J. Pattern of malformations in the children of women treated with carbamazepine during pregnancy. N Engl J Med 1989;320:1661.
22. Kaneko S, Otani K, Fujushima Y, et al. Teratogenicity of antiepileptic drugs. Epilepsia 1988;29:459.
23. Johannessen SI. Antiepileptic drugs: pharmacokinetic and clinical aspects. Ther Drug Monit 1981;3:17.
24. Reynolds EH, Chadwick D, Galbraith AW. One drug (phenytoin) in the treatment of epilepsy. Lancet 1975;1:923.
25. Shorvon SD, Reynolds EH, Reduction in polypharmacy for epilepsy. BMJ 1979;2:1023.
26. Reynolds EH, Shorvon SD. Monotherapy or polytherapy for epilepsy? Epilepsia 1981;22:1.
27. Lesser RP, Pippenger CE, Lueders H, Dinner DS. High dose monotherapy in the treatment of intractable seizures: acute toxic effects and therapeutic efficacy. Neurology 1985;33(Suppl 2):233.

28. Pippenger CE, Lesser RP. An overview or therapeutic drug monitoring principles. Cleve Clin Q 1984;51:241.
29. Mattson RH, Cramer JA, Collins JF, et al. A comparison of valproate with carbamazepine for the treatment of complex partial seizures and secondarily tonic-clonic seizures in adults. N Engl J Med 1992;327:765.
30. Messenheimer J, Ramsay RE, Willmore LJ, et al. Lamotrigine therapy for partial seizures: a multicenter, placebo-controlled, double-blind, cross-over trial. Epilepsia 1994;35:113.
31. Matsuo F, Bergen D, Faught E, et al. Placebo-controlled study of the efficacy and safety of lamotrigine in patients with partial seizures. Neurology 1993;43:2284.
32. Sivenius J, Kalviainen R, Ylinen A, et al. Double-blind study of gabapentin in the treatment of partial seizures. Epilepsia 1991;32:539.
33. Sachdeo R, Kramer LD, Rosenberg A, et al. Felbamate monotherapy: controlled trial in patients with partial onset seizures. Ann Neurol 1992;32:386.
34. Malow BA, Blaxton TA, Stertz B, Theodore WH. Carbamazepine withdrawal: effects of taper rate on seizure frequency. Neurology 1993; 43:2280.
35. Holmes GL. Stopping antiepileptic drugs in children: when and why? Ann Neurol 1994;35:509.
36. Shinnar S, Berg AT, Moshe SL, et al. Discontinuing antiepileptic drugs in children with epilepsy: a prospective study. Ann Neurol 1994;35:534.
37. Callaghan N, Garrett A, Goggin T. Withdrawal of anticonvulsant drugs in patients free of seizures for two years. A prospective study. N Engl J Med 1988;318:942.
38. Kaplan PW. Seizure Disorders. In LR Barker, PD Zieve, JR Burton (eds), Principles of Ambulatory Medicine (4th ed). Baltimore: Williams & Wilkins, 1995;1178.

8

Febrile Convulsions

W. Allen Hauser

Definition

Febrile convulsions (FCs) represent a unique category of convulsive disorder that occurs in young children. This class of seizure disorder includes convulsions occurring in children in association with a febrile illness not caused by an infection of the central nervous system. As with most epileptic syndromes, further specificity in definitions is not well agreed on, and a number of inconsistencies exist in the literature.

There has not been consistency in the age limitations for inclusion in this group. A National Institutes of Health consensus conference suggested that children with a first seizure occurring with a febrile illness between the ages 3 months and 5 years (presumably 72 months but not specified) be included in the category,[1] although most studies (and clinicians) seem not to be constrained by these limitations (see Berg et al. [1992],[2] Tsuboi [1988],[3] and Annegers et al. [1987][4]). Most children who experience an FC episode will experience it in their second year of life—primarily between 12 and 15 months of age; very few children will have a first episode after 3 years of age.

There has not been consistent agreement on the temperature elevation a child must have to be included in this category, although minimum rectal temperatures of 38°C or 38.5°C or 101°F (38.3°C) have been stipulated in some studies that have attempted to define this para-

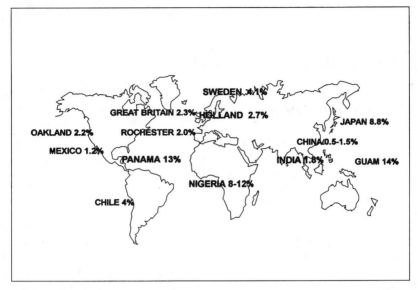

Figure 8-1. *Febrile seizures.*

meter.[2, 4–6] From a practical standpoint, the question is moot, as the child's temperature is rarely known at the time of the seizure. All studies of FCs exclude children who have had recurrent unprovoked seizures before their first FC; some studies have excluded children with prior seizures of any type.[7]

Frequency and Geographic Distribution

Febrile seizures are the most frequently occurring epilepsy syndrome in Europe, the United States, and some Asian countries. Two percent to 5% of all children in the United States and European countries will experience at least one FC.[6, 8–11] There is a striking variation in the cumulative incidence of FCs worldwide (Figure 8-1). A much higher proportion of children experience such episodes in Japan, Korea (8–9%), and the Mariana Islands (up to 14%).[12–14] Interestingly, the proportion of children who experience febrile seizures in China is low—possibly as low as 3 per 1,000.[15] A somewhat lower cumulative incidence has also been reported in some population-based studies in Mexico,[16] Central America,[17] and India.[18] This geographic variation

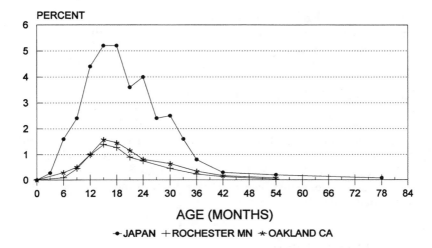

Figure 8-2. *Incidence of febrile convulsions.*

has yet to be explained. It has been suggested that parents may be more cognizant of the occurrence of FCs in Japan and in the Mariana Islands because of the confined living arrangements, with children sleeping in the same room as their parents. A high frequency has also been reported in Africa, although this may be related to cerebral malaria.[19–21] The low frequency of FCs reported in China, Mexico, and Central America, where sleeping conditions are similar to those in Japan and the Marianas, suggests that this is not the sole explanation. In Japan, the use of hot tubs by the entire family (including young children) may allow core temperatures to increase more rapidly or to a greater extent than in populations in Western countries. There also may be basic differences in the genetic pool in these diverse populations.

Age and Sex

Despite major geographic variations in the proportion of children affected with FCs, the age and sex of children affected with FCs seem consistent within populations. FCs occur more often in boys. They are age-related, with the peak incidence of a first FC occurring in the second year of life (Figure 8-2). At this age, 1–2% of the children in western nations experience a convulsion with fever.[8, 10] The patterns of age-specific incidence are similar but considerably higher in Japanese studies.[3] A first FC rarely occurs after a child's third birthday in United States and European populations.

Risk Factors for Febrile Convulsions

All children experience febrile illnesses, but not all children have a convulsion with the fever. There are factors that seem to predispose children to having a convulsion with fever, although there have been few studies of risk factors for a first FC. Most studies have evaluated risk factors for febrile seizure *recurrence*, but most of these are also factors associated with a first event.

Age and Family History

Age is the most obvious risk factor identified for FC; in fact, this variable really defines the syndrome. A second risk factor is family history of febrile seizures. The likelihood of a having a febrile seizure is increased by a factor of three when either a sibling or a parent has experienced a FC. Risk is increased further if multiple family members have been affected.[22–24] This increase in risk is evident in populations with a low incidence (United States) and high incidence (Japan) of FCs.

Maternal and Adverse Perinatal Factors

Several authors have evaluated the effects of prenatal and perinatal factors on the risk of FCs. As with studies of epilepsy, these factors have generally not been associated with an increased risk of febrile seizures in population-based studies after controlling for pre-existing neurologic handicap.[25, 26] Premature birth and neonatal difficulties have been associated with an increased risk in some but not all studies, and the association is weak.[27–29] Eclampsia in the mother and an increased bilirubin level in the child have been associated with an increased risk of FCs in one study, although there was insufficient statistical power to fully evaluate these factors.[24] One might assume that children with "complex" FCs (focal or prolonged) are more likely to have a history of adverse prenatal or perinatal factors of some type, but this was not the case in two case control studies in which this group was independently eval-uated.[24, 30] When taken in aggregate, there is no difference in the fre-quency of all adverse factors in cases or controls in the most recent population-based studies. Verity et al.[31] found a correlation between low birth weight and febrile seizures, but this correlation disappeared after controlling for neurologic handicap before the first FC. Mater-nal smoking during pregnancy, prior pregnancy wastage, breech deliv-ery, and mental subnormality in the mother or sibling have been associated with an increased risk.[31–34]

Day-Care Attendance, Race, and Socioeconomic Status

Day-care attendance has been associated with the occurrence of FCs in one study and with recurrence in several studies.[5, 29] This may reflect a greater exposure to febrile illness, although it may also be a surrogate for socioeconomic status, which has also been shown to be a risk fac-tor for recurrence of FCs.

Only the National Collaborative Perinatal Project (NCPP) has had sufficient sample size to evaluate race as a potential risk factor within the same community. Black children did have a higher frequency of FCs than white children.

Neurologic Status

Children with pre-existing neurologic handicaps—specifically, mental retardation or cerebral palsy—are at a three- to fourfold increased risk for FCs.[7, 9] The inclusion of such cases seems to explain the association with low birth weight in the study of Verity et al.[31] This also seems to explain the association between birth weight and FCs reported from a hospital-based case control study in which 70% of the children were neurologically abnormal.[35]

Immunologic Status

Children with FCs have been reported to have IgA deficiency.[36] Those compromised immunologically may be at increased frequency of infec-tion and thus an increased frequency of seizures. They also have been reported to have an IgG2 deficiency.[37]

Immunization

Two recent studies have specifically addressed the role of pertussis immunization and the subsequent development of seizures, including those occurring with fever. In a study of the relationship between immunization and seizures among children immunized in a health maintenance organization in Seattle, Washington,[38] an increased risk for a febrile seizure within 1 month of the immunization was identified, but there was no increase in risk for unprovoked seizures. A retrospective study of two Danish cohorts, which was characterized by different timing of immunization and different strength of vaccine, was undertaken to evaluate timing of onset of febrile and afebrile seizures.[39] No relationship between vaccination schedule and the onset of epilepsy was identified, although the age of onset of the first FC was significantly different. The overall frequency of FCs did not seem to be increased.

Pertussis vaccine is a pyrogen, and many children develop a low-grade fever in the first 24 hours after immunization (usually 2–7 hours later).[40, 41] These studies suggest that a febrile reaction associated with immunization may trigger a febrile seizure in a susceptible child, thus altering the timing of the occurrence of a febrile seizure but not the incidence of the condition.

Disease Characteristics

There are suggestions that febrile seizures are particularly frequent in children with rosacea. Based on polymerase chain reaction studies and viral cultures,[42] these individuals may in fact have misclassified cases of encephalitis. *Shigella* infection has also been suggested to have a particularly high association with febrile seizures, although no quantitative studies have been undertaken. There is otherwise little evidence of disease specificity. There are clinical suspicions that the rate of temperature increase is important, although there are conflicting data from animal studies and no reliable data from studies on humans.[43]

Genetics of Febrile Seizures

Febrile seizures clearly aggregate in families, although the mode of inheritance remains in question. Whereas dominant, recessive, X-linked, and purely environmental factors have been suggested as underlying mechanisms for the familial aggregation of febrile seizures, recent twin studies seem to confirm a genetic component,[44] but there appears to be genetic heterogeneity.

In studies from Rochester, Minnesota, the majority of cases are clearly accounted for by a polygenic mode of inheritance.[22] Nonetheless, a subgroup characterized by the occurrence of multiple febrile seizures (three or more) in the proband appears to be associated with a dominant mode of inheritance.[45] The relationship between febrile seizures, epilepsy, and unprovoked seizures becomes even more complex. Siblings of children with a febrile seizure have a two- to threefold increase in risk for developing epilepsy. A history of epilepsy in a first-degree relative is associated with an increased risk for febrile seizures.[46] Siblings of children who have both febrile seizures and epilepsy have a sixfold to sevenfold increased risk of also having febrile seizures or epilepsy. This suggests that genetic factors for the two conditions overlap but to some extent are independent.

Electroencephalographic Abnormalities

Closely tied to the question of genetic predisposition for FCs is the aggregation of certain electroencephalographic (EEG) abnormalities within families. The EEG has seldom been of value in the evaluation of children at the time of a febrile seizure. In general, EEG tracings are normal. A focal EEG at this time has the implications of any indicator of localized brain abnormality, and appropriate workup is needed in this situation. There are specific EEG patterns that occur with increased frequency in children with febrile seizures.

Generalized Spike and Wave Pattern

A number of studies have evaluated the frequency of EEG abnormalities among children with a history of febrile seizures, and all have reported an exceedingly high frequency of generalized spike and wave (GSW) patterns—up to 80%.[47-51] In general, these EEG patterns have been recorded not at the time of the FC, but between the ages of 3 and 6 years—generally several years after the initial FC. The highest proportion of cases is reported from studies that include sleeping records. Since the GSW pattern is probably inherited as a mendelian genetic trait, the apparent high concordance suggests some relationship between FCs,

GSW patterns, and possibly the other generalized epilepsies of childhood, for which a GSW pattern is the EEG signature. There also appears to be an increased frequency of GSW patterns in siblings of FC probands.[42]

Doose's Theta

A 4–5 cycles/second rhythm occurring in the parietal regions in children has been described by Doose.[52, 53] The pattern closely resembles the hypersynchronous hypnagogic patterns. This pattern occurs in 5.6% of neurologically normal children and is more prevalent in boys. The prevalence is highest at age 3 years (10%) and decreases with advancing age. The pattern is of interest because of a particularly high prevalence ($\geq$50%) reported in children with FCs.

Prognosis

There are a number of potential adverse outcomes of convulsions with fever that have been explored. The most frequent complication of a FC is a recurrent convulsion at the time of a subsequent febrile illness. The risk for subsequent unprovoked seizures is increased, although only to a modest degree. There is no evidence for an association with permanent brain damage, as manifested by permanent neurologic abnormalities or intellectual difficulties, among children who were normal before their first convulsion with fever.

Recurrence of Febrile Seizures

Approximately 30% of children with one FC will experience a recurrent episode.[54–56] A number of factors have been evaluated as potential risk factors for recurrent episode, although no single factor has been evaluated in every study, and only a few studies have determined risk for recurrence using multivariate analysis.

The most consistent predictor of recurrence is the age at first febrile seizure. Younger age at first episode (younger than 15 months or younger than 18 months of age) is associated with a twofold increase risk for recurrence when compared with those older at the first episode. This increase in risk seems primarily related to a longer duration of exposure during a susceptible age in individuals prone to FC. Some studies have reported complex features of the seizure (focal seizures, repeat episodes with the same illness) to be associated with an increased risk for recurrence, but these factors become less important in multivariable analyses. A family history of febrile seizures (generally a first-degree relative) has been a consistent predictor of recurrence.[57] A family history of epilepsy has been a less consistent predictor. Recurrence is higher in those with a "low" fever at the time of the first febrile seizure (< 40°C). A short duration of fever before the initial convulsion is also related to an increased risk for recurrence. The highest recurrence risk occurs in the first 6 months after the initial episode regardless of age. Factors such as sibship size, day-care attendance, and socioeconomic status have been associated with an increased recurrence risk, all presumably related to a greater frequency of exposure to infectious disease and thus a greater risk for seizures.

Overall, consideration of these risk factors for recurrence can allow the clinician to develop a model allowing prediction of risk for further febrile seizures.[48, 58, 59] For children older than 15 months of age at the time of their first FC who have no family history of seizures, have normal examination findings, and are not in day-care, the risk for another FC is approximately 10%. In children who are younger at their FC and with multiple additional factors, the risk for further seizures approaches 80% or more.

The majority of complex febrile seizures occur at the time of the initial episode. On the assumption that a complex febrile seizure may in some way cause brain damage, some may be concerned about the frequency of and risk factors for complex recurrence. Only about 3% of children with an initial "simple" convulsion will experience a complex recurrence, and there are no data to predict such recurrence.

Approximately 40% of children with two FCs will experience a third episode. Only a few studies have evaluated the risk for a third or more febrile seizure, and the only consistent factor seems to be age of occurrence.[48]

Epilepsy

Children with FCs are six times more likely to develop epilepsy than the general population, but there is wide variation in this risk depending on clinical features. Case control studies have identified febrile seizures as a risk factor for all forms of epilepsy.[60–62] Longitudinal studies of children with FCs have identified an increased risk over that expected in the general population, ranging from less than 3% among children with a simple FC to 50% or more in children with a combination of focal and prolonged FCs.[4, 7, 63]

Different predictors emerge for specific types of epilepsy (generalized versus partial onset).[4] Genetic factors are the major predictors of increased risk for the development of generalized onset epilepsy after FCs. Conversely, there is evidence of localized brain dysfunction at the time of the first FC among those who subsequently develop partial epilepsy.

FCs are frequently assumed to be a cause of epilepsy because of the increased risk for epilepsy in individuals suffering from this condition. While it is possible that prolonged febrile seizures can lead to neuronal damage or death, which in turn leads to residual Ammon's horn sclerosis,[64] such prolonged events are exceedingly rare in the general population (prolonged febrile seizures account for less than 0.5% of all febrile seizures).

Other Adverse Outcomes

A major problem with ascertaining any adverse outcome after a FC is the difficulty in distinguishing the time order of events, particularly in cross-sectional studies. This represents a problem with many studies looking at outcomes and is important in some studies of abnormalities after a FC has occurred. Another difficulty in many studies of outcome after FCs relates to study methodology. Outcome is invariably worse in studies of children admitted to the hospital when compared with studies of children with FCs that are community-based or derived from prospectively followed cohorts.

Intellectual Dysfunction

There have been several studies of intellectual function in children with FCs. In a study of twins discordant for FC, the affected twin had on average a five-point deficit in IQ testing.[65] In a follow-up study of children with FCs, Smith and Wallace reported that recurrent FCs and not treatment therapies were associated with reduced intellectual function.[66] These findings are at odds with data from two large cohort studies. The NCPP in the United States found no evidence of intellectual deficits among probands with FCs when compared with nonaffected siblings.[67] The British National Childhood Development Study found no evidence of a decrement in school performance or intellectual function when children with FCs were compared with controls.

Contrary to the report of Smith and Wallace, a deficit in intellectual function has been reported among children treated prophylactically with phenobarbital in two studies.[79, 80]

Other Neurologic Handicaps

There were no children with permanent new major neurologic sequelae after having a febrile seizure in either the Rochester cohort or the NCPP.[9, 47] In a study of twins discordant for FC, an increased frequency of minor neurologic abnormalities was reported in the affected twin.[56] Although this was interpreted as evidence for dysfunction caused by the FC, time order is again a problem.

Mortality

There are no studies of morbidity or mortality associated with FCs per se. In the population-based study from Rochester, Minnesota, which covered a period of 50 years, no deaths were identified at the time of FCs, and long-term survivorship was not altered from that expected. There were no deaths in association with FCs reported in the NCPP study.[47]

Febrile Seizures as a Prognostic Factor in Patients with Epilepsy

In several studies of the prognosis of patients with epilepsy, a prior history of febrile seizures has been associated with reduced seizure control and reduced likelihood of remission. Among 95 patients with partial seizures (30 patients had complex partial seizures) evaluated in a clinical series from India,[68] 2-year remission occurred in only 27% of those with complex partial epilepsy compared with 45% of those with simple partial seizures. In the complex partial group, there was a trend for those with prior febrile seizures to do less well. In a follow-up of a clinical series of primarily adult patients with complex partial seizures, only 29% of those with prior febrile seizures were seizure-free at 2 years, compared with 69% of those without.[69] In a long-term follow-up of a series of 100 highly selected children with temporal lobe epilepsy, 31% of children with prior febrile status epilepticus were seizure-free off medications and living independently, compared with 55% of those without a febrile status (and presumably with no febrile seizures). In adults and children with intractable temporal lobe epilepsy, a history of a febrile seizure in early childhood has been associated with a good outcome.[70, 71]

Diagnostic Evaluation

The primary focus in the evaluation of children with FCs relates to the determination of the cause for fever. Although a cause may be obvious in some cases, a primary concern is the exclusion of a central nervous system infection. About 5% of all seizures occurring in association with a febrile illness in the age group susceptible to FCs can be attributable to an infection of the central nervous system. Even though an experienced clinician may be able to distinguish those with a meningitis from those without, a lumbar puncture—particularly in very young children, in whom signs of meningitis may be elusive—may be warranted in many children with a first FC.[72] Other diagnostic tests such as EEG, computed tomography, and radiographs of the skull seldom provide information useful in the management of the acute condition.

Treatment

Treatment at the Time of Illness

Antipyretic therapy as well as symptomatic treatment of the underlying illness should be initiated. If the child is still convulsing, diazepam, 0.2 mg/kg, or lorazepam, 0.05 mg/kg, may be administered intravenously. Since diazepam is readily absorbed by the rectum and adequate serum levels are obtained within a few minutes, the rectum may be an alternative route of administration.[73] Diazepam prepared for rectal administration is available in many European countries but is not yet available in North America. Nonetheless, the intravenous form may be administered per rectum. In the study by Knudsen et al.,[73] this method of administration was effective. Since the anticonvulsant effect of diazepam is short, it may be appropriate to administer 10 mg/kg phenobarbital by either an intravenous or intramuscular route to prevent immediate recurrence.[74]

Prophylactic Treatment

While generally benign, FCs are a frightening event to parents and caretakers. Even though only about one-third of children who have had an FC will experience further episodes of FCs, treatment either at the time of a fever or continuous treatment for a specified period of time (2–5 years) had been recommended in the past to prevent FC recurrences and (mistakenly) to modify outcomes other than recurrent FCs. While recurrence of FC may be prevented, there is no evidence that such treatment has any effect on other outcomes.

Antipyretic Therapy

By definition, febrile seizures cannot occur in the absence of fever, and frequency of febrile illness is a definite risk factor for recurrence of FCs. Intermittent antipyretic therapy has been recommended but seldom tested in proper clinical trials. There was no apparent benefit in terms of prevention of FC recurrence in a Canadian trial of antipyretic therapy given at the time of illness.[75]

Anticonvulsant Drug Therapy

Phenobarbital

Although there is no reason to expect phenobarbital administered at the time of fever to be effective in the prevention of FCs, there have been several clinical trials that demonstrate that continuous administration of phenobarbital in a dose sufficient to maintain blood levels of 15 µg/ml will also reduce FC recurrence.[76, 77] Unfortunately, phenobarbital used in this manner is associated with a high frequency of side effects, and few parents continue the regimen.[78] Furthermore, continuous therapy with phenobarbital has been associated with reduction in intellectual performance.[79, 80]

Valproate

Several small clinical trials have demonstrated continuous therapy with valproate to be effective in preventing the recurrence of FCs.[81–84] The hepatotoxicity reported in young children with epilepsy—generally on multiple antiseizure agents—makes this an unlikely choice for long-term therapy for FC prophylaxis in the United States.

Diazepam

A number of studies have demonstrated diazepam administered rectally at the time of fever to be effective prevention for FC recurrence[5, 37, 85, 86] (see Knudsen[87] for a review of these studies). A recent study in the

United States has also demonstrated oral diazepam to be an effective prophylactic agent against repeat FCs.[88]

Other Interventions

Although antipyretic therapy and short-term or long-term antiepilepsy therapy may be associated with a reduction of subsequent febrile seizures under ideal circumstances, there is no evidence that interventions of this type in any way influence the long-term prognosis in these children.It is generally agreed that, regardless of pharmacologic intervention, parental education is also very important in the management of children with FCs.

Conclusion

FCs are the most frequently occurring neurologic disorder of early childhood, affecting 2–4% of children in the United States and Europe before their fifth birthday. This risk varies worldwide, approaching 10% in Japan but only about 1% in China.

The most frequent complication of an FC is a convulsion with a subsequent febrile illness. About one-third of children with one FC will experience further convulsions, although the risk varies from 10% to almost 90% depending on age, family history, and clinical features of the initial episode. Although chronic antiepileptic administration (using phenobarbital or valproate) on a continuous basis in doses adequate to maintain therapeutic levels has been demonstrated to reduce the risk for febrile seizure recurrence, intermittent treatment with oral or preferably rectal diazepam (when available in the United States) at the time of febrile illness would seem a preferable approach to prevention. Antipyretics and parental education are also important.

Children who have experienced FCs have an increased risk of developing epilepsy when compared with the general population, and by age 20 years, about 6% of these children will be so affected. This risk is greatest in the first 10 years of life, but the risk remains elevated at least through the fourth decade of life. This increase in the risk for epilepsy seems primarily related to either pre-existing neurologic abnormality or to a genetic predisposition for epilepsy. Prophylactic treatment with antiseizure medications—either continuous or intermittent—has not been demonstrated to modify this risk. There are no other long-term neurologic sequelae associated with convulsions with fever, and for most children it represents a benign condition.

References

1. Nelson KB, Ellenberg J (eds). Consensus Statement. In Febrile Seizures. New York: Raven, 1982.
2. Berg AT, Shinnar S, Hauser WA , et al. A prospective study of recurrent febrile seizures. N Engl J Med 1992;327:1122.
3. Tsuboi T. Prevalence and incidence of epilepsy in Tokyo. Epilepsia 1988;29:103.
4. Annegers JF, Hauser WA, Shirts SB, Kurland LT. Factors prognostic of unprovoked seizures after febrile convulsions. N Engl J Med 1987;316:493.
5. Knudsen FU. Recurrence risk after a first febrile seizure and effect of short term diazepam prophylaxis. Arch Dis Child 1985;60:1045.
6. Offringa M, Hazebroek-Kampschreur AA, Derksen-Lubsen G. Prevalence of febrile seizures in Dutch schoolchildren. Paediatr Perinat Epidemiol 1991;5:181.
7. Nelson KB, Ellenberg JH. Predictors of epilepsy in children who have experienced febrile seizures. N Engl J Med 1976;295:1029.
8. Hauser WA, Kurland LT. Convulsive disorders in Rochester, Minnesota, 1935–68. Epilepsia 1975;16:1.
9. Verity CM, Butler NR, Goldring J. Febrile convulsions in a national cohort followed up from birth. I. Prevalence and recurrence in the first 5 years of life. BMJ 1985;209:1307.
10. Van den Berg BJ, Yerushalamy J. Studies on convulsive disorders in young children. I. Incidence of febrile and nonfebrile convulsions by age and other factors. Pediatr Res 1969;3:298.
11. Forsgren L, Sidenvall R, Bloonquist H, K:son H, Heijbel J. A prospective incidence study of febrile convulsions. Acta Neurol Scand 1990;79:550.
12. Hauser WA. The Natural History of Febrile Seizures. In KB Nelson, J Ellenberg (eds), Febrile Seizures. New York: Raven, 1982;5.
13. Stanhope JM, Brody JA, Brink E. Convulsions among the Chamorro people of Guam, Mariana Islands. I. Seizure disorders. Am J Epidemiol 1972;95:292.
14. Fukuyama Y, Kagawa K, Tanaka K. A genetic study of febrile convulsions. Eur Neurol 1978;18:166.
15. Fu Z, Lavine L, Wang Z, et al. Prevalence and incidence of febrile seizures (FBS) in China. Neurology 1987;37(Suppl 1):149.
16. Hauser WA, Ortega, R, Zarelli M. The prevalence of epilepsy in a rural Mexican village. Epilepsia 1990;31:604.
17. Gracia F, Loo de Lar S, Castillo L, et al. 1990 epidemiology of epilepsy in Guaymi Indians from Bocas del Toro Province, Republic of Panama. Epilepsia 1990;31:718.
18. Bharucha NE, Bharucha EP, Bharucha AE. Febrile seizures. Neuroepidemiology 1991;10(3):138.
19. Iloeje SO. Febrile convulsions in a rural and an urban population. East Afr Med J 1991;68:43.
20. Akpede GO, Abiodun PO, Sykes RM. Pattern of infections in children under six years old presenting with convulsions associated with fever of acute onset in a children's emergency room in Benin City, Nigeria. J Trop Pediatr 1993;39:11.

21. Akpede GO, Sykes RM, Abiodun PO. Convulsions with malaria: febrile or indicative of cerebral involvement? J Trop Pediatr 1993;39:350.
22. Hauser WA, Annegers JF, Hauser A, et al. The risk of seizure disorders among relatives of patients with febrile convulsions. Neurology 1985,35:1268.
23. Tsuboi T. Febrile Convulsions. In VE Anderson, WA Hauser, JK Penry, CE Siing (eds), Genetic Basis of the Epilepsies. New York: Raven, 1982.
24. Forsgren L, Sidenvall R, Bloonquist H, et al. An incident case referent study of febrile convulsions in children: genetical and social aspects. Neuropediatrics 1990;21:153.
25. Nelson KB, Ellenberg JS. Prenatal and perinatal antecedents of febrile seizures. Ann Neurol 1990;27:127.
26. Zhao F, Emoto SE, Lavine L, et al. Risk factors for febrile seizures in the People's Republic of China: a case control study. Epilepsia 1991;31:510.
27. Sofijanov N, Emoto S, Kuturec M, et al. Febrile seizures: clinical characteristic and initial EEG. Epilepsia 1992;33:52.
28. Forsgren L, Sidenvall R, K:son H, et al. Pre- and perinatal factors in febrile convulsions. Acta Pediatr Scand 1991;80:218.
29. Bethune P, Gordon KG, Dooley JM, et al. Which child will have a febrile seizure? Am J Dis Child 1993;147:35.
30. Blakley SA. Pre- and perinatal risk factors as antecedents of complex febrile seizures. Submitted in partial fulfillment of requirements for Ph.D. University of Texas. 1987.
31. Verity CM, Butler NR, Goldring J. Febrile convulsions in a national cohort followed up from birth. II. Medical history and intellectual ability at 5 years of age. BMJ 1985;209:1311.
32. Wallace SJ. The reproductive efficiency of parents whose children convulse when febrile. Dev Med Child Neurol 1974;16:465.
33. Vanden Berg B, Yerushalamy J. Studies on convulsive disorders in young children. IV. Pediatr Res 1969;3:298.
34. Wallace SJ. Etiologic aspects on febrile convulsions. Pregnancy and perinatal factors. Arch Dis Child 1972;47:171.
35. Wallace JS. Febrile Convulsions. Boston: Butterworth, 1988.
36. Eeg-Olofsson O, Wigertz A, Link H. Immunoglobulin abnormalities in cerebrospinal fluid and blood in children with febrile seizures. Neuropediatrics 1982;13:39.
37. Lenti C, Masserini C, Barlocco A, et al. IgG2 deficiency in children with febrile convulsions: a familial study. Ital J Neurol Sci 1993;14:561.
38. Walker AM, Jick H, Perera DR, et al. Neurologic events following diphtheria-tetanus-pertussis immunization. Pediatrics 1988;81:345.
39. Shields WD, Neilsen C, Buch D, et al. Relationship of pertussis immunization to the onset of neurologic disorders: a retrospective epidemiologic study. J Pediatr 1988;113:801.
40. Griffith AH. Pertussis vaccine and convulsive disorders of childhood. Proc R Soc Med 1974;67:372.
41. Hirtz DG, Nelson KB, Ellenberg JH. Seizures following childhood immunization. J Pediatr 1983;102:14.
42. Caserta MT, Hall CB, Schnabel K, et al. Neuroinvasion and persistence of human herpesvirus 6 in children. J Infect Dis 1994;170:1586.

FEBRILE CONVULSIONS **161**

43. Berg AT. Are febrile seizures provoked by a rapid rise in temperature? Am J Dis Child 1993;147:1101.
44. Corey LA, Berg K, Pellock JM. The occurrence of epilepsy and febrile seizures in Virginian and Norwegian twins. Neurology 1991; 41:1433.
45. Rich SS, Annegers JF, Hauser WA, Anderson VE. Complex segregation analysis of febrile convulsions. Am J Hum Genet 1987;412:249.
46. Annegers JF, Hauser A, Anderson VE, Kurland LT. The risks of seizures disorders among relatives of patients with childhood onset epilepsy. Neurology 1982;32:174.
47. Tsuboi T. Seizures in childhood. A population based and clinic based study. Acta Neurol Scand 1986;74(Suppl 110):1.
48. Franzten E, Lennox-Buchthal M, Nygaard A. Longitudinal EEG and clinical study of children with febrile convulsions. Electroencephalogr Clin Neurophysiol 1968;24:197.
49. Degan R, Degan HE, Hans K. A contribution to the genetics of febrile seizures: waking and sleep EEG in siblings. Epilepsia 1991;32:515.
50. Hauser WA, Rich SS, Anderson VE. Epileptiform EEG patterns in children with febrile seizures. Epilepsia 1991;32:71.
51. Thorn I. Prevention of Recurrent Febrile Seizures: Intermittent Prophylaxis with Diazepam Compared with Continuous Treatment with Phenobarbital. In KB Nelson, JH Ellenberg (eds), Febrile Seizures. New York: Raven 1981;119.
52. Doose H, Gerken H, Volzke E. On the genetics of EEG-anomalies in childhood. I. Abnormal theta rhythms. Neuropaediatrie 1972;3:386.
53. Doose H, Baier WK. Theta rhythms in the EEG: a genetic trait in childhood epilepsy. Brain Dev 1988;10:347.
54. Nelson KB, Ellenberg JH. Prognosis in children with febrile seizures. Pediatrics 1978;61:720.
55. Annegers JF, Blakley S, Hauser WA, Kurland LT. Recurrence of febrile convulsions in a population based cohort. Epilepsy Res 1990;5:209.
56. Berg AT, Shinnar S, Hauser WA, Leventhal JM. Predictors of recurrent febrile seizures: a meta-analytic review J Pediatr 1990;116:329.
57. van Esch A, Steyerberg EW, Berger MY, et al. Family history and recurrence of febrile seizures. Arch Dis Child 1994;70:395.
58. Offringa M, Derksen-Lubsen G, Bossuyt PM, Lubsen J. Seizure recurrence after a first febrile seizure: a multivariate analysis. Dev Med Child Neurol 1992;34:15.
59. Offringa M, Bossuyt PM, Lubsen J, et al. Risk factors for seizure recurrence in children with febrile seizures: a pooled analysis of individual patient data from five studies. J Pediatr 1994;124:574.
60. Rocca WA, Sharbrough FW, Hauser WA, et al. Risk factors for absence seizures: a population-based case-control study in Rochester, Minnesota. Neurology 1987;37:1309.
61. Rocca WA, Sharbrough FW, Hauser WA, et al. Risk factors for complex partial seizures: a population-based case-control study. Ann Neurol 1987;21:22.
62. Rocca WA, Sharbrough FW, Hauser WA, et al. Risk factors for generalized tonic-clonic seizures: a population-based case-control study in Rochester, Minnesota. Neurology 1987;37:1315.

63. Verity CM, Golding J. Risk of epilepsy after febrile convulsions: a national cohort study. BMJ 1991;303:1373.
64. Falconer M. Genetic and related aetiologic factors in temporal lobe epilepsy. A review. Epilepsia 1971;12:13.
65. Schiottz-Christensen E, Bruhn P. Intelligence, behavior, and scholastic achievement subsequent to febrile convulsions: an analysis of discordant twin-pairs. Dev Med Child Neurol 1973;15:565.
66. Smith JA, Wallace JS. Febrile convulsions: intellectual progress in relation to anticonvulsant therapy and to recurrence of fits. Arch Dis Child 1982;57:104.
67. Ellenberg JH, Nelson KB. Febrile seizures and late intellectual performance. Arch Neurol 1978;35:17.
68. Kaliapeumal VG, Sundararaj N, Mani KS. Seizure prognosis for partial epilepsies in India. Epilepsy Res 1989;3:86.
69. Schmidt D, Tsai J, Janz D. Febrile seizures in patients with complex partial seizures. Acta Neurol Scand 1985;72:68.
70. Fish DR, Smith SJ, Quesney LF, et al. Surgical treatment of children with medically intractable frontal or temporal lobe epilepsy: results and highlights of 40 years experience. Epilepsia 1993;34:244.
71. Doderill CB. Correlates of generalized tonic-clonic seizures with intellectual, neuropsychological, emotional, and social function in patients with epilepsy. Epilepsia 1986;27:399.
72. Lorber J, Sunderland R. Lumbar puncture in children with convulsions associated with fever. Lancet 1980;1:785.
73. Knudsen FU. Rectal administration of diazepam in solution in the acute treatment of convulsions in infants and children. Arch Dis Child 1979;54:855.
74. Knudsen FU. Recurrence risk after a first febrile seizure and effect of short term diazepam prophylaxis. Arch Dis Child 1985;60:1045.
75. Camfield PR, Camfield CS, Shapiro SH, Cummings C. The first febrile seizure—antipyretic instruction plus phenobarbital or placebo to prevent recurrence. J Pediatr 1980;97:16.
76. Wolf SM, Carr A, Cavis DC, et al. The value of phenobarbital in the child who has had a single febrile seizure: a controlled prospective study. Pediatrics 1977;59:778.
77. Faero O, Kastrup KW, Lykkegaard Nielsen E, et al. Successful prophylaxis of febrile convulsions with phenobarbital. Epilepsia 1972;13:279.
78. Wolf SM, Forsythe A. Behavioral disturbance phenobarbital and febrile seizures. Pediatrics 1978;68:728.
79. Farwell JR, Lee YJ, Hirtz DG, et al. Phenobarbital for febrile seizures: effects on intelligence and on seizure recurrence. N Engl J Med 1990;322:364.
80. Camfield CS, Chaplin S, Doyle AB, et al. Side effects of phenobarbital in toddlers: behavioral and cognitive aspects. Pediatrics 1979;95:361.
81. Newton RW. Randomized controlled trials of phenobarbitone and valproate in febrile convulsions. Arch Dis Child 1988;63:1189.
82. Wallace SJ, Smith JA. Successful prophylaxis against febrile convulsions with valproic acid or phenobarbitone. BMJ 1980;280:353.

83. Ngwane E, Bower B. Continuous sodium valproate or phenobarbitone in the prevention of simple febrile convulsions. Arch Dis Child 1980;55:171.

84. Lee K, Taudorf K, Hvorslev V. Prophylactic treatment with valproic acid or diazepam in children with febrile convulsions. Acta Paediatr Scand 1986;75:593.

85. McKinlay I, Newton R. Intention to treat febrile convulsions with rectal diazepam, valproate, or phenobarbitone. Dev Med Child Neurol 1989;31:617.

86. Autret E, Billard C, Bertrand P, et al. Double blind randomized trial of diazepam versus placebo for prevention of recurrence of febrile seizures. J Pediatr 1990;119:490.

87. Knudsen FU. Intermittent diazepam prophylaxis in febrile convulsions: pros and cons. Acta Neurol Scand 1991;83(Suppl 135):1.

88. Rosman NP, Colton T, Labazzo JL, et al. A controlled trial of diazepam administered during febrile illness to prevent recurrence of febrile seizures. N Engl J Med 1993;329:79.

9

Prognosis of People with a First Unprovoked Seizure

W. Allen Hauser

Introduction

The majority of individuals with a newly identified seizure disorder have an obvious precipitant (e.g., a high fever in children).[1-3] For these individuals with "provoked" or acute symptomatic seizures, the clinician's roles are the identification of the underlying cause and the initiation of appropriate therapy for the underlying condition. The seizures are a secondary consideration, and seldom is antiseizure medication (ASM) warranted.

Only about one-third of those with newly identified seizures have unprovoked seizures. Of these, more than three-fourths have experienced multiple unprovoked seizure episodes before their first medical contact.[4] These individuals must be considered to have epilepsy, a condition characterized by the tendency to experience recurrent, unprovoked seizures. Eighty percent or more of these individuals can be expected to have further seizures, and for most, treatment with ASM should be initiated.[5]

Less than 10% of all newly identified seizure patients and only about one-fourth of patients with a newly identified unprovoked seizure are identified at the time of a first unprovoked seizure. Unlike individuals with multiple unprovoked seizures at presentation, a considerably lower proportion of cases can be expected to experience additional episodes. Although the exact proportion of patients who experience recurrence is controversial for reasons to be discussed, it appears that, on average, about one in three individuals identified at the time of a first unprovoked seizure go on to have additional seizures, even if followed over a prolonged period of time. Because of this relatively low proportion of people who experience further seizures, the need for ASM in these patients is less clear, and decisions may be less obvious.

Regardless of the nature of the presenting seizure (provoked or unprovoked), the most important role of the physician is to undertake an evaluation to identify any remedial condition that may be the cause of seizures. Once such a condition is excluded, a decision about therapy must be made. A seizure is a frightening event. Although many patients with a first generalized major motor seizure are frequently unaware of the event itself—only the end result—there is confusion and concern on the part of patients and their families about what has happened. Whereas most individuals (and their families) would prefer to experience no further episodes, many individuals (and family members) also have concern about both the short-term and long-term effects of ASM. Because of this latter concern, both the patient with a single unprovoked seizure and family members frequently have a tolerance for further seizures that is greater than many physicians anticipate.[6] Thus, it is important for the treating physician to understand and explain the underlying mechanism for the occurrence of seizures, the risks and potential benefits of long-term therapy, and, for the few individuals who truly have experienced a first seizure, the likelihood of experiencing further seizures.

Recurrence After a First Seizure

Prospective studies of patients identified at the time of their first unprovoked seizure indicate that about 40% can be expected to have further seizures over a 3- to 5-year follow-up period.[4, 7–10] Higher recurrence frequencies have been reported in retrospective studies and studies limited to a first unprovoked generalized tonic-clonic seizure.[11, 12]

Even in studies of similar design, there is considerable variation in summary estimates of the risk for recurrent seizures after a first unprovoked seizure. This is because a wide array of predictors have been identified that modify the risk of recurrence. Thus, differences in the proportion of cases with a factor associated with modification of recurrence risk explain some of these apparent differences in summary recurrence risks.[13] Because of this, a single figure for prediction of recurrence is not meaningful. It is necessary (and possible) to develop a profile to predict risk of recurrence in individual patients based on an array of clinically identified characteristics.

At an individual level, the likelihood of experiencing an additional seizure within a 5-year period after the first seizure varies from 20% for individuals with no identified risk factor for recurrence to nearly 100% for those with multiple risk factors. It might be expected that the proportion of patients who experience a recurrence may be higher at referral or tertiary centers, because, even with only a single seizure, more complex cases or a higher proportion of cases with combinations of risk factors may be expected to be included.

In part because of the tendency for specialization within age groups at academic centers, studies of prognosis after a first seizure have generally been limited to patient samples consisting primarily of adults or primarily of children. Luckily, age does not seem to be an important discriminator for recurrence, and there are few differences in risk across studies that include different age groups and have similar design. In studies that have included individuals of all ages, age alone has not been shown as a predictor of further seizures. Where differences in risk factors between adults and children exist, the discrepancies may be related more to sample size and statistical power considerations than to biology.

History of Neurologic Insult

The most consistent predictor of seizure recurrence is the presence or absence of a history of an insult associated with an increased risk for epilepsy. This classification separately categorizes as "remote symptomatic" those individuals with a history of severe head injury, stroke, central nervous system infection, or other central nervous system pathologic processes associated with a static or a progressive lesion and individuals with no identified historical insult (idiopathic).[4, 7, 8, 10, 13] Individuals with a first remote symptomatic seizure are two to three times more likely to have additional seizures compared with individuals with a first "idiopathic" seizure. A special subset of the remote symptomatic cases are individuals with neurologic abnormalities identified from birth. This group is composed primarily of individuals with mental retardation or cerebral palsy. Only one study has separately evaluated recurrence in such cases and reported it to be virtually 100%.[7]

Neurologic Examination Findings

Individuals with a remote symptomatic first seizure have a presumed structural lesion, and neurologic examination findings may be expected to be abnormal. It seems reasonable to assume that abnormal neurologic examination findings per se may be a predictor of recurrence, but this seems not to be the case. Abnormalities on neurologic examination seem at best a weak predictor of recurrence and may represent a surrogate for other factors associated with classification into a "remote symptomatic" category. In multivariate analysis, once controlling for etiology, an abnormal examination result does not further increase risk for seizure recurrence. When analysis is limited to idiopathic cases, an abnormal neurologic examination result is not associated with an increased risk for recurrence.

Electroencephalographic Findings

Most studies of patients identified at the time of a first seizure have reported individuals with electroencephalographic (EEG) abnormalities to be at higher risk for further seizures than those with normal EEG patterns.[4, 14] It appears that the risk is highest among individuals with epileptiform abnormalities (60–80% recurrence), intermediate in those with slowing or other abnormalities but without epileptiform activity (30–40% recurrence), and lowest in those with a normal EEG pattern (10–25% recurrence).[15] Some EEG abnormalities, particularly patterns such as the generalized spike and wave EEG pattern, are age-dependent—at least in the general (nonseizure) population. One might expect some differences in the predictive value within categories of first seizure patients when stratified by age of onset. In fact, the EEG has been predictive in some (but not all[9]) studies in adults but has been consistently predictive in children. In only a few studies have stratified or multivariable analyses been performed, evaluating EEG concurrently with other predictor variables such as etiology.

As with neurologic examination, one may expect to find EEG abnormalities, frequently focal, in those with a structural or progressive abnormality, and an abnormal EEG pattern is a less important predictor for seizure recurrence among remote symptomatic first seizure cases than among idiopathic cases.[4, 14]

Seizure Type

The prognosis for complete control and for remission of seizures is clearly less favorable in those with partial onset seizures compared with those with generalized onset epilepsy, As a corollary, it is frequently assumed that those with a partial first seizure are more likely to have a recurrence. It is not clear that this same assumption holds true in those with only one partial seizure. Most truly "first" partial seizures are identified because of secondary generalization or because they are prolonged. Brief partial seizures generally must recur before one can be certain that they are truly a seizure. Although it may be very difficult to study the recurrence risk of a first brief partial seizure, one might assume that that the recurrence risk for those with first brief partial seizures would be similar to those with secondary generalization.

Three studies in children have evaluated seizure type as a risk factor for recurrence after a first seizure and report a modest increase in risk for children with a first partial onset seizure when compared with those with a generalized onset seizure.[8, 10, 12, 16] Unlike the findings in studies of children, in studies limited to adults[9] or consisting primarily of older children and adults,[4] seizure type has not been an important predictor of recurrence. There is a clinical perception that truly generalized onset epilepsy is rare in the adult population.[17, 18] It is possible that in the studies of adults, individuals classified as having generalized onset seizures actually experienced a partial seizure with secondary generalization. This misclassification could obscure an effect of seizure type. On the other hand, it is possible that a true difference exists between children and adults.

Family History

Several studies (most in children) have evaluated a family history of epilepsy or of seizures as a possible predictor of seizure recurrence. Only one study reported an increased risk for those with a family history.[4] In this study of adults and older children, a history of unprovoked seizures or epilepsy in a sibling was associated with a significant increase in the risk of recurrence in older children and adults. Definitions of "family history" and of criteria to be included as affected with seizures or epilepsy have not been consistent in all studies. The farther one gets from first-degree relatives, the less reliable is family history. The study reporting family history to be a risk factor was done concomitantly with a genetic study of epilepsy. Thus, it is possible that family history was more reliably obtained. It is also possible that the influence of family history represents another factor for which recurrence risk differs between children and adults.

Prior Acute Symptomatic (Provoked) Seizures

People who experience acute symptomatic seizures have consistently been shown to have an increased risk for subsequent epilepsy compared with appropriate comparison groups without acute symptomatic seizures. Those with neonatal seizures[19] or with febrile seizures[20, 21] also have an increased risk for subsequent epilepsy compared with those in the general population or an unaffected population. It is also true for those with acute symptomatic seizures associated with insults such as head injury, stroke, or infection of the central nervous system when compared with those with similar insults but without acute symptomatic seizures.[22-24]

The effect of prior neonatal seizures on the risk of first seizure recurrence has been evaluated in three studies limited to children. In one study, a modest increase in risk was identified;[12] in two studies, no evidence of an increase in risk was identified, although the number of children with neonatal seizures was small in both studies.[8, 16]

The effect of a history of febrile seizures as a predictor of recurrence was evaluated in three studies limited to children and one study of older children and adults. The studies limited to children with a first unprovoked seizure did not identify an increase in recurrence risk for those with febrile seizures, although a febrile seizure preceding a first unprovoked seizure did seem predictive for an increase in recurrence risk in children with mental retardation or cerebral palsy in one study.[8, 10, 12, 16] The study of adults and older children reported a significant increase in risk in idiopathic first seizure cases, although this effect was not significant in multivariable analysis.[4] At 5 years after the first seizure, recurrence risk was 50% in those with prior febrile seizures, compared with 20% in the comparison group. This may again represent a difference in the predictive value in adults when compared with children.

Only one study has evaluated the effect of other acute symptomatic seizures.[4] In the analysis limited to those falling into a remote symptomatic first seizure group, those with an acute symptomatic seizure associated with the insult have a fourfold increase in risk for seizure recurrence compared with those without such seizures. Although numbers were small, in that study all cases with a remote symptomatic first seizure and a prior acute seizure experienced a recurrent event.

Status Epilepticus

In general, seizures are brief, lasting no more than a few minutes. A measure of severity of seizure may be the duration of continuing convulsions or the tendency to experience repeated episodes in a brief period of time. As with other events that may be construed as a measure of severity, some have assumed that those with more severe seizures (as measured by duration) may be more likely to experience further seizures. The association of a first unprovoked seizure fulfilling criteria for status epilepticus (SE), defined as continuing seizures for 30 minutes or more, and recurrence of unprovoked seizures has been examined in two studies. In children, there is no association between SE and risk for recurrence, although the recurrence risk in children with a first remote symptomatic seizure that met the criteria for SE was 80%, compared with 50% in children with a brief remote symptomatic seizure.[8] In adults, an increased recurrence risk could be identified in those with SE, but the effect disappeared when multivariate analysis was used to evaluate risk.[4] It would seem that SE is not an independent predictor for seizure recurrence but is associated with other factors associated with an increased risk for seizure recurrence, for example, etiology. Whereas a prolonged seizure in and of itself does not alter the risk for further seizures, it may be associated with an altered timing of recurrence. When seizures did recur, the time interval between the first and second seizure was shorter for those with SE than for those without.

Circadian Timing and the Wake-Sleep Cycle

The influences of time of day and of state of alertness have been evaluated as predictors of seizure recurrence. In adults, those who experience a first seizure that occurs nocturnally have an increased risk for seizure recurrence compared with those who experience a first seizure during waking hours.[9, 25] In children with a first idiopathic seizure, those who had a seizure during sleep had an increased risk for recurrence compared with those who had a seizure in a waking state.[26] In children with a first remote symptomatic seizure, state of alertness was not a predictor of recurrence. There appears to be some consistency in the state of alertness in which seizures occur. Second seizures tend to occur in the same sleep state as the first seizure, raising the possibility that children and adults who experienced a first recognized seizure during sleep may have had previous unrecognized episodes.

Other Predictors

Two studies reported a Todd's paresis to be associated with an increased risk for recurrence of a first unprovoked seizure.[4, 10] This effect was primarily accounted for by an increased recurrence in those with a remote symptomatic first seizure.

Factors Unassociated with Recurrence

Age and sex have been evaluated as potential predictors of recurrence and have not been shown to be important predictors of seizure recurrence.

Seizure Recurrence and Predictors of Recurrence After a Second Seizure

Only one study has thus far evaluated the risk for a third or fourth seizure after a second seizure.[27] Once a second seizure has occurred, the risk for further seizures is substantial. In this study, which followed a group from the date of their first seizure for a mean of 6 years or until a fourth seizure, about 85% of subjects experienced a recurrence. The only predictor for differential recurrence was etiology. At least 90% of those with two remote symptomatic seizures experienced a third seizure, compared with 65% of those with a second idiopathic seizure.

Costs and Benefits of Treatment

There are a number of effective ASMs that may be prescribed to reduce the risk of seizures. For most seizure types and epilepsy syndromes, there seems to be little difference between any of these ASMs in terms of efficacy. All of the currently available medications have the potential for idiosyncratic (and potentially fatal) side effects as well as dose-related side effects. Thus, the introduction of a chronic therapy can be done only at some potential discomfort to the patient. Thus, the decision about which ASM to use seems based on the side effect profile of each medication and the potential impact on the patient, taking sex and age into account.[28, 29]

Effectiveness of Antiseizure Medication in Preventing Further Seizures in Persons with a First Unprovoked Seizure

In studies of patients with epilepsy (recurrent unprovoked seizures), clinical trials have demonstrated the effectiveness of all ASMs currently available in the United States. Despite this, in observational studies of seizure recurrence after a first seizure, no definite benefit was noted in terms of preventing seizure recurrence. In fact, a paradoxical effect of an increase in recurrence among treated individuals was observed in some studies.[6, 30] This paradoxical effect is probably related to two factors, both of which have clinical implications.

The first is related to the differential selection of individuals at high risk for recurrence for treatment with ASMs. In general, treatment was initiated in individuals whom clinicians believed were "worse" and thus more likely to have further seizures. Even when multivariate analyses were used in an attempt to control for factors possibly associated with an increased risk for seizure recurrence, no positive effects of treatment could be demonstrated. Nonetheless, it seems likely that the lack of effectiveness of ASMs could be in part related to such selection. The second factor relates to aggressiveness of treatment. In those in whom treatment with an ASM was initiated, seldom was dosage adequate to ensure that "therapeutic" levels of drug were attained.

The effectiveness of ASMs in the prevention of recurrence was well demonstrated in two recent studies. An Italian study of seizure recurrence after a first unprovoked seizure randomized patients to early or delayed treatment after a first seizure, but physicians were required to see that individuals in the treatment arm received doses of ASM adequate to attain therapeutic levels within 1 month of entry into the study. In this study, there was clearly a beneficial effect of ASM in terms of prevention of seizure recurrence in the treatment arm.[31] A small study of randomization in children also demonstrated a beneficial effect of early treatment.[32]

Modification of the Ultimate Course of Epilepsy

It has been suggested that epilepsy is a progressive illness. In this paradigm, each seizure increases the likelihood of additional seizures. Furthermore, subsequent seizures will increase in severity.[33–35] As a corollary, it has been suggested that early treatment of a seizure disorder may prevent progression of the disease. The concept is presumably related in some way to the kindling phenomenon (a research paradigm not yet demonstrated in humans) and its inhibition by some but not all ASMs.

It is difficult at best to evaluate the phenomenon of progression in humans. A retrospective study evaluating the influence of timing of seizures up to the time of presentation to medical care has been interpreted as demonstrating this phenomenon, but the study design is fatally flawed primarily because of the retrospective assessment.[36] Two prospective studies that have attempted to address this question have failed to demonstrate such a phenomenon. In the Italian trial of randomization of initial treatment, there was no difference in the proportion of individuals who reached seizure freedom in either treatment arm.[37] In an analysis of the timing of seizures in a follow-up of individuals identified from their first seizure, no evidence of increasing risk for further seizures could be demonstrated after the second seizure had occurred.[27] In addition, there seemed to be no association of early treatment with any ASM and prognosis for remission or responsiveness to medications once treatment was started in studies of largely untreated populations in developing countries.[38, 39]

Side Effects of Antiseizure Medication

In the debate regarding relative type and severity of side effects of individual drugs, it is agreed that all ASMs have side effects. In some individuals these side effects are intolerable, and, while tolerated by others, they invariably have some impact on day-to-day functioning.[40, 41] In addition, idiosyncratic reactions such as drug-related rashes occur in 10–15% of individuals exposed to ASMs, and a small proportion will suffer side effects that may be potentially life-threatening. The actual proportion of cases in whom the specific nature of side effects is known varies with individual ASM, but a substantial proportion of cases have complaints regardless of drug used. This "cost" associated with side effects occurring in more than the 30–40% of cases likely to experience seizure recurrence over a 3- to 5-year period represents part of the cost–benefit equation in those with only one seizure.

Conclusions

Approximately 50,000 people in the United States will have a first seizure each year; about 20,000 will have a second seizure within a 5-year period. There is a wide array of predictors for recurrence. Only about 20% of individuals with a first idiopathic seizure who have normal EEG findings and no family history of epilepsy have further seizures. Between 40% and 60% of individuals with one of the identified risk factors have a recurrence; when more than one of the predictors is identified in an individual, the risk is additive, particularly in idiopathic cases. The majority of newly identified individuals fall into a low-risk group.

At present, there is no evidence that treatment of the first seizure influences long-term prognosis. Treatment is invariably associated with dose-related side effects and in some cases severe idiosyncratic side effects. While nonmedical considerations may enter into treatment decisions, it would seem that for most individuals who have clearly had only one seizure, a cost–benefit assessment favors delaying treatment until a second seizure has occurred.

References

1. Commission on Epidemiology and Prognosis, International League Against Epilepsy. Guidelines for epidemiologic studies on epilepsy. Epilepsia 1993;34:592.
2. Hauser WA, Annegers JF, Kurland LT. Prevalence of epilepsy in Rochester, Minnesota, 1940–1980. Epilepsia 1991;31:429.
3. Annegers JF, Hauser WA, Lee JR-J, Rocca WA. Acute symptomatic seizures in Rochester, Minnesota, 1935–1984. Epilepsia 1995;36:327.
4. Hauser WA, Rich SS, Annegers JF, Anderson VE. Seizure recurrence after a first unprovoked seizure: an extended follow-up. Neurology 1990;40:1163.
5. Hauser WA, Rich SS, Jacobs MP, Anderson VE. Pattern of seizure occurrence and recurrence risks in patients with new diagnosed epilepsy. Epilepsia 1983;24:516.
6. Devinsky O, Penry JK. Quality of life: the clinician's view. Epilepsia 1993;43(Suppl 4):S4.
7. Annegers JF, Shirts SB, Hauser WA, Kurland LT. Risk of recurrence after an initial unprovoked seizure. Epilepsia 1986;27:43.
8. Shinnar S, Berg AT, Moshe SL, et al. The risk of recurrence following a first unprovoked seizure in childhood: a prospective study. Pediatrics 1990;85:1076.

9. Hopkins A, Garman A, Clarke C. The first seizure in adult life: value of clinical features, electroencephalography and computerized tomographic scanning in prediction of seizure recurrence. Lancet 1988;1:721.
10. Shinnar S, Berg AT, Moshe SL, et al. The risk of seizure recurrence following a first unprovoked seizure in childhood: an extended follow-up. Pediatrics (in press).
11. Elwes RDC, Chesterman P, Reynolds EH. Prognosis after a first untreated tonic-clonic seizure. Lancet 1985;2:752.
12. Hirtz DG, Ellenberg JH, Nelson KB. The risk of recurrence of nonfebrile seizures in children. Neurology 1984;34:637.
13. Berg AT, Shinnar S. The risk of seizure recurrence following a first unprovoked seizure: a quantitative review. Neurology 1991;41:965.
14. Shinnar S, Kang H, Berg AT, et al. EEG abnormalities in children with a first unprovoked seizure. Epilepsia 1994;35:471.
15. Van Donselaar CA, Schimsheimer RJ, Geerts AT, Declerck AC. Value of the electroencephalogram in adult patients with untreated idiopathic first seizures. Arch Neurol 1992;49:231.
16. Camfield PR, Camfield CS, Dooley JM, et al. Epilepsy after a first unprovoked seizure in childhood. Neurology 1985;35:1657.
17. Commission on Classification and Terminology of the International League Against Epilepsy. A revised proposal for the classification of epilepsy and epileptic syndromes. Epilepsia 1989;30:268.
18. Commission on Classification and Terminology of the International League Against Epilepsy. Proposal for revised clinical and electroencephalographic classification of epileptic seizures. Epilepsia 1981;22:489.
19. Holden KR, Mellits ED, Freeman JM. Neonatal seizures. I. Correlations of prenatal and perinatal events with outcomes. Pediatrics 1982;70:165.
20. Annegers JF, Hauser WA, Shirts SB, Kurland LT. Factors prognostic of unprovoked seizures after febrile convulsions. N Engl J Med 1987;316:493.
21. Nelson KB, Ellenberg JH. Prognosis in children with febrile seizures. Pediatrics 78;61:720.
22. Annegers JF, Grabow JD, Groover RV, et al. Seizures after head trauma: a population study. Neurology 1980;30:683.
23. Annegers JF, Hauser WA, Beghi E, et al. The risk of unprovoked seizures after encephalitis and meningitis. Neurology 1988;38:1407.
24. So EL, Annegers JF, Hauser WA, et al. Risk of epileptic seizures after cerebral infarction: a population-based study. Epilepsia 1993;34(Suppl 6):29.
25. Van Donselaar CA, Geerts AT, Schimsheimer RJ. Idiopathic first seizure in adult life: who should be treated? BMJ 1993;302:620.
26. Shinnar S, Berg AT, Ptachewich Y, Alemany M. Sleep state and the risk of seizure recurrence following a first unprovoked seizure in childhood. Neurology 1991;41:971.
27. Hauser WA, Annegers JF, Rich SS, Lee JR-J. How many seizures are epilepsy? Epilepsia 1993;34(Suppl 2):164.
28. Mattson RH, Cramer JA, Collins JF, et al. Comparison of carbamazepine, phenobarbital, phenytoin, and primidone in partial and secondarily generalized tonic-clonic seizures. N Engl J Med 1985;313:145.

29. Mattson RH, Cramer JA, Collins JF, U.S. Department of Veterans Affairs Epilepsy Cooperative. A comparison of valproate with carbamazepine for the treatment of complex partial seizures and secondarily generalized tonic-clonic seizures in adults. Study No. 264 Group. N Engl J Med 1992;327:765.

30. Hauser WA, Anderson VE, Loewenson RB, McRoberts SM. Seizure recurrence after a first unprovoked seizure. N Engl J Med 1982;307:522.

31. First Seizure Trial Group. Randomized clinical trial on the efficacy of antiepileptic drugs in reducing the risk of relapse after a first unprovoked tonic-clonic seizure. Neurology 1993;43:478.

32. Camfield P, Camfield C, Dooley J, et al. A randomized study of carbamazepine versus no medication after a first unprovoked seizure in childhood. Neurology 1989;39:851.

33. Elwes RDC, Johnson AL, Reynolds EH. The course of untreated epilepsy. BMJ 1988;297:948.

34. Reynolds EH, Elwes RDC, Shorvon SD. Why does epilepsy become intractable? Prevention of chronic epilepsy. Lancet 1983;2:952.

35. Gowers WR. Epilepsy and Other Chronic Convulsive Disorders. London: Churchill, 1881.

36. Reynolds EH. Early treatment and the prognosis of epilepsy. Epilepsia 1987;28:97.

37. First Seizure Trial Group. Randomized clinical trial on the efficacy of treatment of first unprovoked epileptic seizure Epilepsia 1993;34(Suppl 2):35.

38. Placencia M, Sander JW, Roman M, et al. The characteristics of epilepsy in a largely untreated population in rural Ecuador. J Neurol Neurosurg Psychiatry 1994;57:320.

39. Watts AE. The natural history of untreated epilepsy in a rural community in Africa. Epilepsia 1992;33:464.

40. Vining EPG, Mellits ED, Dorsen MM, et al. Psychologic and behavioral effects of antiepileptic drugs in children: a double-blind comparison between phenobarbital and valproic acid. Pediatrics 1987;80:165.

41. Wolf SM, Forsythe A. Behavior disturbance, phenobarbital and febrile seizures. Pediatrics 1978;61:728.

10

Treatment of Neonatal and Childhood Seizures

Carl E. Stafstrom and Gregory L. Holmes

Introduction

Seizures are one of the most common neurologic conditions encountered by primary care physicians, who are increasingly being called on to manage these disorders. Once diagnosed, seizures can be difficult to treat, and it is sometimes difficult to decide whether or not treatment is even indicated. Another challenging management question is when to discontinue treatment. The goal of this chapter is to provide the primary care physician with a logical and practical approach to the diagnosis and therapy of the common seizure disorders of neonates and children. More detailed discussions of epidemiology and pathophysiology may be found elsewhere.[1–5] Primary care physicians are often in the best position to address the complex needs of children with epilepsy and their families, and we believe that they can handle most common seizure-related problems. Reflecting this practical approach, our reference list emphasizes reviews and monographs. Certain common childhood seizure disorders are covered in detail elsewhere in this volume, so they are not discussed here (see Chapter 8 for a discussion of febrile seizures and Chapter 12 for a discussion of status epilepticus). Other childhood seizure disorders, not discussed elsewhere in this volume, are covered in greater depth in this chapter (e.g., infantile spasms).

An understanding of definitions is crucial for both diagnostic accuracy and family counseling. A *seizure* is an episode of synchronous, rhythmic firing of a large number of neurons, manifesting as an alteration of motor or sensory function, behavior, or level of alertness. *Epilepsy* is the condition of recurrent seizures. An *epileptic syndrome* is an epileptic disorder characterized by a cluster of signs, symptoms, and electroencephalographic (EEG) findings that usually occur together. Modern classification schemes for seizures and epilepsy syndromes are discussed in Chapter 2.

Most epilepsy begins in childhood. As will become apparent in this chapter, seizures vary dramatically during development, and certain seizure types are restricted to particular age windows (e.g., infantile spasms and febrile seizures). Indeed, the state of brain development at which a seizure occurs often determines the seizure type, neurologic sequelae, and response to particular modes of therapy. Therefore, children, and especially neonates, cannot be considered merely miniature adults; their treatment must be specifically tailored (in terms of medication choice, dosage, duration of therapy, etc.) to reflect the underlying degree of central nervous system maturation.

Neonatal Seizures

In a newborn, seizure recognition is crucial because a seizure may be the only sign of a central nervous system disorder. A neonatal seizure is not a disease but rather a symptom of an underlying cerebral disturbance. The cause of a seizure must be determined promptly, and therapy is usually deferred until a cause is established.

Types and Classification

The International Classification of Epileptic Seizures is not applicable to newborns. The newborn nervous system is unable to sustain organized generalized discharges, and thus generalized tonic-clonic (GTC) seizures and absence seizures are rarely, if ever, seen in neonates. Neonatal seizures were classified by Volpe[6] into four types based solely on clinical manifestations: subtle, tonic, clonic, and myoclonic. The most common type is *subtle seizures*, which may include repetitive sucking or other oral-buccal-lingual movements, pedaling movements of the legs or paddling movements of the arms, blinking, momentary fixation of gaze with or without eye deviation, nystagmus, or apnea. Although clinically unimpressive, subtle seizures are commonly associated with severe central nervous system insults. *Tonic seizures* resemble decerebrate or opisthotonic posturing and consist of intermittent tonic extension of the arms, legs, or all four extremities. Without EEG confirmation, it is virtually impossible to differentiate these movements from nonepileptic motor activity. Tonic seizures are usually associated with severe brain lesions and occur most frequently in preterm infants. *Clonic seizures* consist of rhythmic jerking of groups of muscles in a focal or multifocal pattern. In multifocal clonic seizures, movements may migrate from one part of the body to another. Although focal seizures may be seen with localized brain insults, they may also accompany diffuse cerebral disturbances such as asphyxia, subarachnoid hemorrhage, hypoglycemia, or infection. *Myoclonic seizures* are similar to those seen in older children and consist of rapid, isolated jerks of the trunk, neck, or one or more limbs.

Although this classification system continues to be widely used, many of the behaviors described above, particularly those of subtle seizures, do not have clear EEG correlates. Furthermore, these behaviors frequently do not respond to antiepileptic therapy, which raises the question of whether subtle seizures are really epileptic events.[7]

With the use of cribside simultaneous EEG-video monitoring techniques, it has been demonstrated that focal clonic, focal tonic, and some myoclonic seizures are usually correlated with ictal EEG discharges, whereas generalized symmetric tonic posturing and most behaviors considered to be subtle seizures are not associated with abnormal EEG activity (Table 10-1). Instead, it has been hypothesized that tonic posturing and subtle seizures are "release phenomena" mediated by the brain stem when the usual inhibitory influence of the cerebral cortex is reduced by cortical damage.[8] It remains possible, however, that some epileptic seizures in neonates may simply not be detected using surface EEG electrodes, as it is well recognized that in older patients, some epileptic events, particularly partial seizures, may occur despite a normal EEG pattern.

Etiology and Differential Diagnosis

There are many causes of neonatal seizures, but a few causes account for the majority of cases. The most frequent causes of neonatal seizures

Table 10-1. Electroencephalographic Findings in Neonatal Seizures

---

A. Consistent relation to EEG seizure discharge
  1. Focal or multifocal clonic
  2. Focal tonic (extremity, trunk, eyes)
  3. Myoclonic (generalized or focal)
B. No consistent relation to EEG seizure discharge
  1. Motor automatisms
    a. Oral-buccal-lingual movements
    b. Ocular signs
    c. Pedaling, stepping, rotary arm movements
  2. Generalized tonic (extensor, flexor or mixed)
  3. Myoclonic (generalized or focal)

Source: Modified from EM Mizrahi. Clinical and neurophysiological correlates of neonatal seizures. Cleve Clin J Med 1989;56(Suppl):S100.

are hypoxic-ischemic injury, infection, and hemorrhage. While rare, causes such as hypoglycemia, inborn metabolic errors of metabolism (such as some amino and organic acidopathies), and pyridoxine dependency are important because they are treatable. Because idiopathic seizures are rare in the first months of life, a concerted effort must be made to identify the cause. Determining the cause of a patient's seizures is critical, as it dictates therapy and is highly correlated with outcome.[9] Major causes of neonatal seizures are listed in Table 10-2, and their timing with respect to major etiologic categories is shown in Table 10-3.

As noted above, not all repetitive, stereotyped behaviors in neonates are epileptic seizures. For example, jitteriness, which reflects general nervous system dysfunction,[10] has a similar etiologic spectrum as seizures, including hypoxic-ischemia encephalopathy, drug withdrawal, hypocalcemia, and hypoglycemia. Several clinical clues may help differentiate jitteriness and nonepileptic myoclonus from seizures (Table 10-4). When there is a question about the diagnosis, an EEG recorded during the event can be extremely informative. If an ictal discharge is noted, the clinician has the answer. If no ictal discharges are recorded during a clinical event, the likelihood of an epileptic event decreases but is not entirely eliminated.

Benign familial neonatal convulsions (BFNCs) and benign idiopathic neonatal convulsions (BINCs) ("fifth-day fits") are two syndromes of

Table 10-2. Causes of Neonatal Seizures

Perinatal hypoxia-ischemia

Infections

    Sepsis

    Meningitis: group B *Streptococcus*, *Escherichia coli*

    Meningoencephalitis: herpes simplex, toxoplasmosis, coxsackie B, rubella, cytomegalovirus

Intracranial hemorrhage and ischemia

    Subarachnoid, subdural, or intraparenchymal hemorrhage

    Intraventricular hemorrhage

    Stroke

    Cortical vein thrombosis

Congenital malformations or cortical dysgenesis

Acute metabolic problems

    Hyponatremia and hypernatremia

        Inappropriate fluid therapy

        Sodium bicarbonate therapy in premature infants

        Inappropriate antidiuretic hormone secretion

    Hypoglycemia

        Transient: small for gestational age, prematurity, infant of diabetic mother, perinatal asphyxia or hemorrhage, meningitis, postexchange transfusion

        Persistent: galactosemia, fructosemia, leucine sensitivity, glycogen storage disease, infantile gigantism, Beckwith's syndrome, pancreatic islet tumor, anterior pituitary hypoplasia

    Hypocalcemia

        Early: infant of diabetic mother, small for gestational age, perinatal asphyxia or hemorrhage, postexchange transfusion, DiGeorge syndrome, sepsis, maternal hyperparathyroidism

        Late: low calcium-to-phosphorus ratio in formula (e.g., from improper mixing)

    Hypomagnesemia

        Associated with hypocalcemia

        Magnesium malabsorption syndrome

Other causes

    Inborn errors of metabolism

Table 10-2. *(continued)*

Aminoaciduria: phenylketonuria, maple syrup urine disease, nonketotic hyperglycinemia, congenital lysinuria

Urea cycle defects: carbamyl phosphate deficiency, ornithine carbamyl transferase deficiency, citrullinemia, arginosuccinic aciduria, transient hyperammonemia of prematurity associated with perinatal asphyxia

Organic acidurias: proprionic acidemia, methylmalonic acidemia, methylmalonic-CoA mutase deficiency

Pyridoxine: deficiency; dependency (autosomal recessive)

Biotinidase deficiency

Molybdenum cofactor/sulfite oxidase deficiency

Glucose-transporter protein deficiency

Peroxisomal disorders

Neonatal adrenoleukodystrophy

Cerebrohepatorenal (Zellweger's) syndrome

Mitochondrial diseases

Neurocutaneous disorders (phakomatoses)

Tuberous sclerosis

Sturge-Weber disease

Neurofibromatosis

Incontinentia pigmenti

Toxins

Endogenous: bilirubin

Exogenous: mercury, hexachlorophene, injected penicillin or anesthetics (during labor), maternal isoniazid

Maternal drug dependency(heroin, methadone, barbiturates, or cocaine)

Benign syndromes

Benign familial neonatal seizures

Benign idiopathic neonatal seizures ("fifth-day fits")

Source: Modified from P Kellaway, EM Mizrahi. Neonatal Seizures. In H Luders, RP Lesser (eds), Epilepsy: Electroclinical Syndromes. Berlin: Springer-Verlag, 1987;2; and MJ Painter, LM Gaus. Neonatal seizures: diagnosis and treatment. J Child Neurol 1991;6:101.

Table 10-3. Causes of Seizures in the First Month of Life

0–4 days
 Hypoxia-ischemia
 Meningoencephalitis
 Hypocalcemia
 Hypoglycemia
 Hypomagnesemia
 Trauma
 Pyridoxine dependency
 Incontinentia pigmenti
5–14 days
 Meningoencephalitis
 Hypocalcemia
 Cerebral malformation
 Aminoaciduria
 Hypocalcemia
 Hypomagnesemia
 "Fifth-day fits"
 Hemorrhage
15–28 days
 Cerebral malformation
 Trauma (subdural hemorrhage)
 Infection

neonatal seizures that tend to have good outcomes.[11, 12] BFNCs are usually generalized tonic-clonic convulsions that occur in the first few days of life. A family history of neonatal seizures is always obtained. BFNCs are usually outgrown, although about 15% of children develop seizures after the neonatal period.[12] BINCs usually begin between days 4 and 6 of life (hence the name "fifth-day fits"); no cause or familial basis is uncovered. Both of these neonatal seizure types tend to be benign, but it must be emphasized that they are diagnoses of exclusion.

An entity that may mimic a neonatal seizure is benign neonatal sleep myoclonus.[13] In this disorder, there is bilateral, synchronous, repetitive jerking of the upper or lower extremities. The myoclonus may be quite dramatic but only occurs during non–random eye movement sleep. The

Table 10-4. Differentiation of Involuntary Movements in Newborns

	Jitteriness	Myoclonus	Seizure
Type of movement	Oscillatory	Jerks	Jerks
Movement velocity	Rapid	Rapid	Slow
Periodicity	Rhythmic	Usually non-rhythmic	Usually rhythmic
Involvement of all limbs	Frequent	Occasional	Rare
Response to passive flexion	Diminishes	Variable	None
Stimulus sensitivity	Yes	Often	No
Gaze abnormality	No	No	Often
Altered consciousness	No	No	Often
EEG findings	Normal	Normal or abnormal (see Table 10-1)	Normal or abnormal (see Table 10-1)
Response to antiepileptic medication	Minimal to none	Variable	Frequent

Source: Modified from GL Holmes. Diagnosis and Management of Seizures in Children. Philadelphia: Saunders, 1987; and NP Rosman, JH Donnelly, MA Braun. The jittery newborn and infant: a review. Dev Behav Pediatr 1984;5:263.

myoclonus never occurs during the awake state, and waking the child stops the myoclonus. EEG and neurologic examination findings are normal, and outcome is excellent.

Evaluation

Determining the cause of neonatal seizures is usually more urgent than beginning antiepileptic drug (AED) treatment. The first step in evaluation should be a careful history and physical examination (Figure 10-1). A family history of neonatal seizures is suggestive of benign familial neonatal seizures, whereas a history of maternal drug ingestion may implicate drug withdrawal as a cause of seizures. Maternal infections or a difficult delivery may be helpful in determining the cause of seizures. Chorioretinitis or skin rashes may suggest a congenital infection, whereas needle marks in the scalp raise the possibility of inad-

NEONATAL SEIZURES

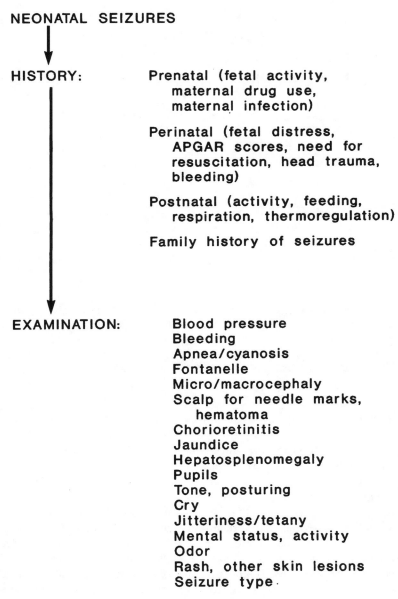

HISTORY:

Prenatal (fetal activity, maternal drug use, maternal infection)

Perinatal (fetal distress, APGAR scores, need for resuscitation, head trauma, bleeding)

Postnatal (activity, feeding, respiration, thermoregulation)

Family history of seizures

EXAMINATION:

Blood pressure
Bleeding
Apnea/cyanosis
Fontanelle
Micro/macrocephaly
Scalp for needle marks, hematoma
Chorioretinitis
Jaundice
Hepatosplenomegaly
Pupils
Tone, posturing
Cry
Jitteriness/tetany
Mental status, activity
Odor
Rash, other skin lesions
Seizure type

Figure 10-1. *Flow diagram for approach to a neonate with seizures. (Modified with permission from MJ Painter. Therapy of neonatal seizures. Cleve Clin J Med 1989;56[Suppl]:S124.)*

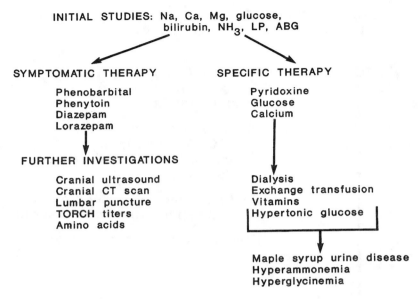

Figure 10-2. *Flow diagram for approach to diagnostic studies and therapy of a neonate with seizures. LP = lumbar puncture; ABG = arterial blood gas; CT = computed tomography; TORCH = toxoplasmosis, other (e.g., syphilis, HIV), rubella, cytomegalovirus, herpes. (Modified with permission from MJ Painter. Therapy of neonatal seizures. Cleve Clin J Med 1989;56[Suppl]:S124.)*

vertent injection of a local anesthetic such as lidocaine during delivery. After the history and physical examination, appropriate diagnostic studies should be performed and a decision regarding treatment made. Figure 10-2 is a flow diagram of recommended diagnostic studies and therapy for a neonate with seizures.

The EEG is an integral part of the workup of a neonate with possible seizures. Interictal EEG abnormalities can offer supportive, but not definitive, evidence that the infant is having seizures, whereas ictal abnormalities are diagnostic of epileptic seizures. Although a detailed discussion of neonatal EEG is beyond the scope of this chapter, it is worth mentioning the prognostic value of certain commonly reported neonatal EEG patterns. Background abnormalities are useful in predicting outcome after a variety of neonatal insults. A background that is isoelectric, shows burst suppression, or is excessively discontinuous or low-voltage with invariant waveforms portends an unfavorable long-term outcome. Essentially all infants with persistent burst suppression or an isoelectric record for 2 weeks will be neurologically impaired. A normal background or a focal abnormality superimposed on a normal background presages a more favorable outlook, even in an infant with seizures. The neonatal EEG rarely suggests a specific disease entity; an important exception is herpes simplex encephalitis (HSE), which is associated with a specific pattern known as periodic lateralized epileptiform discharges (PLEDs). In HSE, PLEDs are seen commonly over the anterior temporal region.[14] One must be cautious when interpreting EEGs performed after phenobarbital or other sedative drugs have been administered.

Treatment

Before treatment of neonatal seizures is initiated, a concerted effort should be made to determine the cause of the seizure as soon as possible. After ventilation and adequate glucose levels are ensured, initial goals are to establish the underlying cause and institute appropriate therapy. The ready availability of accurate and timely chemistry screening panels has largely obviated the need for empiric infusions of glucose and calcium as the first steps in treatment. After correction of metabolic abnormalities, AEDs are given to the infant with recurrent seizures.

There are few data in either the experimental or clinical literature indicating that seizures per se cause damage to the neonatal brain. Recurrent seizures may lead to alterations in autonomic function with hypotension and apnea, however. It is probably not necessary to treat neonatal seizures with antiepileptic medications when they are brief (less than 1 or 2 minutes or so), occur infrequently, and are not associated with autonomic dysfunction.[15] Because there is some evidence that AEDs may be harmful to the developing brain, it is worth attempting to wean the infant from them as soon as possible, preferably before he or she is discharged from the nursery.

The major AED used in the newborn period is phenobarbital (Figure 10-3), a relatively safe and effective medication in neonates. The loading dose is 15–20 mg/kg with a maintenance dose of 3–5 mg/kg/day divided bid. Acutely, we recommend pushing the phenobarbital loading dose up to at least 30–40 mg/kg before adding a second drug. Maintenance phenobarbital may be administered either intravenously or orally. When phenobarbital alone is not effective, phenytoin (Dilantin) (15–20

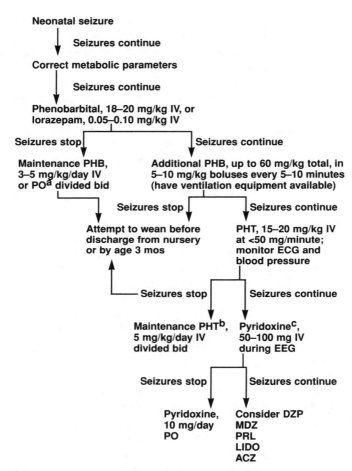

^aCrushed tablets are often tolerated better than elixir.
^bDue to poor absorption, oral PHT is not routinely recommended.
^cPyridoxine may be given at this point or earlier.

Figure 10-3. *Flow diagram for treatment algorithm for neonatal seizures. PHB = phenobarbital; PHT = phenytoin; DZP = diazepam; MDZ = midazolam; PRL = paraldehyde; LIDO = lidocaine; ACZ = acetazolamide. Doses: DZP, 0.1–0.3 mg/kg bolus, may repeat one to three times or begin 0.2–0.8 mg/kg/hour IV drip; MDZ, 0.1–0.4 mg/kg IV load and 1–10 μg/kg/minute IV drip; PRL, 0.3 ml/kg diluted 1:2 in mineral oil PR; LIDO, 2 mg/kg IV load and 4–6 mg/kg/hour IV drip; ACZ, 10–30 mg/kg/day divided bid–tid PO. (Reprinted with permission from CE Stafstrom. Neonatal seizures. Pediatr Rev 1995;16:248.)*

mg/kg) is administered intravenously slowly (< 50 mg/minute or < 1 mg/kg/minute) over several minutes while the blood pressure and electrocardiogram are monitored. The maintenance dose is 5 mg/kg/day intravenously. Because of erratic phenytoin absorption in neonates, it is difficult to maintain a therapeutic level of phenytoin using oral dosing. If seizures continue, 100 mg of pyridoxine should be administered intravenously during EEG monitoring; if the seizures are pyridoxine-dependent, the EEG should improve rapidly (within minutes of infusion).

Other medications that may be used in the acute treatment of neonatal seizures include lorazepam, diazepam, primidone, and paraldehyde. Lorazepam is becoming increasingly used for the short-term treatment of neonatal seizures, especially for status epilepticus. A dose of 0.1–0.3 mg/kg should be administered intravenously and may be repeated once. If the seizures stop, the neonate may not need any additional medication, although it is usually prudent to cover the infant with a longer acting agent such as phenobarbital or phenytoin, at least until the cause is clarified.

The factor that best predicts seizure recurrence is the cause of the seizures. Infants with congenital brain anomalies, severe hypoxic-ischemic injuries, and meningitis or encephalitis are at high risk for recurrence, whereas neonates with seizures secondary to small subarachnoid hemorrhages, transient hypoglycemia, or transient hypocalcemia have a small recurrence risk. Other factors that portend a poor outcome are an abnormal EEG or neurologic examination finding at the time of discharge and a large number of seizures, prognostic features that are intimately related to the cause of seizures.[16]

Childhood Seizures

Most epilepsy begins in childhood (Figure 10-4). Approximately 5% of children experience one seizure, but many of these will not recur; 1–2% have recurrent seizures (i.e., epilepsy). Several epileptic syndromes also have their onset during childhood, with the clinical manifestations being largely dependent on the child's age; these are discussed below. First, we will consider the workup and initial management of a child with a first (unexplained) seizure. The initial goals are to determine the cause of the seizure and classify the event according to criteria established by the International League Against Epilepsy (see Chapter 2). The next step is to determine the appropriate treatment in the context of the individual child's needs.

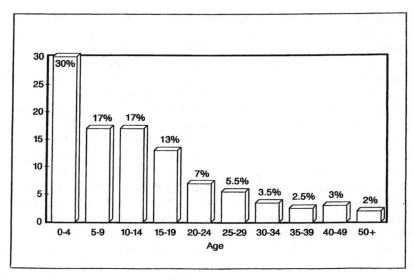

Figure 10-4. *Onset of epilepsy versus age.*

Evaluation

The first step is to obtain a detailed history of the event, to determine whether the event was indeed a seizure, and if so, to get a sense about whether the seizure was generalized or had focal components. In some instances the child may describe warning feelings ("aura"), such as sensory or visual changes, headache, or abdominal discomfort. Parents or other observers of the event should be questioned in detail about the child's level of consciousness, ability to speak or respond to questions, and motor activity during and after the event. Although witnesses may be initially reluctant, we find it very useful to have them "act out" the child's spell. It is also useful to simulate the duration of the event using a stopwatch, since such events are commonly overestimated by observers. Information regarding associated signs, such as urinary or fecal incontinence, head or eye deviation, drooling, facial expression, and vocalizations, should be sought. In children with a known seizure disorder, this seizure should be compared with previous ones. Detailed information about the child's recent health (e.g., fever, how long the fever lasted, how high the child's temperature was, any known reasons for the illness) should be sought and a search made for clues to the cause of the seizures (e.g., recent head trauma, ingestion of medications or toxins, AED noncompliance). In a child with new-onset seizures, detailed family and developmental histories must be obtained to enable accurate diagnosis, accurate determination of the cause of the seizures, and accurate prognosis.

The physical examination may yield important diagnostic and therapeutic clues. If the physician is fortunate enough to witness an event, he or she should make careful note of the patient's level of consciousness—for example, during a suspected partial complex seizure, we ask the child to say something (repetition), do something (follow a command), and remember something (memory function during the event). Concurrently, motor function and tone must be assessed, with particular attention to asymmetry, clonic movements, and deviation of the head or eyes. Increased tone on one side of the body may imply an epileptic focus in the contralateral hemisphere. Similarly, during a seizure, the eyes or head often tonically deviate or beat away from the side of an epileptic focus. During the immediate postictal period, however, the eyes may deviate toward the side of the lesion. Decreased tone or weakness on one side of the body after a seizure (Todd's paralysis) may persist for up to 48 hours and suggests involvement of the contralateral cerebral hemisphere. Therefore, some of these signs may be falsely localizing, depending on whether the seizure is over.

Other physical signs that may help diagnose an epileptic disorder are listed in Table 10-5. Funduscopic examination and Wood's lamp examination of the skin are particularly important. Since the eyes, skin, and central nervous system derive from the same embryonic precursor (ectoderm), a developmental abnormality in one system may predict dysfunction in another.

The initial laboratory evaluation of a child with a seizure should be undertaken with specific questions in mind rather than with a "shotgun" approach.[17] That is, tests should be chosen specifically to rule out treatable metabolic causes of seizures such as low serum glucose, calcium, phosphorus, magnesium, or sodium levels. Blood urea nitrogen and creatinine levels should be obtained, as renal failure may present with seizures in hypertensive encephalopathy. A white blood cell (WBC) count with differential should be obtained, especially if infection is a potential cause or if the child is febrile. A blood culture and spinal fluid examination should be performed if meningitis is suspected. It should be realized, however, that a seizure may cause an increased leukocyte count secondary to stress-induced WBC demargination (in this case, the differential should be normal). One must always consider ingestion of

Table 10-5. Some Important Physical Examination Findings
in Childhood Seizures

Finding	Significance
Asymmetry of tone or strength	Duration <48 hrs: Todd's paralysis Duration >48 hrs: chronic lesion in contralateral hemisphere
Asymmetry of fingernails or toenails	Underdevelopment of contralateral hemisphere
Cranial bruit	Arteriovenous malformation
Eyes	
Cherry-red spot (macula)	Tay-Sachs disease, cherry-red spot myoclonus (neuraminidase deficiency)
Chorioretinopathy	Aicardi's syndrome
Chorioretinitis	Toxoplasmosis, cytomegalovirus, rubella
Cataracts	Rubella, galactosemia
Retinal hamartomas	Tuberous sclerosis
Skin	
Ashleaf-shaped areas of hypopigmentation, shagreen patches, adenoma sebaceum (angiokeratomas)	Tuberous sclerosis
Hemangioma (hemifacial)	Sturge-Weber disease
Cafe-au-lait spots (six spots >1.5 cm after puberty, five spots >0.5 cm before puberty), axillary freckling	Neurofibromatosis
Erythematous bulla (newborn), pigmented whorls (infant), depigmented areas (child)	Incontinentia pigmenti

a toxin in a child with a seizure, and a toxicology screen is mandatory—for example, drugs with such different uses as cocaine and theophylline can cause seizures if ingested in sufficient doses. If the child is already taking an anticonvulsant medication, the serum level of the drug must be checked to determine if it is sufficiently subtherapeutic (e.g., as a result of noncompliance or malabsorption) to explain the seizure exacerbation. A lumbar puncture for cerebrospinal fluid examination is indicated if a child has a fever plus seizure in order to rule out meningitis. An occasional exception to this dictum would be a child with a simple febrile seizure in whom a causative fever source is identified (e.g., otitis media, pharyngitis). A lumbar puncture may not be mandatory in such a child only if there are no neurologic signs or symptoms, there are no meningeal signs, mental function has returned to normal, and the chance of meningitis by clinical criteria is negligible (see Chapter 8). If there is a question of elevated intracranial pressure, a computed tomographic (CT) scan of the head should be obtained before a lumbar puncture is performed. In a child with signs of fulminant meningoencephalitis, antibiotics need not be deferred until after the CT scan and lumbar puncture; in such a case the benefit of immediate antibiotic treatment outweighs that of obtaining an unscathed cerebrospinal fluid sample.

The EEG is an essential part of a seizure workup. Questions often arise about how soon after a seizure to obtain an EEG and whether or not concurrent anticonvulsant medications can alter the EEG. Postictal slowing can persist for several days after a seizure, so it is not necessary (and can even be misleading) to obtain an EEG immediately after the event. The record may normalize later, in which case the early postictal slowing represents a transient abnormality that should not force treatment. (An exception would be when the physician suspects ongoing nonconvulsive status epilepticus, such as absence status.) On the other hand, if a focal EEG abnormality persists 2 weeks or longer after a seizure, it probably represents a real pathologic process. Various AEDs affect EEG findings but do not usually mask underlying electrographic abnormalities. For example, phenobarbital typically increases fast activity, especially in the frontal regions, but this effect is probably clinically irrelevant. Spikes or other signs of epileptiform activity, however, are not usually suppressed by antiseizure drugs. Therefore, if treatment is indicated clinically, it must not be delayed until an EEG is obtained.

In modern practice, a neuroimaging procedure (CT or magnetic resonance imaging [MRI] scan of the brain) should be part of most seizure workups. Such a study is especially important if the child has a focal abnormality during the seizure, on neurologic examination, or on the EEG. Although a CT scan is usually quicker to obtain and can rule out certain major cerebral abnormalities (especially supratentorial), a MRI scan will often detect subtle lesions, such as cortical malformations or low-grade astrocytomas, that are not visible on CT scans. Therefore, a MRI scan is preferred if available. The timing of a neuroimaging study is not rigid; rarely if ever would such a study be emergent in a child with seizure. One exception, alluded to above, would be a child with fever plus focal findings on examination or during the ictal event. In such a case, it is advisable to obtain a CT scan before a lumbar puncture is attempted, because a focal mass lesion such as a cerebral abscess may be responsible for both the fever and the focal abnormalities.

Differential Diagnosis

Because many paroxysmal behavioral events mimic seizures, the task of diagnosing a true seizure is often challenging. Table 10-6 lists several entities commonly mistaken for seizures. Each of these medical conditions shares some clinical characteristics of seizures and must be considered in the differential diagnosis. Because epilepsy carries many social stigmata and because all AEDs have risks and side effects, it is imperative not to misdiagnose a seizure. As described above, history, physical examination, and laboratory investigations all play an important role in the workup of a patient with a suspected seizure. In many cases, however, such information is inconclusive, and the clinician will be forced to make a management decision based on incomplete data. For particularly difficult diagnostic cases, video-EEG monitoring in a specialized epilepsy monitoring unit may be helpful. The goal of such monitoring is to correlate ictal behavior with simultaneous EEG and video recording.

Video-EEG monitoring may be especially useful in differentiating an epileptic seizure from a nonepileptic (psychogenic) pseudoseizure. Table 10-7 offers some clinical clues about their differentiation. Pseudoseizures can often be induced or terminated by suggestion. The etiology of pseudoseizures is often no less serious than that of epileptic seizures (in terms of a child's overall functioning) and is often related to unresolved psychological conflicts and anxiety that are converted into a physical symptom. In children with pseudoseizures, one must always be suspicious of sexual or physical abuse. Many children with a pseudoseizure have witnessed a real seizure, either first-hand or on television. Epileptic and nonepileptic seizures often coexist in the same child. One must approach such patients with a great deal of sensitivity, and it is usually best to avoid confronting them directly with the diagnosis. Therapy must be two-pronged, involving both the child and his or her family. The child's therapy might involve psychotherapy (occa-

Table 10-6. Paroxysmal Events That Mimic Seizures

Apnea
Benign paroxysmal vertigo
Breath holding spells
Cardiac arrhythmias
Cataplexy
Colic
Daydreaming
Episodic dyscontrol (rage attacks)
Gastroesophageal reflux
Hyperekplexia (startle disease)
Hyperventilation
Jitteriness
Migraine
Narcolepsy
Obsessive-compulsive disorder
Pallid infantile syncope
Parasomnias: night terrors
Sleepwalking (somnabulism)
Paroxysmal choreoathetosis
Pseudoseizures (psychogenic seizures), malingering
Shuddering attacks
Spasmus nutans
Syncope
Tics, including Gilles de la Tourette's syndrome

sionally requiring inpatient management), stress management/relaxation therapy, or biofeedback; these therapies are best instituted with the assistance of a psychiatrist or psychologist experienced in this field. The family must be counseled to reduce the secondary gains that the child's behavior is engendering. The child and family should be assured that the symptom (pseudoseizure) is real but does not involve a pathologic process in the brain leading to epileptic neuronal discharges. They should be assured that therapy will be designed to address the underlying cause of the symptom.

Table 10-7. Criteria for Differentiating Epileptic Seizures from Pseudoseizures

Clinical Data	Pseudoseizures	Generalized Tonic-Clonic Seizures	Complex Partial Seizures
Changes in seizures with antiepileptic drugs	Rare	Usual	Usual
Increased seizure frequency with stress	Frequent	Occasional	Occasional
Combativeness	Common	Rare	Rare
Vulgar language	Frequent	Rare	Rare
Self-injury	Rare	Common	Rare
Incontinence	Rare	Common	Unusual
Tongue biting	Rare	Common	Rare
Nocturnal occurrence	Rare	Common	Occasional
Stereotype of attacks	Often variable	Little variation	Not identical but usually have similar patterns
Postictal confusion, lethargy, or sleepiness	Rare	Always	Frequent
EEG activity between seizures (interictal period)	Normal	Frequently abnormal	Frequently abnormal
EEG activity during seizure (ictal period)	Normal	Always abnormal	Usually abnormal

Source: Reprinted with permission from GL Holmes. Diagnosis and Management of Seizures in Children. Philadelphia: Saunders, 1987.

Treatment

General Considerations

In considering therapy for epilepsy, the first modality that probably comes to mind is medication. However, several therapeutic approaches must be considered, only one of which is drugs. Of utmost importance in any medical management decision is the underlying principle of primum non nocere ("first do no harm"). If AEDs are selected as a part of the treatment plan, specific endpoints of therapy should be defined. All

Table 10-8. Common Side Effects of Antiepileptic Drugs in Children

Drug	Dose-Related Side Effects	Idiosyncratic Side Effects
Phenobarbital	Lethargy, hyperactivity, mood changes, irritability, sleep changes	Rash, including Stevens-Johnson syndrome
Phenytoin (Dilantin)	Lethargy, dizziness, ataxia nystagmus, nausea, tremor	Gingival overgrowth, hirsutism, acne, rash, including Stevens-Johnson syndrome
Carbamazepine (Tegretol)	Drowsiness, ataxia, dizziness, nausea, diplopia, hyponatremia	Leukopenia, aplastic anemia, thrombocytopenia, anemia, rash, hepatic dysfunction, involuntary movements
Ethosuximide (Zarontin)	Nausea, vomiting, anorexia, abdominal pain, drowsiness, hiccups	Leukopenia, pancytopenia, rash, systemic lupus erythematosus
Valproic acid (Depakote)	Nausea, tremor, elevation of liver enzymes, sedation	Hepatotoxicity, pancreatitis, thrombocytopenia, anemia, leukopenia, platelet dysfunction, hair loss, weight loss or gain
Benzodiazepines	Drowsiness, nausea, ataxia, headache, increased oral secretions	Hyperactivity, behavior or personality changes, irritability, cognitive dysfunction
Felbamate (Felbatol)	Insomnia, anorexia, nausea	Aplastic anemia, liver failure
Gabapentin (Neurontin)	Lethargy, dizziness, agitation, weight gain	Rash
Lamotrigine (Lamictal)	Lethargy, dizziness, headache, weight gain	Rash

AEDs have side effects (Table 10-8), some serious (see Chapter 13), so one must not rush into drug treatment without first establishing a firm diagnosis and correcting any metabolic disturbance that might have caused or exacerbated the seizure. Keep in mind that general health measures (sufficient sleep, a well-balanced diet, refraining from use of alcohol and nonprescription drugs, reduction of stress) are important in the overall management of epilepsy.

Although some controversy remains, there is an increasing trend among pediatric neurologists not to begin AEDs after a first unprovoked seizure. In a prospective study of 238 children with such seizures, only 26% of children with normal EEG findings and no identifiable cause for the seizures had a seizure recurrence by 30 months, whereas 60% with a history of prior neurologic impairment had recurrent seizures within this time frame.[18] Although each case must be considered individually, given the inherent medical and cognitive risks of anticonvulsant drugs, it is reasonable to delay beginning such treatment until the second seizure.

Once the decision to start AEDs is made, the physician must understand the chosen medication's pharmacokinetics (see Chapter 4) and side effects and convey this information to the family in detail. It should be stressed that dose, interval, and even choice of medication may change with time, based on efficacy as well as the natural history of the seizure disorder. The child and his or her parents must understand the rationale behind dosing schedules and the importance of compliance.

There are few rigid rules regarding the pharmacologic treatment of epilepsy in children (Figure 10-5). Although particular AEDs may be better for treating one seizure type than another, there are no absolutes. In general, monotherapy is preferred. Disadvantages of polytherapy include interaction between AEDs (drugs compete for protein binding sites and can influence each other's metabolism), poorer compliance if multiple drug regimens must be remembered, and a greater chance of drug toxicity with multiple AEDs. Treatment should be initiated with one drug at a dose based on the child's weight. The drug should be started at the lower end of the usual therapeutic range and should be increased gradually until the desired clinical effect is achieved. It usually takes five half-lives for serum levels to achieve the therapeutic range. A specific serum level must not be considered the absolute goal of treatment, however, as the level may differ according to the particular batch of drug, the child's metabolism and liver function, age, the specific analytical method used by the laboratory, and so forth. In addition, some drugs (e.g., valproic acid) have wide and ill-defined therapeutic ranges, and a level that may be effective for one child may be toxic for another. It should rarely be necessary to dose an AED more than three times per day. One should also be sensitive to the timing of the doses; if possible, avoid a dose during school hours. Children are less likely to remember to take their medication at school, and there is a social stigma in being labeled an epileptic.

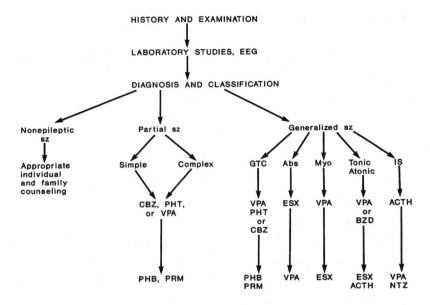

Figure 10-5. *Flow diagram for classification and treatment of childhood seizures. CBZ = carbamazepine; PHT = phenytoin; VPA = valproic acid; PHB = phenobarbital; PRM = primidone; ESX = ethosuximide; BZD = benzodiazepine; ACTH = adrenocorticotropic hormone; NTZ = nitrazepam; GTC = generalized tonic-clonic; Abs = absence; Myo = myoclonic; IS = infantile spasms.*

If the initial AED is ineffective in controlling seizures, a second drug is added using the same approach (begin at the low end of the therapeutic range, increase slowly until efficacy or side effects). The second drug should have a different antiepileptic spectrum than the first. If seizures become controlled on the two-drug combination, one should begin a slow taper of the first drug while closely monitoring the levels of both drugs. Interactions between AEDs are common (Table 10-9) and can lead to erroneous interpretations if not closely observed. AEDs that induce liver microsomal enzymes (phenobarbital, phenytoin, carbamazepine) will tend to decrease levels of other drugs. Enzyme inhibitors such as valproic acid are likely to increase levels of other drugs.

Polytherapy is sometimes required for particularly intractable or mixed-type seizures; this scenario is unfortunately common in children,

Table 10-9. Antiepileptic Drug Interactions in Children

Added Drug	PHB	PRM	PHT	CBZ	VPA	FBM	GP	LTG
PHB	—	V	V or ↓	↓	↓	?	V	↓
PRM	↑	—	V	↓	V	?	V	↓
PHT	V	↓	—	↓	↓	↓	V	↓
CBZ	V	V	↓	—	↓	↓	V	↓
VPA	↑	↑	↓ total ↑ free	V	—	V	V	↑
FBM	?	?	↑	↓	↑	—	?	?
GP	V	V	V	V	V	?	—	?
LTG	V	V	V	V	V	?	?	—

↑ = increased; ↓ = decreased; V = variable or insignificant; ? = unknown; PHB = phenobarbital; PRM = primidone; PHT = phenytoin; CBZ = carbamazepine; VPA = valproic acid; FBM = felbamate; GP = gabapentin; LTG = lamotrigine.
Source: Modified from NP Rosman. Anticonvulsants in childhood seizures: when to start, what to use, when to stop. Int Pediatr 1986;1:85.

who often develop one type of seizure that then evolves into others. We recommend changing only one variable at a time (e.g., drug, dose, interval), otherwise it becomes impossible to determine which variable caused the clinical change.

Drug levels should be used rationally. It is useful to obtain a level once steady state (five half-lives) is reached, when a new drug is added or discontinued, when toxicity is present, if seizure frequency increases, and at 6- to 12-month intervals to assess compliance. AED levels are reported as the total amount in the blood (free plus protein-bound), whereas both efficacy and side effects are determined by the concentration of free drug. In certain clinical situations (e.g., hypoalbuminemia), the proportion of protein-bound AED may be less, although the total level may be within the therapeutic range; thus the child may exhibit toxicity despite a therapeutic AED level.

It is best to obtain trough AED levels if possible, especially for those drugs with short half-lives (carbamazepine, valproic acid). When a drug is first administered, its half-life is often longer than at steady state. Half-lives are often shorter on polytherapy. Children have a higher basal metabolic rate than adults; thus, AED half-lives tend to be shorter, and more frequent dosing may be required to reach steady state. Fever shortens drug half-lives by increasing metabolic rate. Other illnesses, such as liver disease, tend to increase AED half-lives, and toxicity may appear at a formerly stable blood level. If toxic side effects are suspected, it may be more useful to obtain a peak serum drug level, since that is when symptoms are most prominent.

Most AEDs follow first-order kinetics: The level in the blood is proportional to the dose. An important exception is phenytoin, which follows zero-order kinetics. Blood levels increase fairly linearly with dose until binding sites are saturated. After that, all the drug goes directly into the free fraction because there are no more available binding sites. Therefore, a child could rapidly become toxic on phenytoin with only a small increment in dose. This is a situation in which measuring the free and total blood levels would be informative.

Other variables to follow (e.g., complete blood count, determining the aspartate aminotransferase level) are dependent on the specific drug, and are outlined in Table 10-10. It is usually unnecessary to obtain repeat routine EEGs on children with seizures unless seizure frequency or type changes substantially.

There are few absolute guidelines for the discontinuation of AEDs in children.[19-21] A drug should be withdrawn slowly (over weeks to months) unless a severe untoward reaction occurs. One protocol suggests that about 20% of the daily total be tapered every five half-lives.[22] Seizures may occur during AED taper, especially with phenobarbital or benzodiazepines, but these seizures do not necessarily indicate that the drug should be reinstituted. Rather, such breakthrough seizures are often transient;[22] although their occurrence makes it advisable to slow the taper rate, it is not always necessary to stop the taper.

The duration of AED treatment should be determined primarily by length of time the child remains seizure-free. Some controversy exists regarding what seizure-free interval is safest before beginning an AED taper trial; many clinicians favor 2 years, but some recommend 3–4 years. The decision must be based on the individual's seizure type, neurologic history, and to some extent the wishes of the patient and his or her family. It is often advisable to obtain an EEG before tapering AED treatment. Although a principle of epilepsy management states that "the patient should be treated, not the EEG," a persistent paroxysmal abnormality may warrant continued treatment, even if there have been no overt seizures.

In addition to general health measures and pharmacologic therapy, the physician should be sensitive to the child's emotional, psychosocial, and educational needs. Families appreciate inclusion in treatment plan-

Table 10-10. Summary of Commonly Used Antiepileptic Drugs in Children

Drug	Initial Dose (mg/kg)	Maintenance Dose (mg/kg/day)	Dosing Interval	Time to Steady State (days)	Time to Peak Effect (hr)	Plasma Half-life (hr)	Therapeutic Range (µg/ml)	Routine Monitoring
PHB	<1 yr: 3–5 >1 yr: 2–4	Same as initial dose	qd–bid	14–21	5–15	Children: 37–73 Neonates: 45–173	15–40	None
PRM	12–25	<6 yr: 50 mg qhs >6 yr: 100 mg qhs >12 yr: 150 mg qhs	tid–qid	PRM 1–4 PHB 14–21	1–3	5–18	5–12	CBC once or twice/yr
PHT	Four doses of 5–6 mg/ kg PO q8h	4–8	bid	7–10	4–8	Children: 5–18 Neonates: 10–60	10–20	CBC once or twice/yr
CBZ	<6 yr: 5–10 mg/kg 6–12 yr: 100 mg bid	10–30	bid–tid	3–4	3–6	8–25	6–12	CBC and AST before and at 1, 2, and 6 mos then every yr or if side effects occur
ESX	<6 yr: 10– 15 mg/kg or 250 mg	15–40	bid–tid	7–10	1–7	25–40	40–150	CBC every mo for 2 mos then

	(whichever is less) > 6 yr: 250 mg/day							every 6 mos
VPA	15–20 mg/kg in two to four divided doses	15–60	bid (coated) bid–qid (uncoated)	1–4	4–14	50–150		CBC before, at 2 wks, every 2 mos twice, then every 4–6 mos; NH$_3$ before
CLZ	>10 yr: 1–1.5 mg/day in 2–4 divided doses >10 yr or >30 kg: 0.01–0.03 mg/kg/day in two to four divided doses	0.1–0.3	bid–qid	4–8	1–4	20–40	0.02–0.08	CBC twice/yr

Table 10-10. *(continued)*

Drug	Initial Dose (mg/kg)	Maintenance Dose (mg/kg/day)	Dosing Interval	Time to Steady State (days)	Time to Peak Effect (hr)	Plasma Half-life (hr)	Therapeutic Range (µg/ml)	Routine Monitoring
FBM	15 mg/kg/day in three to four divided doses	14–45	tid–qid	4–5	1–4	20	Not established	Not established; AST, BUN, CBC should be followed
GP	10 mg/kg/day in increments of 5 mg/kg	20 (upper limit not established)	tid	1–2	2–4	5–8	Not established	None
LTG	If on VPA: wk 1–2: 0.2 mg/kg wk 3–4: 0.5 mg/kg If on other AED: wk 1–2: 2 mg/kg wk 2–3: 5 mg/kg	If on VPA: 1–5 mg/kg/day If on other AED: 5–15 mg/kg/day	bid	4–8	2–4	On VPA: 37–48 hr On other AED: 6–32 hr	Not established	Not established

PHB = phenobarbital; PRM = primidone; PHT = phenytoin; CBZ = carbamazepine; ESX = ethosuximide; VPA = valproic acid; CLZ = clobazepam; FBM = felbamate; GP = gabapentin; LTG = lamotrigine; CBC = complete blood count; AST = aspartate aminotransferase; AED = antiepileptic drug; BUN = blood urea nitrogen.

ning and need constant education and re-education about the disorder and its therapy. Questions about participation in sports, driving, and vocational planning are particularly important to children with epilepsy. It is crucial to make families aware of available resources such as support groups and Epilepsy Foundation of America services. The child's understanding of epilepsy will change as he or she grows and matures, and the clinician should be cognizant of the child's needs over development.[23]

Specific Seizure Types and Syndromes

Most children can be medically managed with one or more of seven common AEDs: phenobarbital, phenytoin, primidone, carbamazepine, ethosuximide, valproic acid, and clonazepam. A summary of pharmacokinetics, doses, and side effects is found in Tables 10-8, 10-9, and 10-10. A role of the recently approved AEDs gabapentin and lamotrigine has not yet been established in children.[24] For particularly intractable seizures, several centers are conducting trials of experimental AEDs (see Chapter 14). In addition, a variety of surgical options may be considered, depending on the site and extent of the seizure focus, type of seizure, and degree of impairment. This section is restricted to the more common seizure types likely to be seen and managed by primary care physicians, with emphasis on practical aspects of treatment. A detailed discussion of primary and adjunctive AEDs is found in Levy et al.[24]

Generalized Seizures

Generalized Tonic-Clonic Seizures. The stereotyped nature of the motor activity in most GTC seizures (formerly called grand mal seizures) makes them fairly easy to recognize. Typically, GTC seizures consist of a reproducible clinical sequence: tonic extension and flexion, clonic jerking, and postictal state. GTC seizures may be preceded by an aura or focal component; in these cases, it is likely that the seizure began focally then secondarily generalized, and the child may respond best to a medication regimen aimed at the partial component (e.g., carbamazepine). Once treatable metabolic causes of GTC seizures are ruled out, AED treatment is begun. The literature does not clearly support a single drug as the AED of choice for GTC seizures. Phenytoin, carbamazepine, phenobarbital, and valproic acid all seem equally effective in controlling GTC seizures. Therefore, the drug can be chosen on the basis of the experience and preference of the physician and the known side effects of each agent. Phenobarbital may be better tolerated by infants and young children, but its tendency to cause hyperactivity in a significant percentage (up to 50%) of preschool- and school-age children limits its usefulness in this group. Phenytoin is quite effective, but its chronic use may lead to undesirable cosmetic effects such as gingival hyperplasia, hirsutism, and coarsening of facial features. Therefore, phenytoin should be used sparingly in children and teenagers, especially girls. Many of the presumed adverse cognitive effects of phenytoin and phenobarbital may actually be caused by the slowing of motor response time rather than impairment of mental ability per se. Carbamazepine is particularly useful for secondarily generalized seizures and tends to have fewer cognitive side effects. Valproic acid should be used if the child has absence or myoclonic seizures as well as GTC seizures. Because of its potential hepatotoxicity, valproic acid should be used with caution in children younger than 2 years of age, especially if used in conjunction with other AEDs.

Absence Seizures. Absence seizures, formerly called petit mal seizures, are an example of an epileptic syndrome—that is, absence seizures have characteristic clinical and electrographic manifestations and a hereditary pattern that suggests a genetically determined abnormality of brain that predisposes the individual to this type of seizure. Absence seizures are typically seen in school-age children and are often noticed by parents or teachers as brief episodes of staring or spaciness, lasting only a few seconds, without postictal impairment. This scenario (simple absence), however, is actually seen in only about 10% of children with absence seizures. It is more common for the staring to be accompanied by mild clonus, automatisms (chewing, grimacing, lip smacking), or eyelid fluttering. Absence seizures can often be subtle; thus, their true frequency may be underestimated. Absence seizures tend to exacerbate during periods of fatigue or sustained attention (e.g., at school). They can be difficult to differentiate from daydreaming or complex partial seizures (Table 10-11), but this distinction is crucial because each of these entities requires a different therapeutic approach. On EEG tracings, a pattern of three-per-second spike and wave activity is diagnostic of the absence epilepsy syndrome. Although this pattern may be seen on the baseline record, it is characteristically induced by having the child hyperventilate for 3–5 minutes (a mandatory part of the evaluation). The spike and wave discharges are often but not always associated with clinical absences. The physician should attempt to reproduce the child's absence spell in the office by having him or her hyperventilate for at least 3 minutes. Even young children can be encouraged to hyperventilate by blowing on a pinwheel or pretending to inflate a balloon or blow out a candle.

Table 10-11. Differential Diagnosis of Absence Seizures in Childhood

Clinical Data	Absence	Complex Partial	Daydreaming
Frequency/day	Multiple	Rarely 1–2	Multiple, situation-dependent
Duration	Usually <10 secs, rarely >30 secs	Average about 1 min, rarely <10 secs	Seconds to minutes
Aura	Never	Frequent	No
Eye blinking	Common	Occasional	No
Automatisms	Common	Frequent	No
Postictal impairment	None	Frequent	No
Seizures activated by hyperventilation	Very frequent	Occasional	No
Seizures activated by photic stimulation	Frequent, generalized spike and wave	Rare	No
EEG: ictal period	3 per sec generalized spike and wave	Usually unilateral or bilateral temporal or frontal discharges	Normal
EEG: interictal period	Usually normal	Variable; may be spikes or sharp waves in frontal or temporal lobes	Normal

Source: Reprinted with permission from GL Holmes. Diagnosis and Management of Seizures in Children. Philadelphia: Saunders, 1987.

Although absence seizures are not life-threatening, they may interfere with normal function and learning. The goal of treatment is to maximize seizure control with minimal side effects. Most authorities recommend starting with ethosuximide, which is quite effective in controlling absence seizures. The drug should be tried for a sufficient time (several weeks) before concluding that it is ineffective. Valproic acid is also effective against absence seizures and is the drug of choice if the child has myoclonic or GTC seizures in addition to absence spells.

(Approximately 10–20% of children with absence seizures will develop GTC seizures over time.) Although monotherapy is desirable, some children whose absence seizures are not fully controlled on ethosuximide alone will respond favorably to the combination of ethosuximide and valproic acid. Clonazepam is another alternative and seems equally effective, but its sedative side effects and tolerance with prolonged use place it squarely into third place as the drug for treating absence seizures.

Absence seizures are most common in school-age children, and many children "outgrow" their seizures by puberty. A significant minority of children, however, continue to have absences into adulthood. The general guideline is to discontinue AEDs in a child with absence seizures after a 2-year seizure-free interval plus normal EEG findings (including hyperventilation provocation). Even a single spike and wave complex indicates the potential for seizure recurrence; this is one occasion where "the EEG must be treated" as well as the patient.

Brief mention must be made of "atypical" absence seizures, which differ from the above-described typical absence seizures in several ways. Atypical absences are typically longer (minutes), have a less abrupt onset, and are commonly seen in mentally retarded children (e.g., in the Lennox-Gastaut syndrome). The EEG tracing shows slow spike and wave (1.5–2.5 Hz) discharges, and the interictal record is commonly abnormal as well. Treatment of atypical absence seizures is discussed in the section on Lennox-Gastaut syndrome.

Myoclonic Seizures.   Myoclonus, the brief, involuntary, lightning-like contraction of one or more muscles, has multiple possible causes involving any level of the nervous system. There are several myoclonic epilepsies that must be distinguished from movement disorders such as tics, choreoathetosis, and tremor. A complete discussion of myoclonic epilepsies is beyond the scope of this chapter (see Aicardi[25]). However, one syndrome—juvenile myoclonic epilepsy (JME)—deserves discussion, because it is being recognized and treated with increasing frequency by primary care physicians.

JME is a type of primary generalized epilepsy that typically begins during early adolescence in people with normal intelligence and neurologic examination findings.[26] The initial manifestations may be subtle: clumsiness, dropping objects, or jitteriness (which may actually represent myoclonic seizures), especially soon after awakening. The myoclonic seizures may continue throughout the day; they are exacerbated by tiredness, sleep deprivation, alcohol, or emotional stress.

Therefore, general health measures are particularly important in these teenagers. There is often a strong family history; the gene for JME has been mapped to chromosome 6. The interictal EEG pattern is distinctive, with fast spike and wave (3.5–6.0 Hz) and multiple spike and wave discharges. JME is very responsive to valproic acid monotherapy, with various series citing 73–86% of patients satisfactorily controlled. Unfortunately, the myoclonic seizures of JME rarely remit, and most patients will need to remain on AED therapy indefinitely. It is crucial to stress compliance in this group of patients, who by virtue of their age tend to be noncompliant.

Infantile Spasms. Infantile spasms are an age-specific disorder beginning predominantly during the first year of life.[27, 28] The three characteristic features of this syndrome are myoclonic seizures, hypsarrhythmic EEG patterns, and mental retardation, a triad referred to as West syndrome. The clinical manifestations of infantile spasms may vary considerably, however. Some seizures are characterized by brief head nods, whereas other seizures consist of violent movements of the trunk, arms, and legs in a flexor, extensor, or mixed pattern. Spasms are occasionally asymmetric, resembling a "fencing" posture. Infantile spasms are frequently associated with eye deviation or nystagmus, which may precede the onset of the actual spasms by days or weeks or occur independently from the muscular contractions. Spasms may also be accompanied by autonomic dysfunction such as pallor, flushing, sweating, pupillary dilation, lacrimation, and changes in respiratory and heart rate. Akinesia and impaired responsiveness sometimes follow spasms and last as long as 90 seconds. The majority of children with infantile spasms have more than one subtype of spasm.

Infantile spasms may occur as a single myoclonic jerk but more frequently occur in clusters of two to hundreds of single seizures, with as many as one hundred clusters per day. Seizures are sometimes very brief and may be missed by a casual observer. Clusters of spasms commonly occur during sleep or especially on awakening. Crying or irritability during or after a flurry of spasms is commonly observed.

In the child with clusters of flexion or extensor spasms, there is usually no difficulty in making the diagnosis. The biggest error is not considering this diagnosis and attributing the spasms to colic or some other nonepileptic phenomenon. Occasionally, the clinical course will be atypical, and the spasms will not occur in clusters or may involve only slight movements or episodes of akinesia. In these patients, the EEG findings will be helpful, as they are invariably abnormal.

Infantile spasms are usually associated with a markedly abnormal EEG finding called *hypsarrhythmia*, which consists of very high voltage, random slow waves and spikes or sharp waves diffusely throughout the cerebral cortex. The spikes vary from moment to moment in duration, location, and voltage. This chaotic appearance gives the impression that cortical voltage and its regulation are totally disorganized. The hypsarrhythmic pattern may be absent, at least initially, in up to one-third of cases of infantile spasms.

Infantile spasms have been classified historically into those in which there is no apparent preceding neurologic disorder or identified etiologic factor (idiopathic or cryptogenic cases) and those in which a pre-existing, presumptively responsible pathologic event or disorder is demonstrated (symptomatic cases). As our ability to detect subtle dysgenetic lesions improves with MRI and other diagnostic modalities, the proportion of cryptogenic cases is declining. Virtually any insult to the developing brain can be associated with infantile spasms. Common etiologic factors include hypoxic-ischemic encephalopathy; neonatal intracranial hemorrhage, congenital infection, meningitis, encephalitis, congenital abnormalities of the central nervous system, and metabolic diseases such as phenylketonuria. Aicardi's syndrome, which occurs only in girls, consists of infantile spasms, absence of the corpus callosum, and ocular abnormalities. There is a very high association between infantile spasms and tuberous sclerosis; up to 25% of children with infantile spasms in some series have tuberous sclerosis.[30]

One disorder that may be confused with infantile spasms is *benign myoclonus of early infancy*, in which infants have clusters of tonic or myoclonic movements. The movements consist of rapid flexion or extension of either axial or limb musculature or head nods. Unlike infantile spasms, the infants are neurologically and developmentally normal and have normal EEG findings. In all cases, the movements stop by age 18 months.

Also in the differential diagnosis of infantile spasms are two severe epileptic encephalopathies, early infantile epileptic encephalopathy (EIEE) and early myoclonic epileptic encephalopathy (EMEE), which typically begin within the first month of life.[29] EIEE (Ohtahara's syndrome) presents with recurrent tonic seizures and a burst suppression pattern on EEG, whereas patients with EMEE typically have recurrent myoclonic seizures. Both syndromes are associated with a severe neuronal pathologic process and carry a very poor prognosis with regard to seizure control and neurologic development; many affected patients die in infancy.

There is a controversy about whether immunizations, in particular the pertussis component, can cause infantile spasms. This issue has significant medical as well as legal implications. It is very difficult to prove that the pertussis vaccine results in infantile spasms. The vaccine is given at the time of peak incidence of infantile spasms, and therefore a temporal coincidence would be expected in a large number of cases. In addition, the onset of infantile spasms is often insidious, making determination of the exact time of onset difficult. It is possible that in a very small number of patients a causal relationship exists, especially when a striking neurologic reaction occurs within 24 hours after the immunization. It is also possible that in some cases the vaccine acts in conjunction with other unidentified factors to precipitate the clinical onset of symptoms in children already predisposed to the disease.

The majority of patients with the above-mentioned disorders do not develop infantile spasms. The fact that some infants have infantile spasms while others with similar brain disturbances do not develop them suggests that genetic factors may be important. Although there are a number of theories regarding the pathophysiology of infantile spasms, none has been proven.

Unfortunately, the prognosis of infantile spasms is very poor. A large number of infants will demonstrate psychomotor retardation and continue to have seizures. More than two-thirds of these children are mentally retarded, and many develop neurologic impairment such as hemiplegia, diplegia, or quadriplegia. Many children with infantile spasms later develop myoclonic seizures, GTC seizures, or other seizure types, and progression into the Lennox-Gastaut syndrome is common (see section on Lennox-Gastaut syndrome). Prognosis is directly related to the cause of the seizures, with symptomatic cases faring worse.

An infant with infantile spasms requires a thorough developmental evaluation, neurologic examination, and laboratory studies to determine a cause. The physical examination should include an ophthalmologic evaluation to determine if the ocular abnormalities of Aicardi's syndrome are present, such as chorioretinopathy (areas of depigmentation), coloboma, iris synechiae, or microphthalmia. In addition, congenital infections may be associated with chorioretinitis, and retinal hamartomas near the optic nerve head can occur in tuberous sclerosis. The skin should be closely inspected for the hypopigmented, leaf-shaped lesions of tuberous sclerosis, which can often be seen only when the infant is examined with a Wood's lamp in a darkened room.

As with all seizure workups, laboratory studies will be determined by the clinical history and physical examination. Infants with frequent vomiting, lethargy, failure to thrive, developmental regression, peculiar odors, and unexplained neurologic findings should undergo urine amino and organic acid screening and serum ammonia, pyruvate, lactate, and liver function tests. Electrolyte, calcium, phosphorous, and glucose levels and urinalysis should be obtained, since most children will be placed on adrenocorticotropic hormone (ACTH). Unless there is concern about an active infection, examination of the spinal fluid is not usually necessary. An EEG should be obtained on every child suspected of having infantile spasms; a normal EEG finding would raise questions about the diagnosis and might suggest that the child has benign myoclonus of early infancy instead. Because pyridoxine dependency has been reported in association with infantile spasms, an intravenous infusion of 100 mg pyridoxine during the EEG is indicated. In infants with pyridoxine dependency, the EEG should improve within several minutes of administration of pyridoxine.

A CT or MRI scan is recommended in the management of every patient with infantile spasms, because it may provide valuable information regarding the cause of the seizures. For example, cranial calcifications may indicate tuberous sclerosis or a congenital infection. In addition, brain anomalies such as agenesis of the corpus callosum, porencephaly, and hydranencephaly will be apparent.

Several aspects of treatment of infantile spasms are controversial, but it is well accepted that ACTH or corticosteroids are the most effective medications (although the antiepileptic mechanism of action of these agents is unknown). Some physicians consider ACTH to be superior to prednisone;[31] others consider them equally efficacious.[32] In a double-blind, placebo-controlled crossover study, Hrachovy and colleagues[33] compared ACTH (20–30 IU/day) with prednisone (2 mg/kg/day). No major difference between the effectiveness of ACTH and prednisone was found, and children who failed to respond to ACTH sometimes responded to prednisone and vice versa.

In addition to controversy regarding the advantages of ACTH versus prednisone, the optimum dose of ACTH remains uncertain. Snead and colleagues[34] have recommended the use of high-dose ACTH (150 IU/m^2/day) for maximal effectiveness, while Hrachovy and Frost[32] report equivalent effectiveness and fewer side effects with a lower dose of ACTH (20 IU/day). In view of the lack of consensus regarding dosage and treatment duration, the following approach is necessarily empiric. We recommend a starting dose of 40 IU/day of intramuscular ACTH. A nonsynthetic form of ACTH gel should be used. The ACTH is given 2–4 weeks after the cessation of seizures, at which time it can be tapered by 10 IU/week. If the seizures do not completely resolve by 2 weeks, the dose should be increased in increments of 10 IU/week until the seizures cease or a maximum dose of 80 IU/day is reached. If at that point the spasms persist, a trial of valproic acid or nitrazepam (see below) is recommended. If children relapse during tapering or after discontinuation of ACTH, the drug should be restarted at the dose that originally stopped the spasms. After control of the seizures, the ACTH should be continued for a minimum of 1 month before tapering is attempted again. The response to ACTH is sometimes very dramatic, with cessation of seizures and marked improvement of EEG findings within a few days. The timing of treatment has been disputed, with some studies suggesting that early treatment (i.e., within 1 month of diagnosis) gives a more favorable long-term outcome but others finding no difference in ultimate neurologic status. We advise beginning treatment as soon as possible after diagnosis but not to deny therapy to children diagnosed long after spasms began.

The effects of ACTH and other therapies on long-term outcome are also controversial. Many authors have found no developmental differences between patients who did or did not receive treatment.[35, 36] For the large number of infants who exhibit pre-existing brain damage, it is unlikely that any form of therapy will greatly influence the long-range outcome in terms of mental and motor development. It remains unclear whether treatment can improve the outcome in children who were normal before spasms began.

Although ACTH and corticosteroids can be very effective in stopping spasms, they can cause many side effects. Steroid therapy is invariably associated with cushingoid obesity. Growth retardation, acne, and irritability may ensue. With short-term use of ACTH, these side effects are of no major concern, but serious side effects may occur with prolonged use, including infection, arterial hypertension, intracerebral hemorrhage, gastrointestinal bleeding, osteoporosis, hypokalemic alkalosis, and other electrolyte disturbances.

The ketogenic diet[37] has been used with some success in infantile spasms as well as seizure types seen in the Lennox-Gastaut syndrome (see section on Lennox-Gastaut syndrome). Its exact mechanism of action is unknown, but some feel that the diet's high ketone content exerts an antiepileptic effect. The diet consists of foods high in fat but low in protein and carbohydrate and should be formulated with the aid of a nutritionist experienced with its use. Preparation of the diet is difficult and time-consuming for parents. Although the food seems quite unpalatable, many children tolerate them well. The diet is initiated with a 2- to 3-day period of fasting, until the urine becomes positive for ketone bodies. During the fast, transient hypoglycemia may ensue; it does not require treatment unless the child becomes symptomatic. The child must remain ketotic throughout the diet, which the parents can monitor by checking urine ketone levels daily. Daily vitamin supplements, including 500 IU of vitamin D, are recommended to prevent osteomalacia. Care must be exercised regarding administration of other drugs during the ketogenic diet. Many medications are ordinarily manufactured in a carbohydrate base, but carbohydrate-free medications must be used in the ketogenic diet. Serum levels of phenytoin and phenobarbital may increase; acetazolamide can lead to metabolic acidosis (and is best discontinued 2 weeks before starting the diet). Valproic acid can lead to free fatty acidemia, which increases the potential for a Reye's syndrome–like illness. Despite these caveats, children have been safely maintained on the ketogenic diet for months or years, and this modality is worth a try in a child refractory to ACTH and other medications.[38] The diet should be tapered by gradually reducing the ratio of fats to carbohydrates until a normal diet is restored.

A slightly more palatable diet with similar efficacy is the medium-chain triglyceride (MCT) diet, which similarly causes ketosis but involves less severe carbohydrate restriction. It is recommended that the MCT oil be mixed with skim milk in a blender in a 1 to 2 volume ratio and given at mealtimes three times daily.[22, 39] The long-term usefulness of the MCT diet is sometimes limited by side effects such as diarrhea, nausea, and abdominal cramping.

Nitrazepam has been the most effective benzodiazepine used for the treatment of infantile spasms. It is not yet approved for use in the United States. The most commonly reported side effects are drowsiness, hypotonia, exacerbation of generalized seizures, and increased nasopharyngeal and bronchial secretions. The latter two side effects are the most limiting, especially in the developmentally retarded child who is at risk for aspiration. Clonazepam and diazepam have also been used, although neither drug appears to be as effective as nitrazepam.

Valproic acid has been used with some success in the treatment of infantile spasms. Some of the published cases had already been treated unsuccessfully with steroids, and hence the efficacy in these refractory patients is not directly comparable with reports of cases treated with other drugs. Because of the lack of controlled studies comparing valproic acid, benzodiazepines, and steroids, the first-line drug for infantile spasms remains ACTH or prednisone, with nitrazepam and valproic acid used adjunctively in unresponsive cases. Vigabatrin is a promising new AED that has enjoyed considerable success in Europe and Canada in the treatment of infantile spasms and may be available in the United States soon.

Lennox-Gastaut Syndrome. Formerly called petit mal variant (because of the presence of atypical absence seizures) or minor motor seizures, Lennox-Gastaut syndrome is another age-specific epileptic disorder, with the age at onset from 1 to 6 years. It is characterized by mental retardation, a characteristic EEG pattern of slow spike and wave (1.5–2.5 Hz), and several seizure types including absence, tonic, atonic (drop attacks), myoclonic jerks, head drops, and GTC seizures. The seizures tend to be intractable, and children with this syndrome frequently receive multiple AEDs, none of which is particularly effective. The slow spike and wave electrographic pattern worsens during sleep and may or may not be associated with clinical symptoms. Although the syndrome may arise de novo in a previously normal child, most cases occur in children with prior neurologic handicap. Causes are multiple, ranging from congenital brain anomalies to perinatal hypoxia-ischemia or intracranial hemorrhage to such acquired causes as head injury or meningoencephalitis. The causes of Lennox-Gastaut syndrome parallel those of infantile spasms, and in fact many children with infantile spasms progress into Lennox-Gastaut syndrome. Most cases of Lennox-Gastaut syndrome are static and nonprogressive, but some degenerative diseases (e.g., neuronal ceroid lipofuscinosis) may present with the syndrome.

Seizure severity varies over time, with periods of unexplained worsening that probably represent the natural history of the disorder. Such exacerbations inevitably lead to drug switching and dosage manipulations, which are frustrating because they often do not alter the seizures but do produce toxic side effects. Treatment should begin with a single drug even if the child is having several types of seizures. The initial AED choice should be based on the most prominent seizure type. Valproic acid may be the best first choice, with good efficacy against myoclonic and atypical absence seizures and at least fair efficacy against tonic and GTC seizures; the latter two seizure types often respond well to phenytoin as well. Ethosuximide can be effective for drop attacks. Clonazepam is useful for myoclonic, atypical absence, and atonic seizures, although tolerance to benzodiazepines develops quickly and limits their long-term usefulness. A recently marketed anticonvulsant, felbamate, showed considerable promise in children with the multiple seizure types of Lennox-Gastaut syndrome,[40] but the drug has been associated with several cases of aplastic anemia and liver failure. Its use is now restricted to those with severe refractory seizures whose seizures cannot be controlled in any other way. For intractable cases, ACTH or the ketogenic diet may be tried (see protocols above). Carbamazepine may exacerbate atypical absence or atonic seizures of children with Lennox-Gastaut syndrome.[41]

One should avoid switching drugs too rapidly if an immediate response is not achieved—for example, it may take several weeks for valproic acid to demonstrate its maximum potency. AED levels should be used as general guides only, since many children may not respond to levels in the usual therapeutic range. With polytherapy, one must be vigilant about monitoring for toxic side effects. It should rarely be necessary to treat a child with more than two AEDs. Despite vigorous anticonvulsant treatment, the long-term prognosis in this syndrome is poor; seizures usually persist throughout life, and patients are rarely able to lead independent lives. Since children with Lennox-Gastaut syndrome with atonic seizures are at high risk for head injury, we recommend that they wear a protective helmet and that measures be taken to ensure a safe environment. Some children with intractable atonic seizures benefit from corpus callosotomy.[42]

Partial Seizures
Partial (focal) seizures are those that originate from a restricted area of the brain. The clinical and electrographic manifestations of partial seizures reflect this focal onset, with ictal symptoms corresponding to the cortical area activated. For example, seizures arising from the precentral gyrus involve motor phenomena, whereas those originating from the occipital area may be associated with visual symptoms. Partial seizures are divided into those in which consciousness is preserved (simple partial) or impaired (complex partial). Complex partial seizures, which often originate from the temporal lobe, can be associated with a wide array of involuntary behaviors (automatisms), such as lip smacking, staring, picking at clothes, hallucinations, or emotional reactions such as laughter or fear. Complex partial seizures usually have an abrupt onset, stereotyped ictal phase and are followed by postictal confusion. Partial seizures are described in detail in Chapter 7; this section deals with aspects of partial seizures of particular importance in children.

It is important to differentiate partial seizures from other paroxysmal behaviors of childhood that also produce confusion and stereotyped movements. Childhood migraine, which may present with visual or sensory symptoms in the absence of significant headache, can mimic partial seizures. Interictal EEG abnormalities may be present in both conditions, and AEDs often improve both migraine and partial seizures. An ictal EEG may provide definitive evidence, but such a fortuitous recording is not usually obtained. A family history of migraines lends some support to this diagnosis, but often a definitive diagnosis must await the appearance of unequivocal migrainous or epileptic symptoms. Other conditions that may be mistaken for partial seizures are tics, which are sudden-onset sequences of nonpurposeful movements, and choreic movements, which are brief irregular contractions of multiple muscle groups. The movements in both of these conditions are multifocal and less stereotyped than those of partial seizures, although differentiation is often challenging.

Periodic behavior disturbances such as affective psychoses and episodic dyscontrol (rage attacks) can be difficult to distinguish from complex partial seizures. Both complex partial seizures and affective psychosis can be associated with fear, hallucinations, and confusion; however, these symptoms are usually brief and stereotyped in complex partial epilepsy, and epileptic patients often have some realization of the odd nature of their symptoms. One must be aware, however, that both conditions may coexist in the same child. Nonepileptic rage attacks are usually precipitated by an identifiable event or provocation, and the ensuing violence is often directed at a specific target. Symptoms of complex partial epilepsy are shorter, more stereotyped, and not elicited by a specific precipitant, and violence is rarely directed at a specific person. In all paroxysmal behavioral events for which partial seizures are in the differential, long-term video-EEG monitoring to correlate the behavior with the ictal EEG may be helpful.

A key distinction is whether a partial seizure in a child is benign/idiopathic or associated with an underlying lesion. Compared with adults, brain tumors account for relatively few cases of childhood partial epilepsy. Common causes include congenital anomalies, vascular malformations (especially Sturge-Weber syndrome), perinatal asphyxia or trauma, meningoencephalitis, head trauma, and stroke. Herpes simplex encephalitis shows a predilection for the temporal lobe. In the setting of fever, mental status changes, and seizures, it is essential to obtain electrographic, serologic, and radiographic evidence of this devastating necrotizing encephalitis and to institute specific antiviral therapy promptly. Because limbic structures such as the hippocampus and amygdala are especially vulnerable to hypoxic insults, and because these areas of brain also have a low seizure threshold, particular interest has focused on the role of perinatal asphyxia and recurrent febrile seizures on the later development of an epileptogenic temporal lobe pathologic entity. A causal relationship between these early life insults and later temporal lobe epilepsy has not been proven, however. A specific neuropathologic lesion, termed mesial temporal sclerosis, is thought to be responsible for many cases of temporal lobe epilepsy, and such sclerotic tissue is often excised from the temporal lobes of people undergoing surgical resection for intractable seizures. It must be emphasized that, although most cases of complex partial epilepsy are the result of a temporal lobe pathologic entity, seizures with similar clinical characteristics can also arise from other brain areas, particularly the frontal lobe. The differentiation between temporal and frontal lobe complex partial seizures can be quite difficult,[43, 44] although, in general, frontal lobe seizures tend to be briefer, involve more complex motor automatisms, more frequent head turning, and fewer affective symptoms.

Benign rolandic epilepsy (BRE) (benign epilepsy with centrotemporal spikes) is a partial epilepsy syndrome that deserves special mention both because of its relatively high incidence and its favorable prognosis.[3, 45, 46] BRE is characterized by nocturnal partial seizures that may secondarily generalize and daytime partial seizures that do not usually generalize. The seizures arise from the lower rolandic area at the junction of the central sulcus and sylvian fissure. Initial symptoms include twitching and clonic movements of the mouth and face, often with salivation or gurgling noises. Speech is sometimes garbled because of pharyngeal muscle involvement, and occasionally clonic arm movements are present. These initial symptoms are easily missed at night, and parents may first become aware of the seizure after it generalizes. During daytime seizures, consciousness is ordinarily maintained. Automatisms, affective symptoms, and postictal manifestations such as confusion are rare.

Because of the focal origin of rolandic seizures from the lower central gyrus, the syndrome is associated with a characteristic EEG pattern: high-amplitude spike and slow wave discharges localized at the midtemporal and central electrodes. The discharges can occur unilaterally, bilaterally (synchronously or asynchronously), or even shift between hemispheres. Discharges increase dramatically during sleep, accounting for the common nocturnal occurrence of seizures.

BRE most often affects children in the 5- to 10-year-old range. Its incidence is 0.02–0.13% in children from birth to age 15 years, making it four times more common than typical absence seizures. Seizures disappear spontaneously and are virtually never seen after age 16 years, and progression into other seizure types is distinctly rare. Most evidence suggests that the syndrome is transmitted as an autosomal dominant trait with low penetrance. If a child has clinical and electrographic evidence characteristic of BRE and normal neurologic examination findings, further workup is not essential. The seizures usually respond well to a single anticonvulsant with efficacy against partial seizures (see next paragraph). Some authorities recommend no treatment, especially for the first seizure or two.

The primary AEDs for treatment of partial seizures are carbamazepine, phenytoin, phenobarbital, and primidone. Although carbamazepine and phenytoin have roughly equivalent efficacy, many epileptologists start with carbamazepine. As discussed above, phenobarbital (and primidone) are associated with behavioral and cognitive side effects, and chronic phenytoin usage can lead to unpleasant cosmetic changes and may affect cognition. Phenobarbital and phenytoin are appropriate and useful for many patients in whom carbamazepine is not well tolerated. Other medications useful as second-line drugs for partial seizures are methsuximide, clonazepam, and valproic acid. Gabapentin and lamotrigine, new AEDs with good efficacy against partial seizures, will probably play an increasingly important role in the treatment of partial seizures in children.[24, 47]

Many children with complex partial seizures eventually become refractory to multiple AEDs. They experience an increase in seizure frequency or severity after years of relatively good seizure control. For such patients, surgical resection of the epileptogenic focus offers some hope for seizure control. Evaluation of potential candidates for epilepsy surgery is performed in specialized epilepsy centers. Presurgical evaluation and surgical options are discussed in Chapters 15 and 16. It is important to realize that even young children develop medically intractable partial seizures and often respond favorably to surgical resection.[48, 49]

References

1. Dreifuss FE. Pediatric Epileptology. Boston: John Wright, 1983.
2. Aicardi J. Epilepsy in Children (2nd ed). New York: Raven, 1994.
3. Holmes GL. Diagnosis and Management of Seizures in Children. Philadelphia: Saunders, 1987.
4. Wasterlain CG, Vert P (eds). Neonatal Seizures. New York: Raven, 1990.
5. Dodson WE, Pellock JM (eds). Pediatric Epilepsy: Diagnosis and Therapy. New York: Demos, 1993.

6. Volpe JJ. Neonatal seizures: current concepts and revised classification. Pediatrics 1989;84:422.
7. Tuchman RF, Moshe SL. Neonatal Seizures: Diagnostic and Treatment Controversies. In M Sillanpaa, SI Johannessen, G Blennow, M Dam (eds), Paediatric Epilepsy. London: Wrightson Biomedical, 1990;57.
8. Mizrahi EM. Clinical and neurophysiological correlates of neonatal seizures. Cleve Clin J Med 1989;56(Suppl):S100.
9. Rust RS, Volpe JJ. Neonatal Seizures. In WE Dodson, JM Pellock (eds), Pediatric Epilepsy: Diagnosis and Therapy. New York: Demos, 1993.
10. Rosman NP, Donnelly JH, Braun MA. The jittery newborn and infant: a review. Dev Behav Pediatr 1984;5:263.
11. Plouin P. Benign Neonatal Convulsions (Familial and Non-Familial). In J Roger, M Bureau, C Dravet, et al. (eds), Epileptic Syndromes in Infancy, Childhood, and Adolescence (2nd ed), London: John Libbey, 1992;3.
12. Miles DK, Holmes GL. Benign neonatal seizures. J Clin Neurophysiol 1990;7:369.
13. Coulter DL, Allen RJ. Benign neonatal sleep myoclonus. Arch Neurol 1982;39:191.
14. Mizrahi EM, Tharp BR. A characteristic EEG pattern in neonatal herpes simplex encephalitis. Neurology 1982;32:1215.
15. Stafstrom CE. Neonatal seizures. Pediatr Rev 1995;16:248.
16. Legido A, Clancy RR, Berman PH. Neurologic outcome after electroencephalographically proven neonatal seizures. Pediatrics 1991;88:583.
17. Snead OC. Epilepsy in children: a practical approach. Semin Neurol 1988;8:24.
18. Shinnar S, Berg AT, Moshe SL, et al. Risk of seizure recurrence following a first unprovoked seizure in childhood: a prospective study. Pediatrics 1990;85:1076.
19. Shinnar S, Kang H. Discontinuing Antiepileptic Drugs in Children with Epilepsy. In WA Hauser (ed), Current Trends in Epilepsy (Vol. 3). Landover, MD: Epilepsy Foundation of America, 1988;43.
20. Tennison M, Greenwood R, Lewis D, Thorn M. Discontinuing antiepileptic drugs in children with epilepsy: a comparison of a six-week and a nine-month taper period. N Engl J Med 1994;330:1407.
21. Shinnar S, Berg AT, Moshe SL, et al. Discontinuing antiepileptic drugs in children with epilepsy: a prospective study. Ann Neurol 1994;35:534.
22. Engel J Jr. Seizures and Epilepsy. Philadelphia: FA Davis, 1989.
23. Freeman JM, Vining EPG, Pillas DJ. Seizures and Epilepsy in Childhood: A Guide for Parents. Baltimore: Johns Hopkins University Press, 1990.
24. Levy RH, Mattson RH, Meldrum BS, Penry JK (eds). Antiepileptic Drugs (4th ed). New York: Raven, 1995.
25. Aicardi J. Myoclonic epilepsies in childhood. Int Pediatr 1991;6:195.
26. Ferrendelli J (ed). Juvenile myoclonic epilepsy. Epilepsia 1989;30(Suppl 1):S1.
27. Dulac O, Chugani HT, Dalla Bernadina B (eds). Infantile Spasms and West Syndrome. Philadelphia: Saunders, 1994.
28. Hrachovy RA, Frost JD Jr. Severe Encephalopathic Epilepsy in Infants: Infantile Spasms. In WE Dodson, JM Pellock (eds), Pediatric Epilepsy: Diagnosis and Therapy, New York: Demos, 1993.

29. Lombroso CT. Early myoclonic encephalopathy, early infantile epileptic encephalopathy, and benign and severe infantile myoclonic epilepsies: a critical review and personal contributions. J Clin Neurophysiol 1990;7:380.

30. Curatolo P. Tuberous Sclerosis. In O Dulac, HT Chugani, B Dalla Bernadina (eds), Infantile Spasms and West Syndrome. Philadelphia: Saunders, 1994;192.

31. Snead OC III, Benton JW, Myers GL. ACTH and prednisone in childhood seizure disorders. Neurology 1983;33:966.

32. Hrachovy RA, Frost JD Jr. Infantile spasms. Pediatr Clin North Am 1989;36:311.

33. Hrachovy RA, Frost JD Jr, Kellaway PR, Zion TE. Double-blind study of ACTH vs prednisone therapy in infantile spasms. J Pediatr 1983;103:641.

34. Snead OC, Benton JW Jr, Hosey LC, et al. Treatment of infantile spasms with high-dose ACTH: efficacy and plasma levels of ACTH and cortisol. Neurology 1989;39:1027.

35. Jeavons PM, Harper JR, Bower BD. Long-term prognosis in infantile spasms: a follow-up report on 112 cases. Dev Med Child Neurol 1970;12:413.

36. Kurokawa T, Goya N, Fukuyama Y, et al. West syndrome: a survey of natural history. Pediatrics 1980;65:81.

37. Freeman JM, Kelly MT, Freeman JB. The Epilepsy Diet Treatment. An Introduction to the Ketogenic Diet. New York: Demos, 1994.

38. Kinsman SL, Vining EPG, Quaskey SA, et al. Efficacy of the ketogenic diet for intractable seizure disorders: review of 58 cases. Epilepsia 1992;33:1132.

39. DeVivo DC. How to Use Other Drugs (Steroids) and the Ketogenic Diet. In PL Morselli, CE Pippenger, JK Penry (eds), Antiepileptic Drug Therapy in Pediatrics. New York: Raven, 1983;283.

40. The Felbamate Study Group in Lennox-Gastaut Syndrome. Efficacy of felbamate in childhood epileptic encephalopathy (Lennox-Gastaut syndrome). N Engl J Med 1993;328:29.

41. Snead OC, Hosey LC. Exacerbation of seizures in children by carbamazepine. N Engl J Med 1985;15:916.

42. Carmant L, Holmes GL. Commissurotomies in children. J Child Neurol 1994;9(Suppl 2):S50.

43. Williamson PD, Spencer DD, Spencer SS, et al. Complex partial seizures of frontal lobe origin. Ann Neurol 1985;18:497.

44. Bass N, Wyllie E, Comair Y, et al. Supplementary sensorimotor area seizures in children and adolescents. J Pediatr 1995;126:537.

45. Holmes GL. Benign focal epilepsies of childhood. Epilepsia 1993;34(Suppl 3):S49.

46. Kotagal P, Rothner AD. Localization-Related Epilepsies: Simple Partial Seizures, Complex Partial Seizures, Benign Focal Epilepsy of Childhood, and Epilepsia Partialis Continua. In WE Dodson, JM Pellock (eds), Pediatric Epilepsy: Diagnosis and Therapy. New York: Demos, 1993;183.

47. Weiser H-G, Dreifuss FE, Heinemann U (eds). Zurich Consensus Conference on New Antiepileptic Drugs. Epilepsia 1994;35(Suppl 4):S1.

48. Goldring S, Bernardo KL. Surgery of Childhood Epilepsy. In WE Dodson, JM Pellock (eds), Pediatric Epilepsy: Diagnosis and Therapy, New York: Demos, 1993.
49. Adelson PD, Black PMcL (eds). Surgical treatment of epilepsy in children. Neurosurg Clin North Am 1995;6:419.

11

Management of Pregnancy and Epilepsy

Stephen D. Collins and Mark S. Yerby

Nearly a million women with epilepsy in the United States are of child-bearing age. Because of the risks to mother and child from seizures as well as from anticonvulsant medications, pregnant women with epilepsy are considered to have high-risk pregnancies. Multiple problems, both medical and social, exist for pregnant women with epilepsy. This chapter deals with the effects of pregnancy on epileptic women as well as the effects of epilepsy and anticonvulsant medications on women and their children.

Effect of Pregnancy on Seizures

Although no significant change in seizure frequency occurs during many pregnancies, approximately one-third of patients will have an increased number of seizures at some point during their pregnancy.[1] Predicting an individual patient's seizure risk in pregnancy is difficult, because no one type of epilepsy has an increased risk of worsening and the prior duration of epilepsy or seizure frequency during previous pregnancies is not a useful predictor.

It is important to be able to predict which women are at risk for increased seizures during pregnancy because of the significant risks to mother and child of even single seizures. Whereas all seizure types may pose a risk to mother or fetus, generalized motor convulsions (tonic-clonic seizures) are particularly worrisome because they can result in trauma and possible hypoxia. The leading cause of nonobstetric death in pregnant women with epilepsy is trauma. Maternal trauma highly correlates with fetal death. Trauma may result in premature rupture of fetal membranes, with its increased risk of infection, and in premature labor or abruptio placentae, with potential fetal hypoxia, acidosis, and even death.[2]

Numerous reports have documented fetal injuries secondary to generalized tonic-clonic seizures and have described intracranial hemorrhages,[3] heart rate suppression,[4, 5] and miscarriage.[6, 7] It is more difficult to discern the risk of partial seizures to the fetus, but since they may generalize or put the mother at risk during a confusional state, it is, in general, best to control all seizures during pregnancy.

Potential Mechanisms of Seizure Increases

Variations in plasma sex hormones levels have been linked to both seizures and electroencephalographic (EEG) abnormalities. Estrogen increases and progesterone decreases seizure susceptibility.[8] No correlation of plasma sex hormone levels has been found to correlate with changes in seizure frequency during pregnancy, however.[9] Even women with a prior history of catamenial epilepsy, wherein susceptibility to variations in plasma sex steroid levels is presumed to contribute to seizures, do not have an increased risk of seizures during pregnancy.[10, 11] Various authors have found increases in seizures during the first[10–12] and third trimester,[1, 13] and therefore no clearly consistent time during gestation is more likely to be associated with seizure breakthroughs.

The most common factor identified in women with increased seizure frequency in pregnancy has been a trend toward subtherapeutic anticonvulsant levels. This is most probably a result of deliberate noncompliance on the part of women stemming from their concerns of medication effects on the fetus[14–16] and of the decreases in serum anticonvulsant concentrations in pregnancy caused by a multitude of physiologic factors.[17–21] Some of these factors include malabsorption, nausea, increases in drug elimination, and increases in volume of distribution. Primary malabsorption has been described in at least one case.[22] As a general explanation for decreases in serum concentrations, however, it is probably a rare factor. Because serum valproic acid levels exhibit a fairly steady decrease throughout pregnancy[23] and carbamazepine levels decrease primarily in the third trimester,[15, 24] simple dilutional effects secondary to increases in blood volume[25] cannot completely account for all decreases in anticonvulsant levels that are observed.[24] Decreases in serum levels caused by increases in drug clearance have been postulated. The clearance of markers such as antipyrine are decreased in pregnancy,[26, 27] however, and since the clearance of carbamazepine and phenobarbital does not change during pregnancy, it would seem unlikely that clearance is a significant factor in decreases in serum levels.[15]

The physiologic factors that seem to correlate best with gestational changes of anticonvulsant concentrations are the alterations in plasma protein binding that occur during pregnancy. Levels of free drug, that which is unbound to plasma protein, increase as gestation proceeds. Because the free drug is that which is metabolized, increases in the free fraction will result in high rates of metabolism and therefore result in declines in total drug concentration. Free phenobarbital levels significantly decrease, whereas carbamazepine and phenytoin show less significant decreases. Free valproic acid levels increase during the third trimester.[24, 28] These alterations in anticonvulsant concentrations dictate regular monitoring of drug levels during pregnancy. In a patient in whom a past therapeutic range of free drug level is available, monitoring of free drug levels is highly useful. *Therapeutic* refers to a clinical state of seizure control and freedom from clinical signs of toxicity, not any particular serum drug concentration. In all pregnant women, careful monitoring of drug levels with increases in prescribed dosage when levels decrease significantly is an essential element in seizure prevention.

Complications of Pregnancy

Several studies have documented the increased obstetric complications in women with epilepsy compared with the general population.[29–31] Vaginal bleeding,[32] anemia,[33] and hyperemesis gravidarum[29, 32] occur more frequently in women with epilepsy. The latter makes compliance with anticonvulsants particularly difficult. Some studies have found an increased frequency of pre-eclampsia in women with epilepsy.[29, 32, 34]

Several retrospective series have analyzed complications during labor and delivery and noted an increased frequency in women with epilepsy.

These problems have included premature labor[35, 36] and increases in obstetric interventions such as artificial induction of labor; mechanical rupture of membranes, the use of mechanical assistance, or both; and cesarean sections.[29, 37–39] Some of these complications may have been a result of anticonvulsants causing a decrease in uterine contractile force.[39]

Adverse Outcomes of Pregnancy

A multitude of adverse outcomes of pregnancy have been noted in the children of mothers with epilepsy. Most noticeably, stillbirth rates and rates of neonatal and perinatal death are approximately twice the rate found in the general population.[6, 11, 32, 40–42] Premature delivery[29, 35, 40, 42] and low birth weight (less than 2,500 g)[29, 32, 39, 42, 43] occur in 4–11% and 7–10% of women with epilepsy, respectively. Low Apgar scores have been noted in multiple studies,[29, 39, 42, 43] although outcome studies on these patients have not been performed on a long-term basis.

Hemorrhage

Neonatal bleeding, including intracranial hemorrhage, has been associated with in utero exposure to anticonvulsants, and a unique neonatal hemorrhagic disorder with bleeding in the first 24 hours of life has been associated with a deficiency of the vitamin K–dependent clotting factors II, XII, IX, and X.[14, 34, 42, 44–47] In infants, prolonged prothrombin and partial thromboplastin times have been noted, whereas in their mothers these clotting variables are in the normal range. The initial association of neonatal bleeding of this sort linked in utero exposure to phenobarbital or primidone and the condition.[45] Subsequent case reports have noted the same association with the use of phenytoin, carbamazepine, diazepam, methobarbital, amobarbital, and ethosuximide. Usually, this condition has been noted in women on polypharmacy. The frequency of neonatal bleeding is difficult to determine because of a lack of prospective studies; it may be as high as 7%.[48]

The mechanism of this vitamin K–dependent clotting deficiency is presumably the result of competitive inhibition of vitamin K transport across the placenta. Maternal administration of vitamin K_1 in the last week or weeks of pregnancy is prophylactic.[49] It is important to note that intramuscular administration of vitamin K to the infant at birth will not prevent hemorrhage if any two of the coagulation factors have levels below 5% of normal values and will obviously not reverse hemorrhage that has already occurred. If neonatal hemorrhage is noted, these patients need immediate treatment with fresh frozen plasma as well as intramuscular administration of vitamin K.

Seizures

Children of women with epilepsy have a risk of experiencing seizures that is two to three times higher than that of children of normal women,[50] whereas the risk of paternal association is more equivocal. Case studies describe both maternal seizures in pregnancy[51] and multiple drug therapy of the mother[52] as risk factors for the development of epilepsy in offspring of women with epilepsy.

Mental Retardation

Although mental retardation has been associated with maternal epilepsy[32, 42, 53, 54] and directly or indirectly ascribed to anticonvulsant effect, most studies have not taken into account parental intelligence or other contributory factors. By using prospective, blinded study methods with correction for levels of education and other socioeconomic factors, minimal and probably insignificant differences were found between subjects and controls.[54]

Congenital Malformations

Because of the relative ease with which major malformations are diagnosed and the heightened attention brought to pregnancies of women with epilepsy, congenital malformations are the most frequently reported and most discussed adverse outcome of pregnancy. Major malformations have straightforward definitions (e.g., spina bifida or the tetralogy of Fallot). Minor malformations are less well characterized and thus more subject to interobserver variation. The prevalence rates of both major and minor defects are estimates based primarily on retrospective or very small prospective studies and are therefore liable to significant error.

At this time, the best estimate of major and minor birth defect risk predicts that children exposed to anticonvulsants in utero have twice the number of birth defects as unexposed children.[40, 42] We will review selected reports of teratogenicity associated with anticonvulsant use by mothers or fathers. It is hoped that this reiteration of studies will make the impression that an association of malformations and anticonvulsant use definitely exists and is particularly strong when the maternal epilepsy is severe and multiple drugs are prescribed. What is far less clear with regard to most anticonvulsants is a clear association of a single malformation syndrome and a particular drug. Given the potential for serious adverse outcomes to mother and child from seizures, the decision to use any one drug must weigh risk of seizures with risks of malformations.

Malformation rates in the general population generally are in the range of 2–3%;[36] estimates for malformation rates in the offspring of women with epilepsy range from 1.25% to 11.5%.[55-57] An average of the studies (Table 11-1) estimates the risk for an individual epileptic pregnancy at 4–6%, that is, double the rate for the general population.

The initial report correlated anticonvulsant use and malformation occurring in a child exposed to mephenytoin who suffered microcephaly, cleft palate, malrotation of the intestine, and severe mental retardation.[58] After this case, an analysis of 426 pregnancies in 246 mothers with epilepsy[59] disclosed an increase in miscarriages and stillbirths but no difference in malformation rate from that of the general public. A number of investigators reported anomalies such as orofacial clefts associated with barbiturates and cardiac anomalies associated with phenytoin-phenobarbital combination therapy.[55, 60, 61] The first specific association of an anticonvulsant linked first-trimester use of trimethadione with significant teratogenicity in 8 of 14 pregnancies.[62] Speidel and Meadow[42] demonstrated a twofold increase in risk of malformation in a retrospective study of 427 pregnancies of women with epilepsy. They discerned no specific abnormality associated with any one drug and described a subgroup of children with a pattern of anomalies with somewhat broad scope. Children with the most complete pattern demonstrated trigonocephaly, microcephaly, hypertelorism, low-set ears, shortened necks, transverse palmar creases, and minor skeletal anomalies.

After these studies, a plethora of case reports described nearly every type of congenital malformation in association with all anticonvulsants. Three observations have been substantiated by multiple authors: (1) Malformation rates are higher in women with epilepsy treated with

Table 11-1. Examples of Malformation Rates in the Offspring of Epileptic and Control Mothers

	Controls		Epileptic Mothers	
	Malformation Rate (%)	Number of Pregnancies	Malformation Rate (%)	Number of Pregnancies
Janz and Fuchs[59]			2.3	225
German et al.[62]			5.3	243
Elshove and Van Eck[68]	1.9	12,051	15.0	65
Speidel and Meadow[42]	1.6	483	5.2	427
Bjerkdal and Bah[29]	2.2	12,530	4.5	311
Niswander and Wertelecki[115]	2.7	347,097	4.1	413
Weber et al.[116]	2.2	5011	4.0	731
Seino and Miyakoshi[117]			13.7	272
Majewski et al.[118]			16.0	111
Nakane et al.[56]			11.5	700
Hiilesmaa et al.[43]	2.0	5613	7.7	4795
Stanley et al.[119]	3.4	62,265	3.7	244

anticonvulsants during pregnancy than in women with epilepsy untreated during pregnancy,[30, 42, 50, 56, 63, 64] (2) plasma drug levels are higher in women who bear malformed children,[65] and (3) mothers on multiple drug therapy have greater malformation rates than women on monotherapy.[66] A fourth, less agreed on observation is the lack of correlation with seizures occurring in pregnancy and malformation rates.[40]

The most common major malformations reported are cleft lip/palate and congenital heart disease.[50, 67–69] Orofacial clefts are relatively common malformations in the general populace (0.15% of live births), but in infants of women with epilepsy they occur nine times as often (1.38%).[69–71] These anomalies account for 30% of the excess of malformations reported in epilepsy pregnancies. A contribution of epilepsy per se has been suggested by some studies, while being refuted in others.[72, 73] Congenital heart defects occur in anywhere from 1.5% to 2.0% of children of women with epilepsy, a risk three times higher than that of the nonepilepsy pregnancy group.[70] No anticonvulsant is specifically associated with these major malformations; rather, all anticonvulsants have been implicated as possibly being teratogenic.

The absence of a particular malformation pattern has been held up as evidence that anticonvulsants are not teratogenic. Outcome studies evaluating phenobarbital when used for nonepilepsy conditions disclosed no increase in malformation rates, a situation different from phenobarbital use in pregnancies complicated by epilepsy.[74] Studies have also shown increased rates of malformations in children of fathers with epilepsy,[75, 76] again suggesting a linkage of epilepsy "genes" and malformations. Other studies have not replicated these findings,[77] and a prospective study has not been performed that might decide this issue. Given the numbers of children with major malformations with a history of in utero anticonvulsant exposure and the clear-cut evidence of other drug classes yielding major malformations, it is most likely that anticonvulsants do increase the risk of malformation by themselves or in addition to the presence of epilepsy.

"Minor" malformations are deviations from a less well described "norm" that do not cause substantive risk to health. Every major anticonvulsant has been proposed to induce a specific fetal complex (Table 11-2).[62, 78-82] It is important to note that careful examination of all family members has not been performed in the overwhelming majority of syndromes and that a number of the anomalies are subtle, even for dysmorphologists. Other defects are capable of being unequivocally diagnosed, such as distal digit hypoplasia, yet they have been noted with use of four of the six anticonvulsants (hydantoin, phenobarbital, carbamazepine, and primidone), evidence perhaps for a fetal anticonvulsant syndrome but providing less compelling proof that a specific drug induces a defined syndrome. Brief reviews of the syndromes below illustrate the features described and the particular quandaries associated with interpreting each drug's role in minor anomaly development.

Fetal Trimethadione Syndrome

A retrospective analysis of a small group of women exposed to trimethadione in pregnancy yielded the significant finding of extremely low survivorship (3 of 14 infants).[62] Children who were live-born exhibited a number of abnormal characteristics, including V-shaped eyebrows, short stature, and hypospadias.[83] In a review of 53 pregnancies associated with trimethadione use, 87% fetal loss or congeni-

Table 11-2. Syndromes of Minor Anomalies Associated with Anticonvulsants

Fetal trimethadione syndrome
  Developmental delay
  V-shaped eyebrows
  Low-set ears
  Intrauterine growth retardation
  Cardiac anomalies
  Speech difficulties
  Epicanthal folds
  Irregular teeth
  Microcephaly
  Inguinal hernia
  Simian creases
Primidone embryopathy
  Hirsute forehead
  Thick nasal root
  Distal digital hypoplasia
  Antiverted nostrils
  Long philtrum
  Straight, thin upper lip
  Psychomotor retardation
Fetal hydantoin syndrome
  Craniofacial anomalies
  Broad nasal bridge
  Short upturned nose
  Low-set ears
  Prominent lips
  Epicanthal folds
  Hypertelorism
  Wide mouth
  Ptosis or strabismus
  Distal digital hypoplasia
  Intrauterine growth retardation
  Mental deficiency

Fetal carbamazepine syndrome
  Upslanting palpebral fissures
  Epicanthal folds
  Short nose
  Long philtrum
  Hypoplastic nails
  Microcephaly
  Developmental delay
Fetal valproate syndrome
  Craniofacial anomalies
  Epicanthal folds inferiorly
  Small antiverted nose
  Shallow philtrum
  Flat nasal bridge
  Long upper lip
  Down-turned mouth
  Thin vermilion border
  Protruding lips
  Prognathism
  Distal digital hypoplasia
Fetal phenobarbital syndrome
  Developmental delay
  Short nose
  Low nasal bridge
  Hypertelorism
  Epicanthal folds
  Ptosis
  Low-set ears
  Wide mouth

tal abnormality of some type occurred. Surviving children were shown to be mentally retarded at much higher frequencies than the general population.[71] Given the very high fetal and infant loss associated with this drug and the availability of more effective anticonvulsants for generalized seizures, trimethadione is contraindicated for use in women with child-bearing potential.

Fetal Hydantoin Syndrome

Fetal hydantoin syndrome is probably the most widely known syndrome. In actuality, a clear and singular role of hydantoin in production of the distal digital hypoplasia and other anomalies described by Hanson and Smith[78] has never been proven. In that report and others[84, 85] describing digital hypoplasia, multiple drug therapy with barbiturates was nearly a uniform finding. Subsequent researchers have differed significantly in their findings. One study of 98 women taking hydantoin in pregnancy found 30% of children to have distal digital hypoplasia with no other features of the syndrome.[48] Another study[72] found zero incidence of the syndrome but did find evidence of hypertelorism, distal digital hypoplasia, or dermal arches in some children. An association with mental retardation seems untenable, since only 1.4% of infants born to women taking hydantoin had evidence on formal neuropsychiatric testing of mental deficiency, which is not significantly different from the general experience.[54]

The case report of Koerner et al.[86] illustrates the necessity of examining entire families when describing dysmorphisms. Four siblings exhibited the craniofacial characteristics of the hydantoin syndrome; however, only two of the four had intrauterine exposure to the drug. The other two had been treated with barbiturates on the supposition that hydantoins had induced the dysmorphisms in the older siblings.

Our view of the above data is that exposure to hydantoins, especially in combination with barbiturates, may be a necessary but not sufficient cause of minor anomalies. This may occur in a subset of children with a presumed genetic risk for expressing such a phenotype.

Primidone Embryopathy

A variety of craniofacial abnormalities, psychomotor retardation, and heart defects have been described with primidone use.[80, 87] As mentioned above, many of the patients with the so-called fetal hydantoin syndrome were on barbiturates, including primidone, which argues more for a multiple drug syndrome than an individual drug syndrome.

Fetal Phenobarbital Syndrome

The range of abnormalities observed with fetal exposure to phenobarbital mirrors both those seen in fetal hydantoin and fetal alcohol syndromes. Given the similarities, Seip[82] made two recommendations: (1) that the features not be referred to as the fetal phenobarbital syndrome and (2) that all three drugs might act to decrease folate levels, therefore exerting similar dysmorphic effects on infants.

Fetal Valproate Syndrome

DiLiberti et al.[79] described a small group of infants with a number of facial and distal digital abnormalities. Other authors have noted other facial abnormalities and difficulties in labor.[88] In a group of 344 women exposed to valproate in the first trimester, Jeavons[89] found abnormal deliveries but no dose-related effect. A relationship with spina bifida has been noted with valproate use in the first trimester and is discussed in the section on drug-specific teratogenicity.

Fetal Carbamazepine Syndrome

One study has noted craniofacial abnormalities, hypoplastic nails, and microcephaly in a group of infants exposed to carbamazepine monotherapy.[81] They also used a battery of neuropsychiatric tests to measure development and noted a 20% reduction in these abnormalities in 25 of 37 infants when defining one standard deviation from the mean as significantly abnormal. More commonly, differences on intelligence tests are not believed to have significance until two standard deviations are achieved. Other studies have noted small head size at birth[43] but within the normal range, and follow-up studies of the same children failed to find significant differences later in life.[90]

Summary of Minor Anomaly Syndromes

Although craniofacial abnormalities and digital abnormalities are certainly found with higher frequency in infants exposed to anticonvulsants in utero, specific drug syndromes have not been confirmed in the literature to date. There are multiple reasons for this, including the difficulty in accurately diagnosing and quantifying facial dysmorphism, lack of follow-up into adult life, and inadequate parental evaluation for dysmorphism. Last, few prospective studies have been performed. In one prospective study of 172 deliveries of children with mothers with epilepsy, no specific defect could be associated with a specific anticonvulsant, and no clear dose relationship could be ascertained.[91]

Perhaps a better term to describe the variety of abnormalities seen in a small group of children exposed to anticonvulsants is *fetal anticonvulsant syndrome*. Certainly, a large, multicenter prospective study is indicated to better define the role of anticonvulsants in major and minor congenital malformations.

Mechanisms of Teratogenicity

Two specific mechanisms have been postulated to induce major malformations with anticonvulsant exposure. The first centers on arene oxide/epoxide metabolites or free radicals and the second on defects of enzymes responsible for clearing toxic metabolites.[92–103] Because these remain hypotheses, we will not pursue the issue other than to say a number of other possible mechanisms such as alterations in glucocorticoid receptors[104] and folate deficiencies[105–107] have been proposed to exert effects on malformations in infants exposed to anticonvulsants.

Drug-Specific Teratogenicity

A true teratogen has a clearly defined adverse outcome associated with use, such as phocomelia in thalidomide exposure. Valproic acid has a specific malformation associated with its use, namely neural tube defects. In the first report warning of this association, 34% of infants exposed to valproic acid had a malformation, and five of nine with valproate monotherapy had spina bifida.[57] These cases were identified by review of a birth defect registry. Some of the mothers had a prior pregnancy complicated by spina bifida without valproate exposure. A later study conducted by questionnaire[108] yielded a 13% rate of malformations in all anticonvulsant exposures and a higher than expected rate of spina bifida in children exposed to valproate. Various risk rates have been stated for spina bifida; the one neural tube deficit associated specifically with valproate. The estimate by Lindhout and Schmidt[109] is an overall risk of 1.5% per infant, although this number was generated on a small number of actual events and is subject to all the problems of a small sample base. The mechanism of induction is unknown.

Although phenobarbital is recommended by the American College of Obstetrics and Gynecology as the drug of choice in pregnancy, there is no evidence supporting its safety and it appears to have a rate of malformations as high or higher than every other anticonvulsant. Seip[82] has described infants exposed to phenobarbital monotherapy with the same craniofacial stigmata ascribed to the fetal hydantoin syndrome.

In the original papers describing the hydantoin syndrome, 5 of 6 and 4 of 5 infants were also exposed to a barbiturate. Rodents exposed to barbiturates display an increase in the rate of cleft lip/palate[110] and alterations of neuronal structure.[111] After delivery, infants exposed to barbiturates may display withdrawal symptoms for up to 3 months.[112] Breast-feeding may lead to infant sedation in women taking barbiturates, and use of the drug may need to be discontinued.[113] In general, other anticonvulsants are found in such relatively small concentrations in breast milk that their use can continue.

Conclusions and Recommendations

All anticonvulsants cross the blood–placenta barrier,[114] and all have been associated with congenital malformations. The best current estimates of malformation rates in infants exposed to anticonvulsants places a 4–6% overall risk on each pregnancy. A group of children will have a variety of alterations of craniofacial and digital structure, the frequency of which is unknown at this time. A specific defect, spina bifida, has been associated with valproate use. Multiple genetic and environmental factors appear to cooperate in the induction of malformations, and much more research will be necessary to determine and obviate these factors.

Although congenital malformations are serious consequences of anticonvulsant use in pregnancy, the clear and well documented risks of seizures to mother and fetus cannot be forgotten. The clinician must balance these risks by reducing drug dosage to the minimum consistent with seizure control. This translates to monotherapy with seizure control at dosages that do not produce clinical signs of toxicity. Because anticonvulsant levels will change in most women as a result of the physiologic changes of pregnancy, regular and frequent visits are necessary. Monitoring drug levels at these visits assumes a more important role in pregnant patients than in nonpregnant patients, and, if possible, levels of free drug should be determined instead of total drug levels. Alteration of anticonvulsant type or halting anticonvulsant administration is usually not indicated because of the risk of poor seizure control and the risk of trauma to the developing organ systems in the fetus in the early portion of the first trimester. The use of folate supplementation in all women has been shown to be beneficial in reducing malformations and may be doubly important in pregnant women with epilepsy. A recent study has shown a defect in methionine synthase function in women bearing children with neural tube defects.[106] This deficiency can be overcome by oral supplementation with the enzymes cofactor vitamin B_{12}. Although these findings have not been corroborated in women with epilepsy, it would appear that preconceptual "co-therapy" with vitamin B_{12} and folate in women with epilepsy may provide greater protection from fetal neural tube defects than supplementation with folate alone. Vitamin K_1 supplementation in the final weeks of pregnancy should reduce maternal and fetal hemorrhagic risk.

The best drug for a woman with epilepsy is the drug that controls her seizures with a minimum of toxicity.

Because the physiologic changes of pregnancy reverse in the days and first few weeks after delivery, it is important to watch for postpartum toxicity caused by the rising anticonvulsant levels and continue close clinical contact.

Women using valproic acid should be educated about the possible risks of spina bifida, and ultrasonography should be performed at an institution capable of the highest resolution (so-called level II ultrasound) and most expert interpretation. In combination with a serum alpha-fetoprotein determination, more than 95% of spina bifida cases can be detected.

Last and perhaps most important, it should be stressed to the patient and family members that complications do arise in pregnancies of women with epilepsy but that at least 90% of such pregnancies are normal, and the infants grow up to be completely healthy.

References

1. Bardy AH. Epilepsy and Pregnancy. A Prospective Study of 154 Pregnancies and Epileptic Women. Dissertation, University of Helsinki, Helsinki, Finland, 1982.
2. Pearlman MD, Tintinalli JE, Lorenz RP. Blunt trauma during pregnancy. N Engl J Med. 1990;323:1609.
3. Millar JH, Nevin NC. Congenital malformations and anticonvulsant drugs. Lancet 1973;1:328.
4. Teramo K, Hiilesmaa V, Bardy A, Saarihosk S. Fetal heart rate during a maternal grand mal epileptic seizure. J Perinat Med 1979;7:3.
5. Yerby MS. Problems in the management of the pregnant woman with epilepsy. Epilepsia 1987;(Suppl 3):529.
6. Beaussart-Defaye J, Boston N, Demarca C, Beaussart X. Epilepsies and Reproduction. II. Grine Lille, France: Nord Epilepsy Research and Information Group, 1986.
7. Higgins TA, Comerford JB. Epilepsy in pregnancy. J Irish Med Assoc 1974;67:317.

8. Holmes GG. Effects of menstruation and pregnancy on epilepsy. Semin Neurol 1988;8:234.
9. Ramsay RE. Effect of hormones on seizure activity during pregnancy. J Clin Neurophysiol. 1987;4:23.
10. Canger R, Avanzini G, Battino D, et al. Modification of Seizure Frequency in Pregnant Patients with Epilepsy: A Prospective Study. In D Janz, L Bossi, M Dam (eds), Epilepsy, Pregnancy and the Child. New York: Raven 1982;33.
11. Knight AH, Rhind EG. Epilepsy and pregnancy: a study of 153 pregnancies in 59 patients. Epilepsia 1975;16:99.
12. Maroni E, Markoff R. Epilepsie und Schwangerschaft. Gynaecologia 1969;168:418.
13. Remillard G, Dansky L, Andermann E, Andermann F. Seizure frequency during pregnancy and the puerperium. In D Janz, L Bossi, M Dam (eds), Epilepsy, Pregnancy and the Child. New York: Raven, 1982;39.
14. Bossi L, Assrel BM, Avanzini G, et al. Plasma Levels and Clinical Effects of Antiepileptic Drugs in Pregnant Epileptic Patients and Their Newborns. In SI Johannessen et al. (eds), Antiepileptic Therapy: Advances in Drug Monitoring. New York: Raven, 1980.
15. Otani K. Risk factors for the increased seizure frequency during pregnancy and puerperium. Fol Psychiatr Neurol Japon 1985;39:33.
16. Schmidt D, Canger R, Avanzini G, et al. Change of seizure frequency in pregnant epileptic women. J Neurol Neurosurg Psychiatry 1983;46:751.
17. Dam M, Christiansen J, Munck O, Mygind KI. Antiepileptic drugs: metabolism in pregnancy. Clin Pharmacokinet 1979;4:53.
18. Eadie MJ, Lander CM, Tyner JH. Plasma drug level monitoring in pregnancy. Clin Pharmacokinet 1977;2:427.
19. Lander CM, Edward VE, Eadie MJ, Tyner JH. Plasma anticonvulsant concentrations during pregnancy. Neurology 1977;27:128.
20. Mygind KI, Dam M, Christiansen J. Phenytoin and phenobarbitone plasma clearance during pregnancy. Acta Neurol Scand 1976;54:160.
21. Perucca E, Crema A. Plasma protein binding of drugs in pregnancy. Clin Pharmacokinet 1982;7:336.
22. Ramsey RE, Strauss RG, Wilder BJ, Willmore LJ. Status epilepticus in pregnancy: effect of phenytoin malabsorption of seizure control. Neurology 1978;28:85.
23. Krauss CM, Holmes LB, Van Lang QC, Keith DA. Four siblings with similar malformations after exposure to phenytoin and primidone. J Pediatr 1984;105:750.
24. Yerby MS, Friel PN, McCormick KB, et al. Pharmacokinetics of anticonvulsants in pregnancy: alterations in plasma protein binding. Epilepsy Res 1990;5:223.
25. Pritchard JA, Changes in the blood volume during pregnancy and delivery. Anesthesiology 1965;26:393.
26. Dam M, Christiansen J, Munck O. Antiepileptic drugs: metabolism in pregnancy. Clin Pharmacokinet 1977;2:427.
27. Nau H, Kuhnz W, Egger HJ, et al. Anticonvulsants during pregnancy and lactation: transplacental, maternal and neonatal pharmacokinetics. Clin Pharmacokinet 1981;7:508.

28. Bardy AH, Hiilesmaa VK, Teramo K, Neuvonen PJ. Protein binding of antiepileptic drugs during pregnancy, labor, and puerperium. Ther Drug Monit 1990;12:40.
29. Bjerkdal T, Bahna SL. The course and outcome of pregnancy in women with epilepsy. Acta Obstet Gynecol Scand 1973;52:245.
30. Monson RR, Rosenberg L, Hartz SC. Diphenylhydantoin and selected congenital malformations. N Engl J Med 1973;289:1049.
31. Montouris GD, Fenichel GM, McLain W. The pregnant epileptic. Arch Neurol 1979;36:601.
32. Nelson KB, Ellenberg JH. Maternal seizure disorder outcomes of pregnancy and neurologic abnormalities in the children. Neurology 1982;32:1247.
33. Svigos JM. Epilepsy and pregnancy. Aust NZ J Obstet Gynaecol 1984;24:182.
34. Vert P, Deblay MF. Hemorrhagic Disorders in Infants of Epileptic Mothers. In D Janz, M Dam, A Richens, L Bossi, H Helge, D Schmidt (eds), Epilepsy, Pregnancy and the Child. New York: Raven, 1982;387.
35. Hill RM, Tennyson L. Premature Delivery, Gestational Age, Complications of Delivery, Vital Data at Birth on Newborn Infants of Epileptic Mothers: Review of the Literature. In D Janz (ed), Epilepsy, Pregnancy and the Child. New York: Raven, 1982;167.
36. Kalter H, Warkany J. Congenital malformations. N Engl J Med 1983;308:481.
37. Egenaes J. Outcome of Pregnancy in Women with Epilepsy—Norway 1967 to 1978: Complications During Pregnancy and Delivery. In D Janz et al. (eds), Epilepsy, Pregnancy and the Child. New York: Raven, 1982;L167.
38. Hill RM, Tennyson LM. Maternal drug therapy: effect on fetal and neonatal growth and neurobehavior. Neurotoxicology 1986;7:121.
39. Yerby MS, Koepsell T, Daling J. Pregnancy complications and outcomes in a cohort of women with epilepsy. Epilepsia 1985;26:631.
40. Fedrick J. Epilepsy and pregnancy: a report from the Oxford record linkage study. BMJ 1973;2:442.
41. Nakane Y. Congenital malformations among infants of epileptic mothers treated during pregnancy. Fol Psychiatr Neurol Japon 1979;33:363.
42. Speidel BD, Meadow SR. Maternal epilepsy and abnormalities of the fetus and newborn. Lancet 1972;2:839.
43. Hiilesmaa VK, Teramo K, Granstrom ML, Bardy AH. Fetal head growth retardation associated with maternal antiepileptic drugs. Lancet 1981;2:165.
44. Monnet P, Rossenberg D, Bovier-Lapierre M. Thérapeutique anticomitière pendant la grossesse et maladie hemorragique du nouveau né. Rev Fr Gynecol Obstet 1968;63:695.
45. Mountain KR, Hirsh J, Gallus AS. Coagulation defect due to anticonvulsant treatment in pregnancy. Lancet 1970;1:265.
46. Traggis DG, Mauz DL, Baroudy R. Hemorrhage in a neonate of a mother on anticonvulsant therapy. J Pediatr Surg 1984;19:598.
47. VanCreveld S. Nouveaux aspects de la maladie hémorragique du nouveau né. Ned Tijdschr Geneeskd 1957;101:2109.

48. Kelly TE. Teratogenicity of anticonvulsants. III: Radiographic hand analysis of children exposed in utero to dyphenylhydantoin. Am J Med Genet 1984;19:445.
49. Deblay MF, Vert P, Andre M, Marchal F. Transplacental vitamin K prevents haemorrhagic disease of infants of epileptic mothers. Lancet 1982;1:1247.
50. Annegers JF, Hauser WA, Elveback LR, et al. Congenital malformations and seizure disorders in the offspring of parents with epilepsy. Int J Epidemiol 1978;7:241.
51. Ottman R, Annegers JF, Hauser WA, Kurland LT. Higher risk of seizures in offspring of mothers than fathers with epilepsy. Am J Hum Genet 1988;43:357.
52. Squier W, Hope PL, Lindenbaum RH. Neocerebellar hypoplasia in a neonate following intrauterine exposure to anticonvulsants. Dev Med Child Neurol 1990;32:725.
53. Hill RM, Berniaum WM, Morning MG, et al. Infants exposed in utero to antiepileptic drugs. Am J Dis Child 1974;127:645.
54. Gaily E, Kantula-Sorsa E, Granstrom ML. Intelligence of children of epileptic mothers. J Pediatr 1988;113:677.
55. Meadow SR. Anticonvulsant drugs and congenital abnormalities. Lancet 1968;2:1296.
56. Nakane Y, Okuma T, Takahashi R, et al. Multi-institutional study on the teratogenicity and fetal toxicity of anticonvulsants: a report of a collaborative study group in Japan. Epilepsia 1980;21:663.
57. Philbert A, Dam M. The epileptic mother and her child. Epilepsia 1982;23:85.
58. von Muller-Kuppers M. Embryopathy during pregnancy caused by taking anticonvulsants. Acta Paedopsychiatr 1963;30:401.
59. Janz D, Fuchs V. Are antiepileptic drugs harmful when given during pregnancy? Ger Med Mon 1984;25(Suppl 1):550.
60. Centra E, Rasore-Quartino A. La sindrome malformatine digitocardiaca forme genetsche e fenocopie. Probl Azione Teratogen Farm Antiepilep Pathol 1965;57:227.
61. Melchior IC, Svenswark O, Trolle D. Placental transfer of phenobarbitone in women and elimination in newborns. Lancet 1967;2:860.
62. German J, Kowal A, Ehlers KH. Trimethadione and human teratogenesis. Teratology 1970;3:349.
63. Lowe CR. Congenital malformations among infants born to epileptic women. Lancet 1973;1:9.
64. South J. Teratogenic effects of anticonvulsants. Lancet 1972;2:1154.
65. Dansky LV, Andermann E, Sherwin AL, et al. Maternal epilepsy and congenital malformations: a prospective study with monitoring of plasma anticonvulsant levels during pregnancy. Neurology 1980;3:15.
66. Lindhout D, Rene JE, Hoppener A, Meinardi H. Teratogenicity of antiepileptic drug combinations with special emphasis on epoxidation (of carbamazepine). Epilepsia 1984;25:77.
67. Anderson RC. Cardiac defects in children of mothers receiving anticonvulsant therapy during pregnancy. J Pediatr 1976;89:318.
68. Elshove J, VanEck JHM. Aangeboren misvormingen, met name gespleten lipmet of zonder gespleten verhemelte, bij kinderen van moeders met epilepsie. Ned Tijdschr Geneeskd 1971;115:1371.

69. Friis ML, Breng-Nielsen B, Sindrup EH, et al. Facial clefts among epileptic patients. Arch Neurol 1981;38:227.
70. Kallen B. Maternal epilepsy, antiepileptic drugs and birth defects. Pathologica 1986;78:757.
71. Goldman AS, Zachai EH, Yaffe SJ. Environmentally Induced Birth Defect Risks. In JL Sever, RL Brent (eds), Teratogen Update. New York: Alan R Liss, 1986;35.
72. Gaily E, Granstrom ML, Hiilesmaa V, Bandy A. Minor anomalies in offspring of epileptic mothers. J Pediatr 1988;112:520.
73. Gatoh N, Millo Y, Taube E, Bechar M. Epilepsy among parents of children with cleft lip and palate. Brain Dev 1987;9:296.
74. Shapiro S, Slone D, Hartz SC, et al. Anticonvulsant and parental epilepsy in the development of birth defects. Lancet 1976;1:272.
75. Dietrich E, Steveling A, Lukas A, et al. Congenital anomalies in children of epileptic mothers and fathers. Neuropediatrics 1980;11:274.
76. Friis ML, Hauge M. Congenital heart defects in live born children of epileptic parents. Arch Neurol 1985;42:374.
77. Grosse KP, Schwanitz G, Rott HD, Wissmuler HF. Chromosomenuntersuchungen bei behandlung mit anticonfulsiva. Humangenetik 1972;16:209.
78. Hanson JW, Smith DW. The fetal hydantoin syndrome. J Pediatr 1975;87:285.
79. DiLiberti JH, Farndon PA, Dennis NR, Curry CJR. The fetal valproate syndrome. Am J Med Genet 1984;19:473.
80. Rudd NL, Freedom RM. A possible primidone embryopathy. J Pediatr 1979;94:835.
81. Jones KL, Lacro RV, Johnson KA, Adams J. Pattern of malformations in the children of women treated with carbamazepine during pregnancy. N Engl J Med 1989;320:1661.
82. Seip M. Growth retardation, dysmorphic facies and minor malformations following massive exposure to phenobarbital in utero. Acta Paediatr Scand 1976;65:617.
83. Zachai EH, Mellman WJ, Niederen B, Hanson JW. The fetal trimethadione syndrome. J Pediatr 1975;87:280.
84. Loughnan PM, Gold H, Vance JC. Phenytoin teratogenecity in man. Lancet 1973;1:7072.
85. Barr M, Pozanski AK, Schmickel RD. Digital hypoplasia and anticonvulsants during gestation: a teratogenic syndrome? J Pediatr 1974;84:254.
86. Koerner M, Yerby MS, Friel PN, McCormick KB. Valproic acid disposition and the protein binding in pregnancy. Ther Drug Monit 1989;11:229.
87. Gustavson EE, Chen H. Goldenhar syndrome. Enteroencephalocele and aqueductal stenosis following fetal primidone exposure. Teratology 1985;32:13.
88. Jager-Roman E, Deichl A, Jakob S, et al. Fetal growth major malformations and minor anomalies in infants born to women receiving valproic acid. J Pediatr 1986;108:997.
89. Jeavons PM. Non dose related side effects of valproate. Epilepsia 1982;23:553.

90. Granstrom ML. Early Postnatal Growth of the Children of Epileptic Mothers. In P Wolf, M Dam, D Janz, FE Dreifuss (eds), Advances in Epileptology. New York: Raven, 1987;573.
91. Kaneko S, Otani K, Fukushima Y, et al. Teratogenicity of antiepileptic drugs: analysis of possible risk factors. Epilepsia 1988;29:459.
92. Nebert DW, Jensen NM. The AH locus: genetic regulation of the metabolism of carcinogens, drugs, and other environmental chemicals by cytochrom P-450 mediated mono-oxygenases. CRC Crit Rev Biochem 1979;6:401.
93. Shum S, Jensen NM, Nebert DW. The AH locus: in utero toxicity and teratogenesis associated with genetic differences in B(a)P metabolism. Teratology 1979;20:365.
94. Pacifici GM, Colizzi C, Giuliani L, Rane A. Cytosolic epoxide hydrolase in fetal and adult human liver. Arch Toxicol 1983;54:331.
95. Pacifici GM, Rane A. Metabolism of styrene oxide in different human fetal tissues. Drug Metab Dispos 1982;10:302.
96. Martz F, Failinger C, Blake DA. Phenytoin teratogenesis: correlation between embryopathic effect and covalent binding of putative arene oxide metabolite to gestational tissue. J Pharmacol Exp Ther 1977;203:231.
97. Strickler SM, Dansky LV, Miller MA, et al. Genetic predisposition to phenytoin induced birth defects. Lancet 1985;1:746.
98. Buehler BA. Epoxide hydrolase activity and the fetal hydantoin syndrome. [Abstract.] Clin Res 1985;33:A129.
99. Buehler BA, Delimont D, VanWass M, Finnell RH. Prenatal prediction of risk of the fetal hydantoin syndrome. N Engl J Med. 1990;322:1567.
100. Dansky LV, Strickler SM, Andermann E, et al. Pharmacogenetic Susceptibility to Phenytoin Teratogenesis. In P Wolf, M Dam, D Janz, FE Dreifuss (eds), Advances in Epileptology. New York: Raven 1987;555.
101. Finnell RH, DiLiberti JH. Hydantion induced teratogenesis: are arene oxide intermediates really responsible? Helv Paediatr Acta 1983;38:171.
102. Kubow S, Wells PG. In vitro bioactivation of phenytoin to a reactive free radical intermediate by prostaglandin synthetase, horseradish peroxidase, and thyroid peroxidase. Mol Pharmacol 1989;35:504.
103. Wells PG, Zubovits JT, Wong ST, et al. Modulation of phenytoin teratogenicity and embryonic covalent binding by acetylsalicylic acid, caffeic acid, and a-phenyl-N-E-butylnitrone: implications for bioactivation by prostaglandin synthetase. Toxicol Appl Pharmacol 1984;97:192.
104. Goldman AS, Van Dyke DC, Gupta C, Katsumata M. Elevated glucocorticoid receptor levels in lymphocytes of children with the fetal hydantoin syndrome. Am J Med Genet 1987;28:607.
105. Dansky LV, Andermann E, Rosenblatt D, Sherwin AL, Andermann F. Anticonvulsants, folate levels, and pregnancy outcomes: a prospective study. Ann Neurol 1987;21:176.
106. Zhu M, Zhou S. Reduction of the teratogenic effects of phenytoin by folic acid and a mixture of folic acid, vitamins, and amino acids: a preliminary trial. Epilepsia 1989;30:246.
107. Biale Y, Lewenthal H. Effect of folic acid supplementation on congenital malformations due to anticonvulsant drugs. Eur J Obstet Gynecol Rep Biol 1984;18:211.

108. Robert E, Lofkvist E, Maugiere F. Valproate and spina bifida. Lancet 1984;1:1392.
109. Lindhout D, Schmidt D. In utero exposure to valproate and neural tube defects. Lancet 1986;1:1392.
110. Sullivan FM, McElhatton PR. Teratogenic activity of the antiepileptic drugs, phenobarbital, phenytoin, and primidone in mice. Toxicol Appl Pharmacol 1975;34:271.
111. Jacobson CD, Autolick CL, Scholey R, Vemura E. The influence of prenatal phenobarbital exposure on the growth of dendrites in the rat hippocampus. Dev Brain Res 1988;44:233.
112. Desmond MM, Schwanecke RP, Wilson GS, et al. Maternal barbiturate utilization and neonatal withdrawal symptomatology. J Pediatr 1972;80:190.
113. Kuhnz W, Koch S, Helge H, Nau H. Primidone and phenobarbital during lactation period in epileptic women. Dev Pharmacol Ther 1988;11:147.
114. Levy RH, Yerby MS. Effects of pregnancy on antiepileptic drug utilization. Epilepsia 1985;26(Suppl 1):525.
115. Niswander JD, Wertelecki W. Congenital malformation among offspring of epileptic women. Lancet 1973;1:1062.
116. Weber M, Schweitzer M, Mur JM, et al. Epilepsie, médicaments antiepileptiques et grossesse. Arch Fr Pediatr 1977;34:374.
117. Seino M, Miyakoshi M. Teratogenic risks of antiepileptic drugs in respect to the type of epilepsy. Fol Psychiatr Neurol Japon 1979;33:379.
118. Majewski F, Raft W, Fischer P, et al. Congenital anomalies in the newborn infant including minor variations. J Pediatr 1964;64:357.
119. Stanley FJ, Prescott PK, Johnston R, et al. Congenital malformation in infants of mothers with diabetes and epilepsy in western Australia. Med J Aust 1985;143:440.

12

Treatment of Status Epilepticus

Douglas R. Labar

Definition

Status epilepticus (SE), as defined by the International League Against Epilepsy, consists of epileptic attacks that are of sufficient length or that recur rapidly enough that recovery between attacks does not occur.[1] For clinical research purposes, SE usually is defined as continuous seizure activity or repeated discrete seizures without recovery to baseline neurologic function between attacks for a period of 30 minutes or more. On a practical day-to-day basis for the clinical care of critically ill patients, continuous or repetitive seizures that show no sign of abating are evaluated and treated as SE, even if the 30-minute mark after the onset has not been passed.

Incidence, Classification, and Etiology of Status Epilepticus

Population occurrence rates for SE are poorly defined, in part because a wide variety of different acute and chronic, symptomatic, and idiopathic underlying epileptogenic processes may cause SE. It is estimated that about 10% of patients with epilepsy develop SE at one time or another[2] and that between 50,000 individuals[3] and 150,000 individuals[4] in the United States develop SE annually.

Table 12-1. Classification of Status Epilepticus

Generalized status epilepticus
    Convulsive
    Tonic-clonic
    Tonic
    Myoclonic
    Nonconvulsive (absence, petit mal)
Partial status epilepticus
    Simple partial
        Focal motor status
        Epilepsia partialis continua
    Complex partial
        Temporal lobe origin
        Frontal lobe origin

SE may be classified by a variety of schemes. A common, useful, and theoretically reasonable scheme is based on the seizure type occurring; thus, SE is divided into generalized and partial.[1] Generalized SE may be convulsive or nonconvulsive; partial SE may be simple or complex (Table 12-1). Other authors elect to classify SE based on easily observed clinical phenomena;[5] thus, SE is also divided into convulsive and nonconvulsive. In the second scheme, convulsive SE may consist of generalized or partial seizures (focal motor SE); nonconvulsive SE may consist of generalized (absence) or partial (complex partial) seizures. Whereas the former classification is more reflective of the underlying epileptic process, the latter scheme is more easily and rapidly applied in the clinical setting.

Generalized Status Epilepticus

Convulsive Tonic-Clonic Status Epilepticus

The type of SE most widely and easily recognized as a medical emergency is generalized convulsive tonic-clonic SE, which consists of repeated generalized tonic-clonic seizures without recovery of consciousness between attacks. The ictal electroencephalogram (EEG) ini-

Table 12-2. Electroencephalic Ictal Pattern in the Five Stages
of Status Epilepticus

---

1. Repetitive but discrete seizures with tonic activity with continuous high-frequency generalized spikes, followed by clonic activity with repetitive individual generalized spikes and interictal slowing
2. Merging pattern of discrete seizures with tonic and then clonic components but with little or no interictal slowing before the next seizure
3. Continuous ictal discharges
4. Continuous ictal discharges disrupted by brief periods of diffused attenuation
5. Repetitive, periodic epileptiform discharges

Source: Modified from D Treiman. A progressive sequence of EEG changes during generalized convulsive SE. Epilepsy Res 1990;5:49; and D Treiman. Electroclinical features of status epilepticus. J Clin Neurophysiol 1995;12:343.

tially shows repetitive generalized spikes at a rate of 10–15 Hz during the tonic phase. This is followed by repetitive spike wave complexes, initially repeating several times per second, each complex associated with a generalized clonic jerk. These subsequently slow to repeat one every several seconds and then cease after 3–5 minutes. Often the ictal EEG is obscured by movement artifacts. Postictally, the EEG shows suppression of all activity, followed by reconstitution of background with excess slow waves. The entire clinical and electrographic sequence then repeats several minutes later.

Treiman[6, 7] characterized a five-stage progression of EEG findings in generalized convulsive SE (Table 12-2). In essence, this progression evolves from the frequent but discrete seizures described above through continuous electrographic seizures with repetitive spikes to slower (1-Hz) periodic repetitive epileptiform discharges on a low-voltage slow EEG background. Lowenstein and Aminoff[8] questioned this orderly progression of EEG stages. In 57 comatose patients who previously had been in clinically obvious convulsive SE, EEG patterns from all of the five stages described by Treiman were seen. All patients were comatose with little motor activity, but the motor manifestations of the SE that were seen did not correlate with EEG pattern. The EEG findings did not correlate with the duration of SE, as might be predicted by the Treiman five-stage progression model. Furthermore, So et al.[9] described 13 patients with continuing electrographic SE after

Table 12-3. Common Acute Precipitants of Seizures and Status Epilepticus

Subarachnoid hemorrhage, subdural hematoma

Meningitis

Encephalitis

Hypo- and hyperglycemia

Hyponatremia

Hypocalcemia

Abrupt antiepileptic medication withdrawal in a patient with preexisting epilepsy

Alcohol withdrawal

Benzodiazepine withdrawal

Medication overdoses, such as in suicide attempts (phenytoin, theophylline)

Febrile seizures in children

Cocaine

---

generalized convulsive SE had been terminated with antiepileptic medications. None showed the sequence of EEG stages described by Treiman.

Acute symptomatic causes of SE include hemorrhagic, metabolic, and infectious processes. Alcohol withdrawal and abrupt discontinuation of antiepileptic medications may trigger SE. Generalized convulsive SE may occur as a febrile seizure manifestation; somewhat surprisingly, the prognosis for the subsequent development of chronic recurrent epilepsy in this manifestation of febrile seizure is no worse than that of any other febrile seizure[10] (Table 12-3).

Convulsive Tonic Status Epilepticus

In generalized tonic SE, repeated tonic seizures lasting seconds occur many times per hour. Clinically the seizures consist of neck and trunk extension or flexion, facial grimacing, and arm extension. If standing, the patient may fall. The EEG accompaniment typically is rapidly repetitive generalized spikes occurring continuously throughout the attack, but sudden attenuation of EEG amplitude with diffuse low-voltage fast activity also may be seen ictally. Generalized tonic SE occurs in children with pre-existing mixed seizure disorders (history of sporadic tonic seizures), static encephalopathy, and a generalized slow spike and wave EEG pattern (Lennox-Gastaut syndrome).[2] Generalized tonic SE has been precipitated by benzodiazepine treatment in such patients;[11] therefore, this is best treated with intravenous phenytoin.

Convulsive Myoclonic Status Epilepticus

Generalized myoclonic SE (status myoclonus) consists of very frequent, repetitive, but discrete myoclonic jerks most frequently involving the arms, with less prominent involvement of the lower extremities and the face. The jerks each last less than a second and have been described as "lightning-like." Typically they recur in a multifocal, chaotic, arrhythmic pattern. The EEG may show generalized bursts of spikes and polyspikes in association with the myoclonus and interictally. Status myoclonus occurs in patients with idiopathic primary generalized epilepsy (juvenile myoclonic epilepsy of Janz), progressive myoclonic epilepsy, and severe metabolic encephalopathies. Common metabolic encephalopathies producing myoclonic SE include uremic and posthypoxic states.[2, 5] Myoclonic SE is difficult to treat, but clonazepam or valproate may be used. Nearly all patients with myoclonus SE after cardiac arrest die.[12]

Nonconvulsive Generalized Status Epilepticus

The clinical picture of generalized nonconvulsive SE (GNSE) is typically the acute onset of confusion in an awake patient with a history of generalized epilepsy. At times, the patient may even appear hypervigilant, but a clouded sensorium or deep stupor is more the rule. The patient usually can follow simple commands and speak but is quite slow to respond. Brief myoclonic twitches of the eyelids and chin may be seen with close observation. The EEG shows continuous repetitive generalized spike waves. In children with petit mal epilepsy, the spikes repeat relatively regularly at around 3 Hz, but in adults, the repetition tends to be slower and more irregular.[2, 5]

GNSE occurs in two age groups. It is seen as a prolonged absence seizure in children with petit mal epilepsy. It occurs in another cluster of patients in the sixth decade of life or older. Clinical settings of GNSE are presented in Table 12-4 (compiled from references 13–19). At best, these clinical settings can be interpreted as associated with the onset of GNSE, rather than specifically causative. Thomas et al.[15] described 11 cases of adults with GNSE and noted a strong association with use of high-dose psychotropic drugs. In eight cases, onset of GNSE occurred in association with benzodiazepine withdrawal. We reported GNSE in

Table 12-4. Clinical Associations with Generalized Nonconvulsive Status Epilepticus[13-19]

Anticonvulsant withdrawal
Baclofen
Benzodiazepine withdrawal
Ceftazidine
Cerebral angiography
Chronic renal failure
Electroconvulsive therapy
Fever
Generalized tonic-clonic seizures
Human immunodeficiency virus infection
Hyperventilation
Hypocalcemia
Ifosfamide
Lithium
Metrizamide myelography
Methohexital activation
Pentylenetetrazol activation
Sleep deprivation
Stroke
Thyroxine

a patient with acquired immunodeficiency syndrome; the GNSE was most likely caused by direct brain infection with human immunodeficiency virus.[16] Granner and Lee[20] emphasized that in approximately 40% of patients with GNSE, evidence for a focal epileptogenic process can be found on previous interictal EEGs or in the EEG after treatment with intravenous benzodiazepines.

Partial Status Epilepticus

Partial SE occurs when the repetitive or continuous seizures involve only a single cortical region and do not encompass the cerebral hemispheres bilaterally. Clinical manifestations depend on the part of the brain involved in the seizure discharge. As with single seizures, partial SE may be classified as simple or complex. In simple partial SE, there is no alteration of consciousness; in complex partial SE (CPSE), consciousness is disturbed.

Simple Partial Status Epilepticus

When a focal epileptogenic process has a restricted cortical topography and does not disturb cerebral function widely by distant projected effects, consciousness may not be altered, even with the continuous seizure activity of SE. This is termed *simple partial SE*.

Focal motor SE consists of repetitive clonic jerking of the face or arm and less frequently the leg, without disturbed sensorium. Repetitive clonic jerking that lasts for more than 30 minutes is termed *focal motor SE*; repetitive clonic jerking that continues for more than 24 hours is termed *epilepsia partialis continua* (EPC). The EEG usually shows focal slow waves or sporadic spikes over the contralateral rolandic area. Typical ictal EEG rhythmic repetitive spike discharges rarely occur, however, even during clinical seizures. Presumably this is because the epileptogenic focus occupies a small region of cortex and is spatially oriented such that the electrical field of the ictal discharges is not well detected by scalp surface EEG electrodes.

EPC occurs in two clinical settings. It may occur in any age group because of symptomatic structural lesions in the rolandic cortical area. In these cases, the clinical picture is one of focal motor SE refractory to antiepileptic medication treatment in conjunction with the neurologic disease expected from the underlying lesion. The other unique clinical setting is EPC in children, which is associated with focal inflammation of the cortex contralaterally. In these children, the seizures of EPC progressively spread unilaterally to involve the face, arm, and leg slowly over years. There is associated development of hemiparesis and atrophy on that side of the body, with cognitive decline.[21] Although this condition predictably is resistant to antiepileptic medications, a remarkable recovery may follow neurosurgical treatment with functional hemispherectomy.

Other types of simple partial SE occur, depending on the area of the brain involved in the seizure. For example, we described global aphasia as the sole manifestation of simple partial SE in a patient with a left temporal brain tumor.[22] Language function normalized when the SE was terminated by intravenous diazepam.

Complex Partial Status Epilepticus

In CPSE, repeated complex partial seizures occur without recovery of a normal level of consciousness and cognitive functions between attacks. Clinically, this is manifest as a confusional state that may be difficult to differentiate from any other cause of encephalopathy. Certain features, however, may be distinctive and suggest the diagnosis. Most important is clinical cycling in and out of discrete complex partial seizures, with a postictal state between attacks. Thus, periods of unresponsive blank staring with oral-alimentary automatisms alternate with periods of normal or mildly impaired responsiveness. On EEG monitoring, ictal patterns of rapidly repetitive focal spiking are seen during the complex partial seizures, and focal or generalized slowing is seen during the interictal periods. A history of localization-related epilepsy with sporadic complex partial seizures often can be obtained. If there is an acute onset of CPSE and no previous history of chronic epilepsy, herpes simplex encephalitis should be considered in the differential diagnosis. This cyclic pattern of CPSE suggests an underlying temporal lobe epileptogenic process.[21]

Noncyclic, continuous CPSE is thought to suggest an underlying frontal lobe epileptogenic process.[21] Temporal lobe CPSE also needs to be contrasted with GNSE. Both cause a confusional state. Automatisms are more prominent in temporal lobe SE. Cycling in and out of discrete seizures occurs in temporal lobe SE, whereas a more invariant encephalopathy characterizes GNSE. On EEG, temporal lobe SE consists of intermittent repeated discrete focal seizures, whereas GNSE is associated with a continuous generalized electrographic ictal discharge.

Outcome of Status Epilepticus

The outcome of SE is reviewed here before discussing treatment because some controversy exists about the outcome of SE, and our concepts concerning outcome have a significant impact on treatment strategies. Most work with human patients suggests that outcome, particularly mortality, is determined by underlying neurologic or medical disease. In contrast, experimental evidence suggests the abnormal excessive electrical activity of SE per se may produce irreversible neuronal damage.

Human Studies

In separate reviews, Hauser[3] and Leppik[23] concluded that the most significant influence on mortality in patients with SE is the underlying neurologic or medical condition. Their assessment of reported SE mortality before 1960 put the death rate at 50%, but they report recent estimates of mortality less than 1%. Mortality rates for several large series of SE cases ranged from 3% to 43%.[24–30] When cases in these series are divided into those with remote or cryptogenic causes for seizures and those with acute symptomatic causes, it can be seen that the mortality rate is much higher in the patients with acute symptomatic seizures. In the prospectively acquired series by Maytal et al.,[28] all deaths occurred in the acute symptomatic group.

We reviewed outcome in 46 patients who developed SE while already hospitalized for a condition other than epilepsy.[31] Mortality in this select group of patients was high (65%). Mortality was not associated with the duration of SE but was determined by the underlying neurologic or systemic process. Lowenstein and Aminoff[8] noted a mortality rate of 55% in their series of patients who were comatose but had electrographic SE. All deaths in that series were attributed to the underlying process. In two series of patients with status myoclonus after cardiac arrest, all died of the underlying process.[12, 32] In a study of prognostic factors for outcome after pentobarbital coma for severe SE, Yaffe and Lowenstein[33] found multiorgan failure to be present before the onset of SE in seven of their nine patients who died, but multiorgan failure was not seen in any of their eight SE survivors. We reported on two patients in generalized convulsive SE or iatrogenic coma treatment for 26 and 56 days.[34] Neither patient had underlying major neurologic or systemic disease, and both survived (with incomplete neurologic recoveries).

On the other hand, several human studies do suggest that SE itself causes brain damage. The most valid data to support this point are from patients who develop new neurologic deficits related to brain regions documented to be focally involved in an episode of partial SE. Surprisingly, few such cases have been reported. Permanent memory deficits have been reported after CPSE.[21, 35] A visual field deficit was noted after occipital lobe SE.[36] We have cared for a 40-year-old woman who developed a permanent right hemiparesis after partial SE of left frontal lobe origin. Electrographically, seizures consisted of repetitive spikes at the FP1 and FPZ electrodes and clinically were manifest by speech arrest, right facial twitching, right arm extension, left arm flexion, head rotation to the right, and clonic movement of the right foot.[37] In general, however, reports of permanent brain damage from partial SE are rare. Also, contradictory clinical reports can be found. For example, Roberts and Humphrey[38] described a patient in CPSE for 202 days who recovered to a normal state.

Experimental Models of Status Epilepticus

During the last several decades, different experimental models of SE have suggested that prolonged excessive neuronal excitation itself produces nerve cell injury and death. Epstein and O'Connor[39] found that 12 of 12 cats put into SE for 4 hours but well maintained with artificial ventilation and perfusion died within 48 hours of the SE. In eight artificially ventilated baboons put into SE lasting as short as 3 hours, ischemic neuronal damage was seen microscopically in the neocortex, thalamus, and hippocampus.[40] Chapman et al.[41] demonstrated free fatty acid accumulation in the brains of well-ventilated rats in biculline-induced SE lasting 30–60 minutes; free fatty acids may elicit cell damage by undergoing oxidative breakdown. Necrosis of the brain stem, basal ganglia, and cortical neurons was induced in well-oxygenated rats by florothyl-induced SE lasting 30–120 minutes.[42] Excitatory cell death from N-methyl-D-aspartate receptor activation and subsequent calcium influx into the neuron may contribute to the production of brain damage by SE.[5] In the future, neuroprotective agents may be used to prevent brain damage from SE.

Treatment of Status Epilepticus

As for any medical emergency, treatment of SE proceeds through rapid assessment and diagnosis based on the history and physical examination, immediate attainment of any critical laboratory studies, institution of therapy, and reassessment and further planning based on early treatment and testing results. Several formal, structured treatment protocols for SE have been published.[2, 5, 21, 23, 43, 44] Some authors believe that such treatment protocols should emphasize a time frame that the interventions should follow.[23, 43, 44]

It is at this point that interpretation of the SE outcome data becomes critical. All workers in this field agree that generalized convulsive SE constitutes a medical emergency with associated mortality. All agree generalized convulsive SE should be treated rapidly and aggressively, even if the treatment itself carries significant risks. The best approach to the treatment of partial SE and GNSE is less clearly defined. Some authors state partial SE causes brain damage and should be treated as aggressively as generalized convulsive SE.[5, 43] This treatment includes high-dose intravenous antiepileptic drugs (AEDs), which carry serious risks of cardiovascular and central nervous system depression; intubation as necessary to artificially support ventilation and general anesthesia if other measures fail. As discussed above, however, definite examples of partial SE producing brain damage are limited to a handful of cases, even though in 1987, Delgado-Escueta and Treiman[21] found more than 100 cases of psychomotor status documented in the literature in the preceding 25 years and believed the condition no longer should be considered rare. A reasonable approach to the treatment of partial SE and GNSE might be using the same protocol as for generalized convulsive SE (see below) but incrementing AED dosing upward more slowly over 24 hours as suggested by Delgado-Escueta and Treiman.[21] Under these circumstances, the goal in mind is the termination of partial SE without incurring the depressant effects of rapid intravenous administration of sedative drugs and without resorting to iatrogenic coma. If after 24 hours partial SE persists, the patient then should be entered into the generalized convulsive SE protocol.

A proposed treatment protocol for generalized convulsive SE is presented in Table 12-5. It should take no longer than 10 minutes to assess the patient clinically, draw samples for appropriate initial blood tests, establish the intravenous line, and begin treatment.[23, 43, 44] Although difficult at times with a critically ill unstable patient, the search for one of the underlying causes of SE as listed in Table 12-3 should not be ignored, despite the attention focused on terminating the ongoing seizures.

Glucose is administered to rapidly reverse hypoglycemia, in case that is present and causative. Thiamine should be administered to prevent the precipitation of Wernicke-Korsakoff syndrome by the administration of 50% glucose. Several points regarding Table 12-5 and SE treatment in general require further comment.

Lorazepam

Lorazepam is a newer benzodiazepine than diazepam and has proved useful in the initial treatment of SE. The antiepileptic effects of

Table 12-5. Treatment Protocol for Generalized Convulsive Status Epilepticus

---

1. Assess vital signs and institute emergency treatment to maintain blood pressure and ventilation as indicated.

2. Make a diagnosis of generalized convulsive SE by history, physical examination, and observation of at least one seizure. SE occurring in the field may end before the patient arrives in the emergency department.

3. Insert an intravenous catheter and establish an infusion of normal saline solution. While placing the catheter, obtain blood samples to determine serum electrolytes levels, blood counts, and AED levels.

4. Intravenously infuse 100 mg thiamine and 50 ml 50% glucose.

5. Administer intravenous diazepam at a maximum rate of 2 mg/min up to 20 mg total or intravenous lorazepam, 0.1 mg/kg, at a maximum rate of 2 mg/min until seizures stop.

6. At this point, if bacterial meningitis is seriously considered in the differential diagnosis, perform a lumbar puncture and a cerebrospinal fluid analysis, and start appropriate antibiotics.

7. Administer intravenous phenytoin, 20 mg/kg, at a rate no faster than 50 mg/min. Monitor blood pressure closely, and if hypotension develops, give intravenous fluids and slow the phenytoin infusion rate.

8. If SE persists, intubate the patient and provide artificial ventilation.

9. Administer intravenous phenobarbital, 20 mg/kg, at a maximum rate of 100 mg/min.

10. When convulsive activity ceases, perform an EEG to assess for ongoing electrographic seizure activity; if present, institute iatrogenic coma with intravenous pentobarbital or lorazepam. Continuous EEG monitoring is needed for iatrogenic coma.

11. If convulsive SE persists, institute continuous EEG monitoring and iatrogenic coma.

12. Administer pentobarbital or lorazepam.

    a. Pentobarbital: Give intravenous pentobarbital loading dose, 5 mg/kg, and institute a continuous infusion of pentobarbital at a rate of 1 mg/kg/hr. Monitor EEG and increase pentobarbital infusion rate until seizures stop. Monitor blood pressure closely, preferably with an intra-arterial pressure transducer. Administer intravenous fluids, vasopressor agents, or both, as indicated.

    b. Lorazepam: Give intravenous lorazepam at 1 mg/hr. Monitor EEG and increase lorazepam delivery rate in increments of 1 mg/hr until seizures stop.

13. Determine blood levels of phenytoin and phenobarbital and establish a standing-dose administration schedule to maintain these levels high.

14. Perform studies such as a computed tomographic scan to determine the underlying process as indicated.

15. Maintain seizure-free on pentobarbital or lorazepam for 24 hours.

16. Titrate pentobarbital or lorazepam infusion rate down and discontinue gradually over 24 hours. Observe for recurrent SE, reinstitute pentobarbital or lorazepam if necessary for another 24 hours.

17. If seizures persist, administer standing dose of carbamazepine via NGT, valproate via NGT or PR, lidocaine,[50] or propofol.[51]

AED = antiepileptic drug; EEG = electroencephalogram; PR = per rectum; NGT = nasogastric tube; SE = status epilepticus.

lorazepam last up to 24 hours, whereas diazepam's effects last 15–30 minutes.[5] In several clinical series, lorazepam has been shown to be effective in the acute termination of SE,[45–48] and the longer effective period after an intravenous dose allows less urgency in the addition of a second agent, such as phenytoin.

Phenytoin

The diluent in which phenytoin for intravenous infusion is prepared is propylene glycol. Propylene glycol is a hypotensive agent that limits the intravenous infusion rate of phenytoin to 50 mg/minute. Phenytoin itself may cause cardiac dysrhythmias, but typically this occurs with very high blood levels of the drug, such as are seen with overdoses in suicide attempts, and not in the setting of controlled medical treatment for SE.[49] Phenytoin tends to be more effective against a generalized epileptogenic process than against focal epileptogenic processes. Thus, if generalized tonic-clonic SE persists despite maximal doses of phenytoin, an acute focal structural lesion should be suspected as causing the secondarily generalized SE.[5]

Intractable Status Epilepticus

Over the years, a variety of agents have been used to treat refractory SE not terminated by high doses of phenytoin and phenobarbital. Agents used included intravenous lidocaine, paraldehyde, thiopentone, and propofol; rectal valproate syrup; and inhalation anesthesia.[2, 21, 23, 50, 51] Pentobarbital coma produced as outlined in Table 12-5 has been widely used. A major difficulty with pentobarbital is induction of systemic hypotension at therapeutic doses, which occurs in the majority of treated patients.[33, 52–54] To avoid this complication, we have used a continuous intravenous infusion of lorazepam to induce coma for refractory SE.[55] This has been effective without producing hypotension. Kumar and Bleck[56] reported success in the treatment of four patients with refractory SE with a continuous intravenous infusion of midazolam, a short-acting, water-soluble benzodiazepine.

No systematic study and only a few case reports describe treatment strategies and outcome in patients with prolonged SE that continues to recur despite repeated coma inductions with pentobarbital and maximal phenytoin and phenobarbital blood levels.[34, 38, 57] Carbamazepine or valproate liquids may be administered via nasogastric tube. This may be ineffective, however, because of poor absorption of these AEDs as a result of impaired gastrointestinal motility in the presence of high-dose pentobarbital. A valproate formulation for intravenous injection is under development.[23] Valproate syrup may be administered rectally, but absorption is slow.[58] Massive doses of phenobarbital may be administered to produce blood levels of more than 60 μg/ml.[57]

Generalized Nonconvulsive Status Epilepticus

When SE has been successfully terminated, consideration of chronic AED treatment needs to be undertaken. Indications, approaches, and complications of the medical management of seizures in general are reviewed elsewhere in this volume. A brief comment about follow-up treatment for GNSE in adults is in order, however.

GNSE in adults typically recurs several times during a patient's life span. With this low recurrence rate, the efficacy of any AED in preventing relapses is difficult to demonstrate. If only absences and no convulsive seizures are present, ethosuximide may be used. If both absences and grand mal seizures are present, valproate should be substituted, or phenytoin or phenobarbital may be added. Surprisingly, phenytoin or phenobarbital alone appears effective in preventing the recurrence of GNSE in adults but is not effective in the treatment of absence seizures in children.[2]

Intermittent Home Treatment of Status Epilepticus

Lombroso[59] reviewed his experience at Boston Children's Hospital in the use of diazepam for intermittent home treatment of SE. The drug is supplied to patients' families in the commercially prepared 2-ml ampules of diazepam for injection. Administration is rectally or orally with a tuberculin or insulin syringe to measure the dose accurately. Rectal administration in control subjects produces therapeutic blood levels in 5 minutes, which are sustained for 6 hours. Peak diazepam blood levels are reached in 7 minutes. Patients with clusters of seizures, prolonged seizures, or repeated bouts of SE were treated; patients included 43 children, 22 adolescents, and 11 adults. In children younger than 5 years of age, the dose was 0.5 mg/kg; for those 6–12 years of age, the dose was 0.3 mg/kg; for those older than 12 years of age, the dose was 0.2 mg/kg. The duration of seizures for the 2-year baseline period before implementation of the intermittent home treatment was compared with the duration of seizures during a 2-year trial of this experimental approach. During the baseline phase, 1.5% of seizures lasted 6–10 minutes, and 75.6% of seizures lasted more than 30 minutes. During the experimental treatment phase, 52.8% of seizures lasted 6–10 minutes, and 3.5% of seizures lasted more than 30 minutes. Thus, intermittent home treatment with rectal diazepam may be used effectively to prevent the evolution of a sporadic single seizure into SE. This approach is appropriate only when SE predictably recurs on a regular basis.

References

1. Commission on Classification. Proposal for revised clinical and EEG classification of epileptic seizures. Epilepsia 1981;22:489.
2. Rothner D, Morris H. Generalized Status Epilepticus. In H Luders, R Lesser (eds), Epilepsy: Electroclinical Syndromes. New York: Springer-Verlag, 1987;207.
3. Hauser W. Status epilepticus: epidemiological considerations. Neurology 1990;40(Suppl):9.
4. DeLorenzo R, Pellock J, Towne A, Boggs J. Epidemiology of status epilepticus. J Clin Neurophysiol 1995;12:316.
5. Treiman D. Status Epilepticus. In S Resor, H Kutt (eds), The Medical Treatment of Epilepsy. New York: Marcel Dekker, 1992;183.
6. Treiman D. A progressive sequence of EEG changes during generalized convulsive status epilepticus. Epilepsy Res 1990;5:49.
7. Treiman D. Electroclinical features of status epilepticus. J Clin Neurophysiol 1995;12:343.
8. Lowenstein D, Aminoff M. Clinical and EEG features of status epilepticus in comatose patients. Neurology 1992;42:100.
9. So E, Ruggles K, Ahmann P, et al. Clinical significance and outcome of subclinical status epilepticus in adults. J Epilepsy 1995;8:11.

10. Maytal J, Shinnar S. Febrile status epilepticus. Pediatrics 1990;86:611.
11. Tassinari C, Gastaut H, Dravet C, Roger J. A paradoxical effect: status epilepticus induced by benzodiazepines. Electroencephalogr Clin Neurophysiol 1971;31:182.
12. Wijdicks E, Parisi J, Sharbrough F. Prognostic value of myoclonus status in comatose survivors of cardiac arrest. Ann Neurol 1994;35:239.
13. Guberman A, Cantu-Reyna G, Stuss D, Broughton R. Nonconvulsive generalized status epilepticus. Neurology 1986;36:1284.
14. Varma N, Lee S. Nonconvulsive status epilepticus following electroconvulsive therapy. Neurology 1992;42:263.
15. Thomas P, Beaumanoir A, Genton P, et al. 'De novo' absence status of late onset. Neurology 1992;42:104.
16. Wong M, Suite N, Labar D. Nonconvulsive status epilepticus in the acquired immunodeficiency syndrome. Ann Intern Med 1992;116:171.
17. Zak R, Solomon G, Petito F, Labar D. Baclofen-induced generalized nonconvulsive status epilepticus. Ann Neurol 1994;36:113.
18. Jackson G, Berkovic S. Ceftazidine encephalopathy: absence status and toxic hallucination. Lancet 1992;340:333.
19. Wengs W, Talwar D, Bernard J. Ifosfamide-induced nonconvulsive status epilepticus. Arch Neurol 1993;50:1104.
20. Granner M, Lee S. Nonconvulsive status epilepticus: EEG analysis in a large series. Epilepsia 1994;35:42.
21. Delgado-Escueta A, Treiman D. Focal Status Epilepticus: Modern Concepts. In H Luders, R Lesser (eds), Epilepsy: Electroclinical Syndromes. New York: Springer-Verlag, 1987;347.
22. Wells C, Solomon G, Labar D. Aphasia as the sole manifestation of simple partial status epilepticus. Epilepsia 1992;33:84.
23. Leppik I. Status epilepticus: the next decade. Neurology 1990;40(Suppl):4.
24. Oxbury J, Whitty C. Causes and consequences of status epilepticus in adults. Brain 1971;94:733.
25. Aicardi J, Chevrie J. Consequences of Status Epilepticus in Infants and Children. In A Delgado-Escueta, C Wasterlain, D Treiman, R Porter (eds), Advances in Neurology, Vol. 34: Status Epilepticus. New York: Raven, 1983;115.
26. Celesia G. Prognosis in Convulsive Status Epilepticus. In A Delgado-Escueta, C Wasterlain, D Treiman, R Porter (eds), Advances in Neurology, Vol. 34: Status Epilepticus. New York: Raven, 1983;55.
27. Phillips S, Shanahan R. Etiology and mortality of status epilepticus in children. Arch Neurol 1989;46:74.
28. Maytal J, Shinnar S, Moshe S, Alvarez L. Low morbidity and mortality in status epilepticus in children. Pediatrics 1989;83:323.
29. Towne A, Pellock J, Ko D, DeLorenzo R. Determinants of mortality in status epilepticus. Epilepsia 1994;35:27.
30. Scholtes F, Renier W, Meinardi H. Generalized convulsive status epilepticus: causes, therapy, and outcome in 346 patients. Epilepsia 1994;35:1104.
31. French J, Labar D, Pedley T, Rowan A. Status epilepticus onset among hospitalized patients [abstract]. Epilepsia 1988;29:704.
32. Young G, Gilbert J, Zochodne D. The significance of myoclonic status epilepticus in postanoxic coma. Neurology 1990;40:1843.

33. Yaffe K, Lowenstein D. Prognostic factors of pentobarbital therapy for refractory generalized status epilepticus. Neurology 1993;43:895.
34. Labar D, Coll R, Solomon G. Intractable status epilepticus. J Epilepsy 1993;6:170.
35. Engel J, Ludwig B, Fettel M. Prolonged partial complex status epilepticus: EEG and behavioral observations. Neurology 1978;28:863.
36. Engel J, Kuhl D, Phelps M, et al. Local cerebral metabolism during partial seizures. Neurology 1983;33:400.
37. Borchert L, Labar D. Permanent hemiparesis due to partial status epilepticus. Neurology 1995;45:187.
38. Roberts M, Humphrey P. Prolonged complex partial status epilepticus. J Neurol Neurosurg Psychiatry 1988;51:586.
39. Epstein M, O'Connor J. Destructive effects of prolonged status epilepticus. J Neurol Neurosurg Psychiatry 1966;29:251.
40. Meldrum B, Vigouroux R, Brierley J. Systemic factors and epileptic brain damage. Arch Neurol 1973;29:82.
41. Chapman A, Ingvar M, Siesjo B. Free fatty acids in the brain in biculline-induced status epilepticus. Acta Physiol Scand 1980;110:335.
42. Nevander G, Ingvar M, Auer R, Siesjo B. Status epilepticus in well-oxygenated rats causes neuronal necrosis. Ann Neurol 1985;18:281.
43. Delgado-Escueta A, Wasterlain C, Treiman D, Porter R. Status Epilepticus: Summary. In A Delgado-Escueta, C Wasterlain, D Treiman, R Porter (eds), Advances in Neurology, Vol. 34: Status Epilepticus. New York: Raven, 1983;537–541.
44. Working Group on SE. Treatment of convulsive status epilepticus. JAMA 1993;270:854.
45. Crawford T, Mitchell W, Shodgrass S. Lorazepam in childhood status epilepticus and serial seizures. Neurology 1987;37:190.
46. Leppik I, Derivan A, Homan R, et al. Double-blind study of lorazepam and diazepam in status epilepticus. JAMA 1983;249:1452.
47. Levy R, Krall R. Treatment of status epilepticus with lorazepam. Arch Neurol 1984;41:605.
48. Walker J, Homan R, Vasko M, et al. Lorazepam in status epilepticus. Ann Neurol 1979;6:207.
49. Labar D. Antiepileptic Drug Toxic Emergencies. In S Resor, H Kutt (eds), The Medical Treatment of Epilepsy. New York: Marcel Dekker, 1992;573.
50. De Giorgio C, Altman K, Hamilton-Byrd E, Rabinowicz A. Lidocaine in refractory status epilepticus: confirmation of efficacy with continuous EEG monitoring. Epilepsia 1992;33:913.
51. Borgeat A, Wilder-Smith O, Jallon P, Suter P. Propofol in the management of refractory status epilepticus: a case report. Intensive Care Med 1994;20:148.
52. Lowenstein D, Aminoff M, Simon R. Barbiturate anesthesia in the treatment of status epilepticus. Neurology 1988;38:395.
53. Osorio I, Reed R. Treatment of refractory generalized tonic-clonic status epilepticus with pentobarbital anesthesia after high-dose phenytoin. Epilepsia 1989;30:464.
54. Rashkin M, Young C, Penovich P. Pentobarbital treatment of refractory status epilepticus. Neurology 1987;37:500.

55. Labar D, Ali A, Root J. High-dose intravenous lorazepam for the treatment of refractory status epilepticus. Neurology 1994;44:1400.
56. Kumar A, Bleck T. Intravenous midazolam for the treatment of refractory status epilepticus. Crit Care Med 1992;20:483.
57. Drury I, Beydoun A. Prolonged convulsive status epilepticus refractory to pentobarbital [abstract]. Epilepsia 1989;30:638.
58. Thorpy M. Rectal valproate syrup and status epilepticus. Neurology 1980;30:1113.
59. Lombroso C. Intermittent home treatment of status and clusters of seizures. Epilepsia 1989;30(Suppl):S11.

13

Anticonvulsant Toxicity

Sudhansu Chokroverty

Introduction

The adverse reactions of antiepileptic drugs (AEDs) continue to remain serious disadvantages in the treatment of patients with epilepsy.[1] The first antiepileptic drug, bromide, was discovered in 1857. Fifty-five years later, phenobarbital (PB), and another 25 years later, phenytoin (PHT) were found to possess effective anticonvulsant properties but not without serious side effects. Continued efforts to find highly efficacious AEDs with little or no side effects resulted in the introduction of a number of AEDs over the years. Some of these have stood the test of time, whereas others have been discarded because of serious adverse reactions. Four promising new AEDs underwent extensive clinical trials for several years, and three of them (felbamate, gabapentin, and lamotrigine) were approved by the Food and Drug Administration for general use in United States between 1993 and 1995. These newer AEDs are thought to have less serious side effects (see Chapter 18), but the extent of their efficacy and their adverse reactions remain to be determined by further use in a larger number of epileptics over a longer period of time.

The clinical toxic effects of the first- and second-line AEDs are described in this chapter. The third-line drugs have the least therapeutic efficacy, display major toxicity, and are rarely used currently (see Chapter 18 for a classification of AEDs). The adverse reactions associated with the first- and second-line AEDs are discussed according to the following categories:[1-4]

Dose-related general adverse effects.

Idiosyncratic or hypersensitivity reactions.

Chronic cumulative effects that are associated with long-standing use and that are not necessarily dose-related.

Specific effects of AEDs, some of which may be dose-related and some of which are not.

Teratogenic effects that are not necessarily dose-related but that definitely increase in incidence with polytherapy.

Drug interactions that may occur not only among the various AEDs but also between AEDs and non-AEDs. Indirectly these interactions cause adverse effects. For drug interactions see Chapters 4, 18, and 19.

Miscellaneous adverse reactions.

General Adverse Effects

Dose-related adverse reactions can be decreased or eliminated by reducing the dose or can be prevented by gradually increasing the dose of AEDs. Some of the effects may be selective for a particular AED. Most of the dose-related side effects produce neurotoxicity as well as oral and gastrointestinal manifestations.

Drowsiness

Toxic doses of all AEDs may produce somnolence, lethargy, and impaired cognition. In the initial stage of treatment, all of the AEDs except PHT may cause drowsiness, which generally decreases or disappears within a few weeks. This symptom is particularly troublesome with PB and primidone (PR); hence these drugs are best administered at bedtime to avoid daytime somnolence. Some patients may have chronic drowsiness, lethargy, and fatigue as a result of high normal or higher than the therapeutic drug levels. PB may sometimes cause dose-related irritability and other behavioral changes associated with somnolence that disappear on dose reduction. PHT may cause drowsiness at a drug level of 40 µg/ml.[5] Somnolence is also a troublesome side effect of clonazepam (CNZ).

Acute Vestibulocerebellar Dysfunction

Of all the AEDs, PHT is mostly associated with acute vestibulocerebellar dysfunction. It occurs before drowsiness or alterations of other brain functions. A linear relationship has been noted between serum PHT level and vestibulocerebellar dysfunction. Nystagmus, which manifests initially in the horizontal and later in the vertical directions, is noted as the drug level increases. Generally, horizontal nystagmus occurs at a drug level of about 20 µg/ml, and ataxia of gait occurs at a level of about 30 µg/ml.[5] PB, PR, carbamazepine (CBZ), and CNZ may also cause vestibulocerebellar dysfunction.

Visual and Eye Movement Disorders

CBZ may cause various eye movement disorders and visual symptoms. Reducing the dose of the medication will decrease the symptoms. Diplopia has been noted with PHT, PR, and CNZ. PHT and CBZ may cause transient ophthalmoplegia.

Encephalopathy

PHT encephalopathy[6] is a reversible neurologic syndrome usually associated with high serum PHT levels (50–100 µg/ml) in patients on chronic PHT treatment but sometimes may occur at therapeutic levels. The encephalopathy is manifested by an insidious decline of intellectual function; drowsiness; ataxia; nystagmus; involuntary movements; elevated cerebrospinal fluid protein levels with pleocytosis; increasing frequency of seizures and diffuse electroencephalographic (EEG) abnormalities; and sometimes focal signs such as hemiparesis, hemisensory defects, or hemianopia. When PHT is stopped or is replaced with another AED, these manifestations generally disappear.

An overdose of CBZ may also cause an acute encephalopathy characterized by increasing seizures, respiratory depression, nystagmus, myoclonus, other orofacial dyskinesias, ophthalmoplegia, ataxia, and later coma.[7] An overdose of PB, PR, or CNZ may cause a similar encephalopathic picture characterized by stupor, respiratory depression, and coma. An acute encephalopathy[8] has also been described when the dose of valproate or valproic acid (VPA) is increased.

Movement Disorders

Several dose-related involuntary movement disorders such as chorea, choreoathetosis, tics, other orofacial dyskinesias, dystonia, ballism, myoclonus, and asterixis have been noted in patients treated with PHT, CBZ, VPA, and ethosuximide (ETS).[1] The hyperkinetic syndromes have been most frequently noted with PHT[9] and in those with pre-existing brain damage or encephalopathy. Asterixis has also been noted with PB and PR. There is no clear relationship between VPA-induced asterixis and blood ammonia level. Akathisia was reported in three patients taking CBZ.[10]

In about 10% of patients taking VPA, postural action tremors similar to essential tremors occur as the dose is increased.[11] Treatment consists of a dose reduction of VPA, the administration of propranolol,[11] or both.

Sleep Disorders After Acute or Short-Term Use of Antiepileptic Drugs

Sleep architecture is often disrupted by anticonvulsants.[12] Sometimes it is difficult to know if the anticonvulsants or the repeated seizures are responsible for sleep disturbances.

A reduction of rapid eye movement (REM) and non–REM stages III and IV and an increase of stage II non–REM sleep have been noted after an acute exposure to anticonvulsants.

There is a lack of well-controlled studies to document the effects of anticonvulsant medications on the sleep architecture separating the effects of seizures and sleep. A sleep study by Touchon et al.[13] of patients with partial complex seizures on CBZ treatment showed an increasing number of awakenings and decreased sleep efficiency. In a later prospective study before and one month after CBZ treatment, these same authors[13] noted an improvement in sleep architecture, however, and they concluded that the abnormal sleep structure may have been related to the seizure itself. Wolf et al.[14] noted a reduction in REM sleep as well as total awake time and an increase in non–REM stage II sleep after short-term use of barbiturates. The short-term effects of PHT included a decrease in non–REM sleep stages I and II and an increase in sleep stages III and IV; however, REM sleep remained unaltered. No relationship between the serum drug levels and the sleep architectural changes was noted.

Oral and Gastrointestinal Manifestations

Mild dose-related alimentary disturbances are noted with CBZ, PB, PR, CNZ, and ETS at the initiation of treatment. These disturbances can be minimized by gradually increasing the dose of the medication.[1] Anorexia, nausea, vomiting, and abdominal discomfort are noted as dose-related effects in patients taking VPA; these symptoms may be minimized by ingesting the drug with or after meals.[15] Both central and local mechanisms are responsible for these effects.

Idiosyncratic Reactions

Idiosyncratic reactions are not dose-related but usually occur within the first 6 months of initiation. Reactions are, for the most part, related to dermatologic, hematologic, hepatic, pancreatic, and renal toxicity.

Hematologic Effects

Megaloblastic anemia with macrocytosis associated with folate deficiency has been noted occasionally with PHT, PB, and PR.[17] Idiosyncratic hematologic toxic effects have rarely been noted with all AEDs.[17] The rare occurrence of leukopenia or myeloid hypoplasia has been noted with PHT.[1, 6, 18] Similarly, PB, PR, ETS, and CNZ may on rare occasions cause leukopenia, pancytopenia, and aplastic anemia.[1, 18] In contrast to some early reports, more recent studies show that serious hematopoietic toxicity with CBZ is not common.[1, 7] In the beginning of treatment with CBZ, transient leukopenia of 2,500–3,000 cells/µl occurs in about 10% of patients, but the number of leukocytes returns to the normal level without any change in the dosage or in the drug itself.[1, 7, 18] If, however, the leukocyte count falls below 2,500 cells/µl, the drug should be discontinued. Rarely, idiosyncratic agranulocytosis has been noted with CBZ. Careful monitoring (e.g., for sore throat, bruising, or overt bleeding) is the best way to avert fatal bone marrow suppression.[18]

Infrequently, thrombocytopenia, bleeding, and inhibition of platelet aggregation have been reported as idiosyncratic reactions to VPA.[19] Sandler et al.[20] ascribed these to an IgM platelet antibody formation.

In infants born to mothers taking PHT or PB, neonatal coagulation defect and bleeding resulting from a vitamin K deficiency have been described.[1, 21] Therefore, vitamin K therapy should be given to these women for 1 to 2 weeks before delivery and to the infants immediately after birth.

Dermatologic Effects

Most AEDs occasionally cause skin rashes, but the highest incidence has been noted with PHT and CBZ.[1, 6, 7] These are usually hypersensitive reactions and may be associated with fever, eosinophilia, lymphadenopathy, and hepatitis; rarely, hypersensitive reactions may be associated with exfoliative dermatitis, Stevens-Johnson syndrome, and erythema multiforme exudativum. These hypersensitive reactions are usually described with PHT, but occasionally such reactions may occur with CBZ. PB-associated skin rashes are uncommon and may present as punctate erythema or macular rashes and rarely may cause exfoliative dermatitis. Skin rashes from VPA and CNZ are unusual. Rarely, PHT-induced toxic epidermal necrolysis resembling scalding of the skin (Lyell's syndrome) has been described as an idiosyncratic reaction with a high mortality.[22]

Pancreatitis and Effects of Hepatic Toxicity

PHT, PB, and CBZ may cause hepatic enzyme induction without any clinically obvious adverse effects.[1, 6, 7] Rarely these drugs may, however, cause acute hepatic failure. A transient hepatic dysfunction characterized by a rise of serum aspartate aminotransferase (AST), alanine aminotransferase (ALT), and alkaline phosphatase levels may occur with PHT. Sometimes a more severe type of PHT-induced hepatic dysfunction, mostly in adolescents and young adults and characterized by hepatic necrosis and jaundice, has been described.[1, 6]

In about 10% of patients on VPA therapy, transient elevation of serum aminotransferase levels without signs and symptoms of hepatic failure is seen.[15, 18, 23] The most serious effect of VPA treatment, although rare, is hepatic failure associated with hyperammonemia, which has been fatal in some patients.[15, 18, 23] This has been noted mostly within 6 months of onset of treatment. A retrospective analysis of the data between 1984 and 1986 by Dreifuss et al.[24] listed an overall incidence of hepatic failure of 1 in 10,000. Children younger than 2 years of age with neurologic dysfunction and on polypharmacy showed an incidence of hepatic fatality of 1 in 500. For patients on VPA monotherapy, the incidence of hepatic fatality in all ages was 1 in 37,000. The risk of hepatotoxicity decreases with age, however. Occasionally, patients on both VPA and aspirin have developed a Reyes-like syndrome.[18] There is a recent report of eight new fatalities from severe hepatotoxicity during valproate therapy.[25]

An acute fatal hemorrhagic pancreatitis has been described as a rare complication of VPA treatment.[1, 26, 27] Most of the cases have been described in children, and clinical monitoring is essential. In patients who develop severe abdominal pain and nausea, this diagnosis should be considered, and serum amylase and lipase levels should be obtained in these patients.

Nephrotoxicity

AEDs may rarely cause nephrotoxicity as part of a severe hypersensitivity reaction. There have been occasional reports of nephritis and reversible renal failure after PHT and CBZ treatment.[1, 6, 7]

Lymphoid Tissue Effects

In a few patients, the occurrence of a pseudolymphoma syndrome within a few weeks of PHT treatment has been described.[1, 6] This syndrome is manifested by painless generalized lymphadenopathy with or without skin rashes and eosinophilia. These features disappear within weeks after cessation of PHT treatment. Rarely, malignant lymphoma and acute leukemia have been reported in patients taking PHT.[1, 6]

Chronic Cumulative Effects

Chronic cumulative effects are associated with a long-standing use of AEDs and are not necessarily dose-related.

Neuromuscular Effects

In many patients on long-term PHT treatment, bilateral distal polyneuropathy, particularly affecting the legs, has been described.[6, 28, 29] This is mostly related to the duration of treatment and is characterized by impaired reflexes and slowing of nerve conduction velocity rather than by overt clinical polyneuropathy. This neuropathy is not related to subnormal serum folate levels, which may be noted in many patients on chronic PHT treatment. Occasionally, chronic CBZ treatment may be associated with mild peripheral neuropathy.[7] PHT, on rare occasions, may cause a myasthenia-like state or may uncover latent myasthenia gravis because of its neuromuscular blocking effect.[29] Lipid storage myopathy associated with carnitine deficiency may occur in patients taking VPA.[30]

Cognitive Impairment and Behavioral Disturbances

Pseudodementia and other cognitive and intellectual impairment associated with behavioral disturbances have been noted with some AEDs as chronic cumulative effects.[1, 6, 18] PB and PR may cause cognitive impairment that is manifested by a lack of attention, an impairment of calculation, and a decline in school performance in children. Quantitative psychometric tests may detect this cognitive impairment. Sometimes paradoxical effects such as hyperkinetic and hyperexcitable syndrome in children, agitation, and confusion in the elderly patients have been noted. PHT may also be associated with pseudodementia and mild impairment of cognitive function.

ETS psychosis[31] consisting of delusions, hallucinations, anxiety, and depersonalization has been described in some patients. These manifestations usually are noted in adolescent patients with a prior history of psychiatric disturbances. If such episodes occur, medication should be discontinued and replaced by another AED. On rare occasions, CNZ may cause behavioral disturbances characterized by hyperactivity and violent behavior.[1] Treatment consists of reducing the dose and even discontinuing medication. A reversible parkinsonism-dementia syndrome has been reported in a few patients on VPA treatment.[32, 33]

Sleep Disturbances

The long-term use of AEDs has been associated with disturbances of sleep architecture.[12] Well-controlled studies to document such effects have not been performed, however. Wolf et al.[14] performed sleep studies in 12 patients on long-term PHT treatment. The polysomnographic (PSG) findings consisted of an increase in non–REM sleep stages I and II and a decrease in stages III and IV without any change in REM sleep. After chronic ETS treatment, PSG findings included an increase in stage I sleep, a decrease in stage III and IV sleep, and increased awakenings. Improved sleep organization and increased slow-wave sleep after long-term VPA treatment have been observed in children.[34] Harding et al.[35] observed a decrease in delta and REM sleep with high doses of VPA. The bulk of the evidence in the literature suggests an overall stabilization of sleep disturbance rather than a deleterious effect of AEDs on the sleep of the epileptics.[12]

Specific Effects Related to a Particular Drug

Specific effects related to a particular drug generally are not dose-related except in occasional cases. For example, tremor, which has been noted specifically with VPA treatment, may be dose-related.

Dysmorphic Features

AEDs may have dysmorphic effects. Excessive growth of hair on the trunk and limbs is peculiar to PHT[1, 6, 18] and is cosmetically disadvantageous. Long-term treatment with PB or CNZ may occasionally cause such hirsutism.[1] Coarsening of the facial features has occasionally been described after long-term PHT or PB treatment.[1, 6, 18] A combination of acne, pigmentation, hirsutism, and hypertrophy of subcutaneous facial tissues after long-term PHT treatment results in a characteristic facial appearance referred to as "Dilantin facies"[36] or "family likeness."[37] VPA may sometimes cause alopecia or hair thinning; rarely this has been noted with PR and CNZ.[1, 38] VPA may also cause curly hair[37] and changes in hair color.[39] A reduction of VPA dose may be helpful, although it is not known whether the hair changes are related to dose or duration of VPA treatment. On rare occasions, Dupuytren's contracture and contracture of the plantar fascia have been described with both long-term PHT treatment and PB treatment.[1, 6, 18]

Long-term PHT and occasionally PB treatment are associated with gum hypertrophy and hyperplasia.[1, 6, 18, 40] It is important for the patient to maintain careful dental hygiene to reduce the severity of this complication. Occasionally, gingivectomy may be needed. Gingival hyperplasia is related to plasma PHT levels. One of the factors for this complication may be repeated infection related to the reduced salivary IgA levels noted after PHT treatment.

Cerebellar Degeneration

Long-term treatment of PHT may be associated with cerebellar atrophy accompanied clinically by chronic cerebellar dysfunction and pathologically by cerebellar Purkinje cell loss.[1, 6, 41–45] This degeneration seems to be related to the duration of treatment, whereas the acute cerebellar syndrome is clearly dose-related. The association between chronic PHT intoxication and permanent cerebellar damage has been somewhat controversial. It has, however, been generally accepted that cerebellar atrophy results directly from long-term PHT treatment rather than from anoxia related to chronic repeat seizures.

Immunologic Disorders

Approximately 25% of patients on PHT treatment may show subnormal IgA levels; a much smaller percentage may show low IgG and IgM levels.[1, 6] Occasionally, a low level of IgG in the cerebrospinal fluid is noted after PHT treatment. Such immunologic abnormalities may be responsible for the increased incidence of lymphoid cancer after PHT treatment.[1, 6] VPA-induced thrombocytopenia may also be an autoimmune response with the development of IgM antibodies against platelets.[20]

Antinuclear antibodies have occasionally been noted in patients taking PHT and ETS.[1] On rare occasions, a reversible systemic lupus erythematosus-like syndrome has been observed in patients taking PHT, PB, PR, ETS, and CBZ.[6, 7, 18]

Skeletal Abnormalities

Osteomalacia has been reported in patients on chronic PHT treatment. Hypocalcemia and elevated serum alkaline phosphatase levels are noted in these patients. These patients are, for the most part, from Europe and India; cases of osteomalacia resulting from chronic PHT treatment have rarely been reported in the United States.[1, 6] Clinically, osteomalacia is usually silent but can be demonstrated on radiologic examination. Suggested mechanisms include a direct effect on calcium metabolism and an alteration of hepatic metabolism of vitamin D. Occasionally, osteomalacia and osteoporosis have been described in patients taking PB and PR.

Weight Gain

Excessive weight gain has been noted in patients on VPA treatment.[46] The mechanism is unknown but may be reversed by reducing caloric intake. A mild to moderate gain in weight has occasionally been reported with CBZ treatment.

Endocrine System Effects

AED treatment may also cause various endocrine system effects. PHT may displace circulating thyroxine from plasma protein-binding sites, causing low protein-bound iodine but without clinical hypothyroidism.[1, 6] Patients on long-term CBZ treatment may also have low serum thyroxine levels.[7] CBZ is known to cause increased release of antidiuretic hormone (ADH) from the posterior pituitary gland, causing hyponatremia and low plasma osmolality.[1, 7, 18] The syndrome of inappropriate ADH secretion may also be related to increased renal tubular sensitivity to vasopressin. The resulting water intoxication may cause neurologic manifestations such as confusion, dizziness, headache, and an increase in seizures. CBZ-induced hyponatremia may[47] or may not[48] be dose-related.

Impotence and decreased libido have been noted in many men taking PB and PR[49] and occasionally in men taking CBZ.[50] The mechanism may include both an altered metabolism of testosterone and a central nervous system effect. There is an increasing incidence of polycystic ovaries, hyperandrogenism, and menstrual disturbances in epileptic women taking VPA.[51]

Respiratory System Effects

CNZ may occasionally cause respiratory disturbances as a result of increased salivary and bronchial secretions.[1] Rarely, chronic PHT treatment may cause decreased pulmonary diffusion capacity associated with respiratory dysfunction.[1]

Cardiovascular Effects

In some patients, particularly in those older than age 50 years, CBZ may cause sinoatrial block and other cardiac conduction disturbances;[1, 7, 52, 53] therefore, this drug should be used with caution in patients with cardiac arrhythmias. PHT treatment has also been reported to cause cardiac arrhythmias in some patients.[1, 6]

Teratogenic Effects

Teratogenic effects are not necessarily dose-related, but these adverse reactions definitely increase in incidence with polypharmacy. Most of the teratogenic effects have been noted with PHT, PB, and PR. VPA has been known to cause neural tube defect in about 1–2% of infants born to epileptic mothers on VPA treatment.[54] Such defects have also been described in less than 1% of infants born to mothers on CBZ treatment.[55] Teratogenic effects are described in detail in Chapter 11.

Miscellaneous Adverse Reactions

The following adverse reactions are mostly rare and long-term cumulative effects and are related to the duration of treatment rather than to the dosage of AEDs.

Subnormal folate levels without associated megaloblastic anemia have been noted after long-term treatment with PHT, PB, PR, and, rarely, CBZ.[1] The significance of subnormal folate level is somewhat controversial. The PHT-induced folate deficiency may result from malabsorption of folic acid, enzyme induction, competitive interaction between PHT and folate coenzymes, or increased metabolic demand for folic acid.[6] An asymptomatic carnitine deficiency has been noted in many patients on VPA treatment.[30, 56] This deficiency is not dose-related and is seen more frequently in children and in those on polytherapy. Whether carnitine deficiency is related to VPA-induced hyperammonemia[30, 57] remains controversial. PHT has occasionally caused hyperglycemia and glycosuria, most likely because it inhibits insulin secretion.[18] Subclinical hyperglycinemia and hyperglycinuria have been described in some patients treated with VPA.[58] Hypersecretion of bronchial mucus and hypersalivation have been noted in children after CNZ treatment.[59]

Precipitation of acute intermittent porphyria[1] after treatment with PHT and PB and rarely after treatment with VPA, CNZ, and CBZ has been noted in occasional reports. There are rare reports of increased serum ceruloplasmin levels after PHT treatment,[1] and impairment of taste has been described rarely after CBZ treatment.[1]

VPA treatment in young women may occasionally cause a transient amenorrhea.[60] A reversible retinotoxic effect was reported in two patients after several years of treatment with CBZ.[61] This improved after CBZ was discontinued.

Anticonvulsant drug toxicity may occur after acute and long-term use of AEDs. It is important to be aware of the various side effects, as some of these may give rise to severe morbidity or may be associated with high mortality. Generally, the dose-related acute side effects can be minimized by reducing the dose or by initiating treatment with a smaller dose and gradually increasing the dosage. There is no way of predicting the idiosyncratic reactions, however. Clinical monitoring is many times better than laboratory monitoring; therefore, it is important to discuss the various side effects with patients and to periodically follow patients on AED treatment. Particular attention should be paid to patients treated with multiple drugs because of the possibility of drug interactions and because of the increasing incidence of the adverse reactions of patients while they are on multiple AED therapy.

References

1. Chokroverty S, Sachdeo R, Khalifeh R. Anticonvulsant toxicity: clinical and EEG effects. Am J EEG Technol 1988;28:197.
2. Levy RH, Dreifuss FE, Mattson RH, et al. Antiepileptic Drugs (3rd ed). New York: Raven, 1989.
3. Dam M, Gram L. Comprehensive Epileptology. New York: Raven, 1991.
4. Wyllie E. The Treatment of Epilepsy: Principles and Practice. Philadelphia: Lea & Febiger, 1993.
5. Kutt H, McDowell F. Management of epilepsy with diphenylhydantoin sodium. JAMA 1968;203:969.
6. Reynolds EH. Phenytoin Toxicity. In RH Levy, FE Dreifuss, RH Mattson (eds), Antiepileptic Drugs (3rd ed). New York: Raven, 1989;241.
7. Gram L, Jensen PK. Carbamazepine Toxicity. In RH Levy, FE Dreifuss, RH Mattson (eds), Antiepileptic Drugs (3rd ed). New York: Raven, 1989;555.
8. Tartara A, Manni R. Sodium valproate "encephalopathy": report of three cases with generalised epilepsy. Ital J Neurol Sci 1985;6:93.
9. Harrison MB, Lyons GR, Landow ER. Phenytoin and dyskinesias: a report of two cases and review of the literature. Movement Disorders 1993;8:19.

10. Sachdev P. Akathisia and Restless Legs. New York: Cambridge University Press, 1995.
11. Karas BJ, Wilder BJ, Hammond EJ, Bauman AW. Treatment of valproate tremors. Neurology 1983;33:1380.
12. Chokroverty S. Sleep and Epilepsy. In S Chokroverty (ed), Sleep Disorders Medicine. Boston: Butterworth-Heinemann, 1994;429.
13. Touchon J, Baldy-Moulinier M, Billiard M, et al. Sleep architecture in epileptic patients with complex partial seizures before and after treatment by carbamazepine [abstract]. Epilepsia 1986;27:640.
14. Wolf P, Roder-Wanner UU, Brede M, et al. Influences of Antiepileptic Drugs on Sleep. In A Martins da Silva, CD Binni, H Meinardi (eds), Biorhythms and Epilepsy. New York: Raven, 1985;137.
15. Dreifuss FE, Langer DH. Side effects of valproate. Am J Med 1988;84(Suppl 1A):39.
16. Reynolds EH. Chronic antiepileptic toxicity: a review. Epilepsia 1975;16:319.
17. Patton WN, Duffull SB. Idiosyncratic drug-induced hematological abnormalities: incidence, pathogenesis, management and avoidance. Drug Safety 1994;11:446.
18. Smith DB. Antiepileptic Drug Selection in Adults. In DB Smith (ed), Epilepsy: Current Approaches to Diagnosis and Treatment. New York: Raven, 1990;111.
19. Loiseau P. Sodium valproate platelet dysfunction and bleeding. Epilepsia 1981;22:141.
20. Sandler WP, Emberson C, Robert GE, et al. IgM platelet antibody due to sodium valproate. BMJ 1978;2:1683.
21. Solomon GE, Hilgartner MW, Kutt H. Coagulation defects caused by diphenylhydantoin. Neurology 1972;22:1165.
22. Gately LN, Lam MA. Phenytoin-induced toxic epidermal necrolysis. Ann Intern Med 1979;91:59.
23. Dreifuss FE, Langer DH, Moline KA, Maxwell JE. Valproic acid hepatic fatalities: US experience since 1984. Neurology 1989;39:201.
24. Dreifuss FE, Santilli N, Langer DH, et al. Valproic acid hepatic fatalities: a retrospective review. Neurology 1987;37:379.
25. König SA, Siemes H, Bläker F, et al. Severe hepatotoxicity during valproate therapy: an update and report of eight new fatalities. Epilepsia 1994;35:1005.
26. Camfield PR. Pancreatitis due to valproic acid. Lancet 1979;1:1198.
27. Rosenberg HK, Ortega W. Hemorrhagic pancreatitis in a young child following valproic acid therapy. Clinical ultrasonic assessment. Clin Pediatr 1987;26:98.
28. Chokroverty S, Sayeed ZA. Motor nerve conduction study in patients on diphenylhydantoin therapy. J Neurol Neurosurg Psychiatry 1975;38:1235.
29. So EL, Penry JK. Adverse effects of phenytoin on peripheral nerve and neuromuscular junction: a review. Epilepsia 1982;22:467.
30. Engel AG. Carnitine Deficiency Syndromes and Lipid Storage Myopathies. In AG Engel, BQ Banker (eds), Myology. New York: McGraw-Hill, 1986;1663.

31. Wolf P, Inone Y, Roder-Wanner UU, Tsai JJ. Psychiatric complications of absence therapy and their relation to alteration of sleep. Epilepsia 1984;25(Suppl 1):556.
32. Armon C, Miller P, Carwile S, et al. Valproate-induced parkinsonism-dementia syndrome: a potential model for acquired chronic neurodegenerative diseases [abstract]. Ann Neurol 1991;30:252.
33. Shin C, Gray L, Armon C. Reversible cerebral atrophy: radiologic correlate of valproate-induced parkinsonism-dementia syndrome [abstract]. Neurology 1992;42:277.
34. Findji F, Catani P. Readjustment des therapeutiques anticonvulsives chez l'enfant. L'Encephale 1982;8:595.
35. Harding GFA, Alfrod CA, Powell TE. The effect of sodium valproate on sleep, reaction times and visual evoked potential in normal subjects. Epilepsia 1985;26:597.
36. Trimble MR, Corbett JA. Some Somatic Consequences of Antiepileptic Drugs. In D Janz, H Meinardi, J Oxley (eds), Chronic Toxicity of Antiepileptic Drugs. New York: Raven, 1983;201.
37. Walshe MM. Cutaneous drug effects in epilepsy. Trans St John's Hosp Derm Soc 1972;58:269.
38. Jeavons PM, Clark JE, Harding GFA. Valproate and curly hair. Lancet 1977;1:359.
39. Herranz JL, Arteaga R, Armijo JA. Change in hair colour induced by valproic acid. Dev Child Neurol 1981;23:386.
40. Angelopoulos AP, Goaz PW. Incidence of diphenylhydantoin gingival hyperplasia. Oral Surg Oral Med Oral Pathol Oral Radiol Endod 1972;34:898.
41. Eadie MJ. Unwanted Effects of Anticonvulsant Drugs. In JH Tyrer (ed), The Treatment of Epilepsy. Philadelphia: Lippincott, 1980;129.
42. Dam M. Adverse Reactions to Antiepileptic Drugs. In J Laidlaw, A Richens (eds), A Textbook of Epilepsy. New York: Churchill Livingstone, 1982;348.
43. Shorvon S. The Treatment of Epilepsy by Drugs. In A Hopkins (ed), Epilepsy. New York: Demos, 1987;266.
44. Ghatak NR, Santoso RA, McKinney WM. Cerebellar degeneration following long-term phenytoin therapy. Neurology 1976;26:818.
45. Selhorst JB, Kaufman B, Horwitz SJ. Diphenylhydantoin-induced cerebellar degeneration. Arch Neurol 1972;27:453.
46. Dinesen H, Gram L, Anderson T, Dam M. Weight gain during treatment with valproate. Acta Neurol Scand 1984;70:65.
47. Rado JP. Water intoxication during carbamazepine treatment. BMJ 1973;3:479.
48. Appleby L. Rapid development of hyponatremia during low-dose carbamazepine therapy. J Neurol Neurosurg Psychiatry 1984;47:1138.
49. Mattson RH, Cramer JA, Collins JF, et al. Comparison of carbamazepine, phenobarbital, phenytoin, and primidone in partial and secondary generalized tonic-clonic seizures. N Engl J Med 1985;313:145.
50. Connell JMC, Rapeport WG, Beastall GH, Brodie MJ. Changes in circulating androgens during short term carbamazepine therapy. Br J Clin Pharmacol 1984;17:347.

51. Isojarvi JIT, Laatikainen TJ, Pakarinen AJ, et al. Polycystic ovaries and hyperandrogenism in women taking valproate for epilepsy. N Engl J Med 1993;329:1383.
52. Boesen F, Andersen EB, Jensen EK, Ladefoged SD. Cardiac conduction disturbances during carbamazepine therapy. Acta Neurol Scand 1983;68:49.
53. Kasarkis EJ, Kuo C-S, Berger R, Nelson KR. Carbamazepine-induced cardiac dysfunction. Arch Intern Med 1992;152:186.
54. Rosa FW. Teratogenesis in Epilepsy: Birth Defects with Maternal Valproic Acid Exposures. In RJ Porter, RH Mattson, AA Ward, M Dam (eds), Advances in Epileptology: XVth Epilepsy International Symposium. New York: Raven, 1984;309.
55. Rosa FW. Spina bifida in infants of women treated with carbamazepine during pregnancy. N Engl J Med 1991;324:674.
56. Smietana S, Frankowski M, Nigro E, Nigro M. Asymptomatic carnitine deficiency in valproic acid monotherapy versus polytherapy [abstract]. Neurology 1991;41:201.
57. Ohtani Y, Eudo F, Matsuda J. Carnitine deficiency and hyperammonemia associated with valproic acid therapy. J Pediatr 1982;101:782.
58. Mortensen PB, Koluraa S, Christensen E. Inhibition of the glycine cleavage system: hyperglycinemia and hyperglycinuria caused by valproic acid. Epilepsia 1980;21:563.
59. Sato S. Benzodiazepines, Clonazepam. In RH Levy, FE Dreifuss, RH Mattson et al. (eds), Antiepileptic Drugs (3rd ed). New York: Raven, 1989;765.
60. Margraf JW, Dreifuss FE. Amenorrhea following initiation of therapy with valproic acid. Neurology 1981;31:159.
61. Nielsen NV, Syvertsen K. Possible retinotoxic effect of carbamazepine. Acta Ophthalmol 1986;64:287.

14

When to Terminate Antiepileptic Drug Therapy

Gregory D. Cascino

Introduction

Antiepileptic drugs (AEDs) are the primary treatment for patients with epilepsy (i.e., recurrent, unprovoked seizures)[1] and are an effective therapy in most patients with epilepsy.[2] AED therapy, however, is not without risks. The potential hazards of AEDs include cognitive, behavioral, and sexual alterations.[3, 4] All AEDs have significant dose-related and idiosyncratic toxicity.[1, 3, 4] They have also been demonstrated to be associated with minor and major malformations in offspring.[5] The financial cost of AEDs may undermine patient acceptance of therapy as well. These concerns affect the selection of the AED(s) and patient compliance. The need for AED therapy is determined by the risk for subsequent seizure activity. Patients who achieve a seizure remission on AED therapy may be candidates for withdrawal of drug therapy.[6] This chapter is devoted to identifying the variables that may affect the success of AED withdrawal and the probability of seizure relapse.

Termination of Antiepileptic Drugs

Selection of Candidates for Antiepileptic Drug Withdrawal

Patients who do not have epilepsy but are receiving AEDs for nonepileptic behavioral events are candidates for withdrawal of medication. Long-term electroencephalographic (EEG) monitoring with or without concomitant video recording of ictal behavior may be useful for classifying seizure type(s).[7, 8] Patients who experience episodic symptoms that are not seizures should not receive AED therapy because of the potential toxicity associated with these medications and because of the diagnostic confusion that the use of this therapy creates. Patients who experience episodic symptoms and are placed on AED therapy may be incorrectly assumed to have an epileptic or a nonepileptic disorder simply because they are on AED therapy. Treatment with AEDs in patients with psychogenic seizures may also defer recognition of the causative factors of the clinical symptoms and initiation of appropriate therapy. The response to AEDs should not be used for diagnostic purposes to determine if paroxysmal symptoms are epileptic in nature. A common diagnostic problem is distinguishing psychogenic seizures from complex partial seizure activity. The lack of response to AEDs may not be diagnostically useful, because 45% of patients with partial epilepsy have seizures that are medically refractory.[3, 9] If clinical and laboratory data (e.g., EEG and neuroimaging studies) do not support the diagnosis of epilepsy, long-term EEG monitoring for diagnostic classification should be considered before initiating AED therapy.[7, 8]

Patients who are experiencing seizures that are unresponsive to AED therapy are also candidates for drug withdrawal. If a medication has been used to maximally tolerated drug levels without benefit, there is no reason for continuing the AED. Substitution of another AED is recommended with the taper and withdrawal of the initial drug. Polypharmacy is more likely to be associated with AED toxicity; therefore, monotherapy is preferred whenever possible.[10–12] AED interactions also alter drug metabolism(s) and make interpretation of drug(s) levels more difficult.[1, 11–13] Production of unmeasured drug metabolites may contribute to neurotoxicity. Addition of a second AED renders only 11–13% of patients seizure-free but creates AED toxicity in 90% of patients.[11, 13] There is at present no definite evidence for a synergistic effect of AEDs in the management of epilepsy. In addition to drug toxicity, multiple drug therapy is also associated with drug compliance problems and an increased expense for AEDs. The methodology for the withdrawal of an AED in a patient with poorly controlled seizure activity is discussed below. Patients with medically refractory seizure disorders may be candidates for alternative treatments such as drug investigational studies or epilepsy surgery.[14]

Patients experiencing significant drug toxicity despite effective seizure control may also be candidates for AED withdrawal. If AED therapy is considered necessary, a less toxic agent should be substituted for the offensive AED.[15] Chronic barbiturate therapy may be associated with neurotoxic effects, such as sedation, that impair a patient's cognitive performance.[12] Depending on the seizure type(s), another AED should be selected that is unlikely to be associated with similar side effects. Initially reducing the drug dosage and serum level of the original drug may be attempted to see if seizure control may be attained with less toxicity. The goal of AED therapy is to improve the quality of the patient's life; therefore, an offensive drug should not be continued even if the seizures are in remission.

Finally, patients who may be candidates for drug withdrawal are those whose seizure disorders have entered remission.[6] Seventy-six percent of the 457 pediatric and adult patients with epilepsy in the Rochester study at 20 years follow-up were seizure-free for 5 years.[2] AEDs may not affect the probability of seizure remission.[2, 6] The longer the duration of follow-up, the greater the probability of seizure remission.[2] The minimum seizure-free duration necessary to initiate AED withdrawal has not been well established. It is important to note that not all patients with epilepsy need be committed to a "life-long sentence" of AED therapy that may be unnecessary and associated with undesirable effects.[6] Identification of appropriate candidates and the likelihood that drug withdrawal will be successful are considered below.

Illustrative Cases

Patient 1

A 23-year-old woman had medically refractory complex partial seizures and was referred to the Mayo Clinic for consideration of ablative surgery. Long-term EEG monitoring revealed localization of the epileptogenic zone in the left anterior temporal lobe. The patient was seizure-free and asymptomatic after a left anterior temporal lobectomy and was maintained on monotherapy carbamazepine (1,200 mg/day). Two years after surgery, the patient was considered for medication withdrawal.

Sleeping and awake EEG monitoring showed only generalized nonepileptiform and nonspecific changes thought to represent medication effect. The serum carbamazepine level before the initiation of AED withdrawal was 10.6 µg/ml, and the drug was tapered 100 mg every 2 weeks. The patient was successfully withdrawn from the medication in 6 months and has subsequently remained seizure-free.

Comment: The necessity of AED therapy in patients undergoing epilepsy surgery may be difficult to determine. Exposing a patient who is rendered seizure-free to a single AED for 1–2 years after surgery appears reasonable. The dose of the AED may be reduced if the patient develops drug toxicity. The subsequent need for AED medication can best be determined by the recurrence of seizure activity during AED withdrawal.

Patient 2

A 19-year-old man with idiopathic generalized epilepsy experienced generalized tonic-clonic seizures. The patient subsequently became seizure-free after administration of sodium valproate at a dose of 1,500 mg/day. Two years after starting valproate, the patient was considered for AED withdrawal. EEG findings at the time of valproate withdrawal revealed generalized atypical spike and wave discharges. The serum valproate level before tapering the drug was 86 µg/ml. The valproate was tapered at 250 mg/month. Eight months after discontinuing valproate, the patient experienced a single generalized tonic-clonic seizure on awakening. Valproate was restarted, and the patient was maintained on valproate therapy at a dose of 1,000 mg/day.

Comment: The recurrence of seizure activity may not indicate the need for long-term AED therapy. Seizure-precipitating factors that may have increased the seizure tendency (e.g., sleep deprivation) should be identified and avoided. A slower withdrawal schedule of valproate may be appropriate if another attempt at AED tapering is considered. Perhaps the EEG findings in this patient may be a useful indicator of the likelihood of seizure recurrence.

Factors Affecting the Success of Antiepileptic Drug Withdrawal

Patients with epilepsy may obtain complete seizure control on AED therapy. A critical question for the patient and the physician is the duration of AED necessary for treatment of the seizure disorder. Not uncommonly, the patient and family members have been instructed previously that the medication should be continued indefinitely. There is a tremendous anxiety associated with withdrawal of medication when seizure control has been achieved ("why rock the boat?"). Reasons to consider AED withdrawal include drug toxicity, expense, difficulty with compliance, and problems associated with administration. The necessity for AEDs should be evaluated in patients contemplating pregnancy because of potential AED-induced teratogenesis.[5] Patients without epilepsy, such as those who have a single seizure episode or who have provoked seizures (e.g., alcohol withdrawal seizures), are not to be considered in the discussion of AED withdrawal.

Studies have been performed to assess the probability of seizure recurrence after AED withdrawal.[15–27] Several factors have been evaluated independently, including seizure type, etiology, duration of seizure remission, duration of drug withdrawal, neurologic examination, and the results of EEG studies. Age at seizure onset, age at withdrawal, sex, and race may not be important predictors of seizure relapse after AED withdrawal.[6]

There is conflicting evidence regarding the effect of seizure type on seizure recurrence with AED withdrawal.[19, 22, 24, 26] Studies have inconsistently suggested that patients with partial epilepsy have a higher risk of seizure recurrence.[27] Patients with generalized tonic-clonic seizures may have a lower rate of seizure relapse.[26] Certain seizure types are age-dependent and may be associated with a reduced risk for seizure activity with maturation.[16] Patients with childhood absence seizures and those with partial epilepsy of the rolandic type may experience seizure activity only and demonstrate the characteristic interictal EEG abnormalities during childhood and adolescence. AED withdrawal would be successful in these patients when the seizure tendency is reduced with maturation. The latency of AED therapy before effective control of seizures and the difficulty obtaining seizure control may be factors that are more important than the specific seizure type.[17, 22, 26] Patients who experience seizures that are initially difficult to control are more likely to relapse after AED withdrawal. The longer the duration of AED therapy necessary to enter a seizure remission, the more likely AED withdrawal will be unsuccessful.[22] Patients on multiple drug therapy and with mixed seizure types have an increased risk of seizure recurrence with medication withdrawal.[16, 18, 22, 26]

The cause of a patient's seizure disorder may be an important predictor of seizure recurrence.[16, 27] Patients with idiopathic seizures may be less likely to experience relapse than patients who have seizures that are symptomatic of an identified neurologic disorder (e.g., cerebral neoplasm or vascular malformation).[19] This is an inconsistent finding, and some studies have failed to show an association.[20]

The duration of seizure remission before AED withdrawal is considered may also be an important variable in determining the possibility of seizure recurrence after AED withdrawal. Most studies have assessed AED withdrawal after an established period of seizure-free time, usually a minimum of 2 years.[17–19, 22, 24–26] The duration of the seizure remission (beyond 2 years) has not been demonstrated to be a significant factor in the success of drug withdrawal. A seizure-free period of less than 2 years has not been adequately evaluated.

The duration of drug withdrawal was only predictive of seizure relapse in one study that demonstrated a higher recurrence rate in patients tapered over less than 6 months.[27] The recurrence rate in one study in which medication was tapered over 2–3 months compared favorably with the rates in other series in which the medication was withdrawn over a 6-month period.[22, 28] Three other studies did not find the duration of drug withdrawal to be an independent factor in the determination of seizure relapse.[20, 21, 23] The necessity for long periods of drug withdrawal (e.g., years) has not been confirmed. Patients on multiple drug therapy may be tapered faster than those receiving only one AED. Adult and pediatric daily dose reductions for the primary AEDs used in one study is summarized in Table 14-1.[22] The total AED dosage and drug serum level should be considered before determining the tapering schedule. If the patient is experiencing drug toxicity, the tapering schedule may need to be accelerated depending on the clinical severity of the drug effect. Patients with poorly controlled seizures who are being withdrawn from an AED that has proven ineffective may need to be tapered slowly as the second AED is being introduced in order to avoid increased seizures.

Abnormalities on neurologic examination (e.g., a neurologic deficit or mental retardation) may indicate an increased risk of seizure recurrence with AED withdrawal.[15, 16, 19, 21, 26] Patients who are mentally retarded or who have cerebral palsy have a higher relapse rate after AED therapy is terminated. Evidence of drug toxicity on examination is not a significant factor in determining seizure relapse.

Finally, specific EEG abnormalities (e.g., spike and spike and wave discharges) that are associated with an increased epileptogenic potential may correlate with a negative outcome with AED withdrawal.[24] Epileptiform EEG patterns that develop during AED withdrawal may also increase the risk of seizure relapse.[17] The presence of generalized spike and wave discharges before or after initiation of drug taper

Table 14-1. Drug Withdrawal Schedule Used in One Study with Decrements Made Every 4 Weeks*

Drug	Adult Dose Decrement (mg)	Children's Dose Decrement (mg/kg)
Phenobarbital	130	1
Phenytoin	50	1.5
Carbamazepine	100	3
Valproate	200	6
Primidone	125	4
Ethosuximide	250	4

*The minimal withdrawal period was 6 months.
Source: Modified from Medical Research Council Antiepileptic Drug Withdrawal Study Group. Randomised study of antiepileptic drug withdrawal in patients in remission. Lancet 1991;337:1176.

appears to indicate an unfavorable seizure outcome associated with AED withdrawal.[24, 27] Other studies have failed to show a significant prognostic effect of the EEG study on seizure recurrence.[16] Focal or generalized nonepileptiform abnormalities (e.g., intermittent slowing in the temporal region) are not predictive of seizure recurrence.

Assessing the Success of AED Withdrawal

It is important to consider the likelihood of seizure recurrence before withdrawing medication for a patient who has achieved a seizure remission from AED therapy. If the patient has acquired "social skills" (e.g., driver's license and employment) while rendered seizure-free on AED(s), there is a reluctance to consider a withdrawal of medication. The patient must become an important part of the decision-making process concerning AED withdrawal. In some individuals, any risk of seizure recurrence is unacceptable, and chronic AED therapy may be preferred. It is important to note that patients in remission who continue to receive AEDs may have a recurrence of seizures.[22] It is easier to discuss with the patient the termination of AED therapy if there is drug toxicity or if there are other problems associated with the medication. Certainly there is little reason to continue multiple AED therapy in the patient who has entered a seizure remission, and tapering to monotherapy should be considered.

The success of AED elimination in patients with seizure disorders in remission has been previously assessed. The risk of relapse has ranged predominantly from approximately one-fourth to one-third of patients during a variable duration of follow-up (several months to several years).[15–19, 21, 23, 24] The relapse rate for patients in seizure remission remaining on AEDs was 22% in one study.[22] Most of the patients who relapse do so in the first or second year after the AED is withdrawn.[6, 22] The percentage of patients seizure-free is even higher if certain higher risk patients (see above) are excluded. Patients with these specific risk factors such as mental retardation may still be successfully tapered and withdrawn from AED(s) but at a higher probability of seizure relapse.

Summary

More information is available about when to initiate AED therapy than about when to terminate treatment. Concern regarding seizure recurrence has resulted in patients receiving multiple drug therapy with medications that potentially could impair cognitive function. It is important to note that patients may be seizure-free because they have entered a seizure remission that is not related to AED(s) medication. A periodic assessment of the continued need for AED therapy should be performed in patients with epilepsy, and a consideration of AED withdrawal may be appropriate in patients who have entered a seizure remission. A favorable profile for AED withdrawal includes a patient receiving a single AED, without a remote symptomatic neurologic disorder, with a short latency after seizure onset until remission occurred, and who has a long duration seizure-free. Unfortunately, most candidates for AED withdrawal have one or several complicating factors, such as multiple drug therapy, which requires careful consideration before eliminating AED therapy.

References

1. Engel J Jr. Antiepileptic Drugs. In J Engel Jr (ed), Seizures and Epilepsy. Philadelphia: FA Davis, 1989;410.
2. Annegers JF, Hauser WA, Elveback LR. Remission of seizures and relapse in patients with epilepsy. Epilepsia 1979;20:729.
3. Dreifuss FE. Goals of Surgery for Epilepsy. In J Engel Jr (ed), Surgical Treatment of the Epilepsies. New York: Raven, 1987;1.

4. Thompson PJ, Trimble MR. Anticonvulsant drugs and cognitive function. Epilepsia 1982;12:531.
5. Hauser WA, Hesdorffer DC. Pregnancy and Teratogenesis. In WA Hauser, DC Hesdorffer (eds), Epilepsy Frequency, Causes and Consequences. New York: Demos, 1990;147.
6. Hauser WA, Hesdorffer DC. Prognosis. In WA Hauser, DC Hesdorffer (eds), Epilepsy Frequency, Causes and Consequences. New York: Demos, 1990;197.
7. Gumnit RJ. Intensive Neurodiagnostic Monitoring: Summary and Recommendations. In RJ Gumnit (ed), Intensive Neurodiagnostic Monitoring. New York: Raven, 1987;291.
8. Mattson RH. Value of Intensive Monitoring. In JH Wada, JK Penry (eds), Advances in Epileptology: Xth Epilepsy International Symposium. New York: Raven, 1980;43.
9. Ward AA Jr. Perspectives for Surgical Treatment of Epilepsy. In AA Ward Jr, JK Penry, D Purpura (eds), Epilepsy. New York: Raven, 1983;371.
10. Lesser RP, Pippenger CE, Luders H, et al. High dose monotherapy in treatment of intractable seizures. Neurology 1984;34:707.
11. Schmidt D. Two anti-epileptic drugs for intractable partial epilepsy with complex partial seizures. J Neurol Neurosurg Psychiatry 1982;45:1119.
12. Theodore WH, Porter RJ. Removal of sedative-hypnotic drugs from the regimens of patients with intractable epilepsy. Ann Neurol 1983;13:320.
13. Mattson RH, Cramer JA, Collins JF, et al. Comparison of carbamazepine, phenobarbital, phenytoin and primidone in partial and secondarily generalized tonic-clonic seizures. N Engl J Med 1985;313:145.
14. Engel J Jr. Alternative Therapy. In J Engel Jr (ed), Seizures and Epilepsy. Philadelphia: FA Davis, 1989;443.
15. Sakamoto Y, Kasahara M, Satouchi H, et al. Long-term prognosis on recurrence of seizures among children with epilepsy after drug withdrawal-elimination. Folia Psychiatr Neurol Japan 1978;32:435.
16. Arts WFM, Visser LH, Loonen MCB, et al. Follow-up of 146 children with epilepsy after antiepileptic therapy. Epilepsia 1988;29:244.
17. Bouma PAD, Peters ABC, Marts RJH, et al. Discontinuation of antiepileptic drug therapy: a prospective study in children. J Neurol Neurosurg Psychiatry 1987;50:1579.
18. Callaghan N, Ganett A, Goggin T. Withdrawal of anticonvulsant drugs in patients free of seizures for two years. N Engl J Med 1988;318:942.
19. Emerson R, D'Souza BJ, Vining EP, et al. Stopping medication in children with epilepsy: predictors of outcome. N Engl J Med 1981;304:1125.
20. Juul-Jensen P. Frequency of recurrence after discontinuation of anticonvulsant therapy in patients with epileptic seizures. Epilepsia 1964;5:352.
21. Matricardi M, Brincoiotti M, Benedetti P. Outcome after discontinuation of antiepileptic drug therapy in children. Epilepsia 1989;30:582.
22. Medical Research Council Antiepileptic Drug Withdrawal Study Group. Randomised study of antiepileptic drug withdrawal in patients in remission. Lancet 1991;337:1175.
23. Overweg J, Binnie CD, Oosting J, Rowan AJ. Clinical and EEG prediction of seizure recurrence following antiepileptic drug withdrawal. Epilepsy Res 1987;1:272.

24. Shinnar S, Vining EP, Mellits ED, et al. Discontinuing antiepileptic medication in children with epilepsy after two years without seizures. N Engl J Med 1985;313:976.
25. Shinnar S, Berg AT, Moshe SL, et al. Discontinuing antiepileptic drugs in children with epilepsy: a prospective study. Ann Neurol 1994;35:534.
26. Thurston JH, Thurston DL, Hixon BB, Keller AJ. Prognosis in childhood epilepsy: additional follow-up of 148 children 15 to 23 years after withdrawal of anticonvulsant therapy. N Engl J Med 1982;306:831.
27. Todt H. The late prognosis of epilepsy in childhood: results of a prospective follow-up study. Epilepsia 1984;25:137.
28. Chadwick D. The Discontinuation of Antiepileptic Therapy. In BS Meldrum, TA Pedley (eds), Recent Advances in Epilepsy (2nd ed). Edinburgh: Churchill Livingstone, 1985;111.

15

Presurgical Evaluation in Complex Partial Seizures

Thaddeus S. Walczak

Epidemiologists estimate that 2,000–5,000 new patients may benefit from surgical treatment of epilepsy every year.[1] Appropriate resections stop or significantly reduce seizures in most patients with medically refractory epilepsy. No more than 500 surgical procedures for control of epilepsy are performed yearly in this country, however. The relatively low number of epilepsy surgeries is in part a result of the poor understanding of the indications for this procedure. In this chapter the indications for epilepsy surgery in complex partial seizures are briefly reviewed, the various tests performed during evaluation for epilepsy surgery are enumerated, and how this information is used to decide whether the patient is an appropriate candidate for epilepsy surgery is discussed. Discussion is limited to focal cortical resections for complex partial seizures.

When to Refer Patients for Epilepsy Surgery

Patients referred for surgical therapy of partial complex seizures must meet several requirements (Table 15-1). The seizures must originate from a limited area of cortex that is not critical for patient function.

Table 15-1. Indications and Contraindications for Focal Resection in Epileptic Seizures

Indications
Epilepsy is localization-related
Epilepsy is medically refractory
Epilepsy significantly interferes with the patient's quality of life
Contraindications
Significant medical illness
Progressive degenerative cerebral disease
Significant psychiatric illness (not absolute)
Age older than 60 years (not absolute)
Intelligence quotient of less than 70 (not absolute)

This means that the seizures must be localization-related in the international classification (see Chapter 2). The distinction between localization-related and generalized epilepsies is occasionally difficult to make on the basis of history and outpatient evaluations. If there are any doubts and the patient meets other requirements, the more extensive evaluations available at comprehensive epilepsy centers usually allow this distinction to be made.

The epilepsy must be refractory to medical treatment. In practice, this means that high therapeutic serum levels of appropriate anticonvulsant drugs have been achieved or the patient has experienced unacceptable toxicity, and seizures have persisted. How many combinations and what combinations of drugs should be used before a patient is considered medically refractory are somewhat controversial. Most centers require that high-dose monotherapy with at least two different anticonvulsants effective against focal seizures should be attempted before surgery is seriously considered for complex partial seizures. The Veterans Affairs Cooperative study[2, 3] demonstrated that only 10–15% of patients who failed two aggressive trials of anticonvulsants in monotherapy benefited from treatment with two anticonvulsants together. Only 5% benefited from treatment with three anticonvulsants. Thus, failure of two monotherapy trials and one duotherapy trial with appropriate anticonvulsants is a reasonable definition of medically refractory. Some centers require more extensive trials of anticonvulsant medications. If aggressively pursued, trials of appropriate anticonvulsants can usually be completed within 2 years. Although it is always possible to try a new combination of anticonvulsant drugs, it is important not to deny the patient a chance for surgical cure when the risk of surgery is minimal.

The epilepsy must be severe enough to significantly interfere with the patient's life. The severity of epilepsy that is acceptable to a patient varies and depends on seizure frequency; pattern; type; and the patient's social, psychological, and vocational situations, among other factors. Many centers require that the seizures occur at least every month, but this may be modified if the seizure is extremely disruptive or if a lesion is present.

Significant medical illness and progressive degenerative cerebral disease are absolute contraindications for epilepsy surgery. There are several relative contraindications. Advanced age may be associated with lower chances of success and decreased duration of potential benefit. Many centers avoid epilepsy surgery in patients older than 60 years of age; epilepsy surgery in patients older than 70 years of age is exceptional. Many centers avoid focal resections for epilepsy in patients with severe psychiatric disorders or an intelligence quotient (IQ) of less than 70. A low IQ often indicates diffuse cerebral damage and thus increases the likelihood that the patient's seizures will emerge from multiple foci. Furthermore, return to work or other useful pursuits is unlikely even if seizures are cured. On the other hand, cessation of seizures may significantly ease the burden patients place on caregivers. Cognitive function may improve if anticonvulsant medication can be reduced after a successful epilepsy surgery. Again, potential benefits must be assessed individually.

Epilepsy surgery is *not* contraindicated in patients with multifocal interictal epileptiform abnormalities, with seizure foci in the dominant temporal lobe, with postictal psychosis, or with moderate psychiatric difficulties. Evaluation in such patients is occasionally more complicated, but many patients with these features are cured by routine epilepsy surgery.

Noninvasive Evaluation for Epilepsy Surgery

The goal of epilepsy surgery is to excise enough cortex to cure the seizure disorder without causing neurologic impairment. Consequently, the goals of the evaluation are to determine whether the patient's seizures originate in one area, to identify that area, and to demonstrate

Table 15-2. Evaluation for Epilepsy Surgery

Noninvasive evaluation
History and neurologic examination
Interictal scalp EEG monitoring
Magnetic resonance imaging of the brain
Positron emission tomography of the brain
Single photon emission computed tomography of the brain
Neuropsychometric testing
Video and scalp EEG monitoring
Intracarotid amytal testing
Invasive evaluation
Video-EEG recording with depth or subdural electrodes
Evoked potential recordings from subdural electrodes
Cortical stimulation studies

that this area can be resected without causing neurologic impairment. Because the area of seizure onset may be structurally, metabolically, electrically, and functionally abnormal, evaluation for seizure surgery examines all of these features. Nonetheless, epilepsy is a disorder of abnormal electrical excitability; therefore, the evaluation must demonstrate that the cortex thought to include the zone of seizure onset is abnormally excitable. Structural, physiologic, or metabolic dysfunction may provide supportive evidence but cannot by itself establish the zone of seizure onset. The evaluation proceeds in a stepwise fashion, with the least risky procedures first (Table 15-2).

History and Neurologic Examination

A precise description of the aura and clinical features of the seizure may provide useful clues regarding the area of seizure onset. Focal simple sensory or visual hallucinations usually provide accurate lateralizing and localizing information. Simple auditory auras suggest onset in Heschl's gyrus but do not provide lateralizing information.[4, 5] The common rising epigastric sensation is usually, but not invariably, associated with temporal lobe onset.[4, 5] Auras may be confined to the early years of a seizure disorder and disappear as the seizures become more frequent.[6]

A history of febrile seizures is often associated with mesial temporal sclerosis (see below) and hippocampal onset. Hippocampal onset of seizures is also much more common if other risk factors for epilepsy are sustained before age 4 years.[7] For example, seizures in patients who experience encephalitis before 4 years of age usually start in the hippocampus, whereas seizures in patients who experience encephalitis later typically start in multiple areas of neocortex.[8] Neurologic examination may point to focal regions of cerebral dysfunction. Unilateral diminished facial movement with spontaneous smiling appears to be a particularly useful lateralizing sign in seizures originating in the temporal lobes.[9] Psychiatric evaluation is important for several reasons. It is important to establish that the patient can cooperate with the extensive evaluation involved, especially when evaluation with intracranial electrodes is considered. Psychiatric disease may be a relative contraindication to epilepsy surgery (see above). Presurgical psychiatric evaluation also establishes a baseline against which to measure any changes that may occur after epilepsy surgery.

Interictal Electroencephalographic Monitoring

Characteristic epileptiform spikes and sharp waves (also known as epileptiform discharges) provide evidence of abnormal electrical excitability. Focal epileptiform discharges confirm that the patient suffers from a partial seizure disorder. Focal slowing or attenuation of background activity indicates focal physiologic dysfunction in those regions. Rarely, a seizure will be recorded during routine electroencephalographic (EEG) monitoring, confirming the presence of epilepsy and often indicating the side or, less frequently, the focus of seizure onset. Information recorded interictally—that is, between seizures—has some limitations, however.

Abnormal excitability in a given region between seizures does not necessarily mean that this region gives rise to the patient's seizures. For example, multiple foci of interictal epileptiform discharges are noted in more than one-fourth of patients cured by epilepsy surgery.[10, 11] Although multiple electrically abnormal regions are present in these cases, only one abnormal area was responsible for all of the patients' seizures. Furthermore, the presence of interictal epileptiform discharges does not necessarily mean that the patient suffers from seizures. Somewhat more than 2% of adult patients with a variety of medical and cerebral disorders but without epilepsy have characteristic interictal epileptiform discharges,[12, 13] and the prevalence is somewhat higher in nonepileptic children.[14, 15] Finally, the presence of interictal epileptiform discharges does not necessarily mean that the patient has experienced seizures recently, although frequency of interictal epileptiform discharges probably increases after a seizure.[16] Sampling is an important limitation of interictal EEG monitoring. The characteristic epileptiform spikes and sharp waves that indicate abnormal cortical excitability occur sporadically, and their distribution in time is not well understood. A routine EEG study, lasting approximately 40 minutes, may not record these abnormalities. Therefore, it is important to review all EEG studies obtained during the course of the patient's disorder. Commercially available software can screen continuously recorded EEG studies for epileptiform spikes and sharp waves.[17] This software allows detection of infrequent epileptiform discharges and is now routinely used in epilepsy monitoring units. Finally, the spatial relationship between the abnormally excitable cortex and the distribution of the resulting epileptiform discharge on the scalp is not always precise. Additional electrodes, including the semi-invasive sphenoidal electrodes, may increase the precision of localization. Even given these limitations, multiple interictal EEG studies confirm the presence of an electrically abnormal cortex and often provide valuable lateralizing and localizing information.

Structural Neuroimaging

Magnetic resonance imaging (MRI) is the preferred imaging technique because of its superior resolution and sensitivity when compared with computed tomography (CT). MRI has allowed detection of subtle lesions such as low-grade gliomas, heterotopias, cavernous hemangiomas, and regions of cortical dysgenesis that are often not visible on CT scans.[18–20] Such lesions are often associated with an abnormally excitable cortex that initiates seizure onset. More important, some minor variations in routine MRI techniques allow the detection of hippocampal atrophy (Figure 15-1). With somewhat more sophisticated analysis, the volume of the hippocampal formation can be calculated and compared with a set of normal controls, allowing quantitative confirmation of atrophy. Hippocampal atrophy has been strongly associated with mesial temporal sclerosis,[21, 22] the most common finding in complex partial seizures arising from the hippocampus. Furthermore, the presence of hippocampal atrophy has been correlated with good surgical outcome.[23, 24] Electrophysiologic studies of this resected tissue both in vivo and in vitro have demonstrated abnormal electrical excitability that may play a major role in generating seizures or interictal epileptiform discharges. Thus, MRI often demonstrates discrete

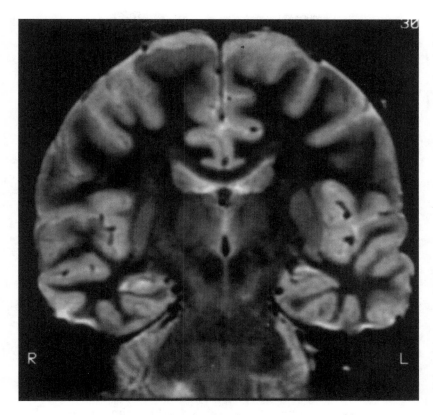

Figure 15-1. *Right (R) mesial temporal sclerosis in a 38-year-old patient. Coronal magnetic resonance imaging scans, performed with a double inversion recovery technique, demonstrate increased signal and decreased size of the right hippocampus. The patient has been seizure-free for approximately 1 year after right temporal lobectomy. (Courtesy of Steve Chan, M.D.)*

structural abnormalities that can be correlated with electrical abnormalities demonstrated with EEG monitoring.

Metabolic Neuroimaging

Positron emission tomography (PET) with fluorodeoxyglucose measures rates of glucose use by cerebral cortex. Resolution is considerably less than with MRI. PET has demonstrated temporal hypometabolism between seizures in 70–80% of patients with seizures originating in the temporal regions[19, 25, 26] and this particular finding has been associated with good surgical outcome.[27] Unfortunately, PET shows hypometabolism less often in patients with extratemporal seizures, and occasionally ipsilateral temporal hypometabolism is seen in these patients.[19, 28] False lateralization with PET has been reported rarely.[28, 29] The region of hypometabolism defined by PET often exceeds the region of anatomic or electrical abnormality defined by structural imaging and intracranial ictal recording, however. For example, PET may show hypometabolism in hippocampal as well as temporal and frontal neocortical regions in patients cured by a minimal temporal neocortical resection and extensive hippocampectomy.[27] Ictal PET demonstrates hypermetabolism that appears to include the zone of seizure onset as defined by other evaluations; however, recording PET during seizures is technically difficult.

Physiologic Neuroimaging

Single photon emission computed tomography (SPECT) with a variety of tracers measures cerebral blood flow. Diminished blood flow is recorded in the interictal state in as much as 80% of patients with temporal lobe seizures. Resolution is poor, however, and false localization and lateralization occur with some frequency.[30–32] Ictal SPECT shows considerably more promise. The tracer substances commonly used are bound to receptor sites on first circulation through the brain and produce signals for a relatively long period thereafter. Thus, if the tracer substance is injected during the seizure, imaging up to an hour later can demonstrate blood flow patterns during the seizure. Several recent studies have demonstrated good localization and lateralization of seizure onset, even in seizures starting outside the temporal lobes.[31–33] Although ictal SPECT is technically feasible, obtaining such studies requires a good degree of specialized training and organization.

Neuropsychometric Testing

Neuropsychometric testing may provide useful clues regarding abnormalities in higher cortical function that may in turn suggest focal dysfunction.[34, 35] For example, deficits in verbal memory suggest dysfunction in the dominant hippocampus, whereas deficits in naming suggest dysfunction in the dominant temporal neocortex. Deficits in executive function, measured with tests such as the Wisconsin Card Sort, Trailmaking Test, or Stroop test, suggest frontal lobe dysfunction. Formal psychological assessments such as the Minnesota Multiphasic Personality Inventory, especially when normalized for epilepsy patients, may support psychiatric impressions of personality disorder. Higher cognitive processes, however, require the functioning of extensive cerebral networks; consequently, deficits detected in these functions probably do not define discrete areas of abnormality. Because evaluation for epilepsy surgery seeks to remove limited areas of cortex that constitute the zone of seizure onset, neuropsychometric testing may not be as useful as some of the other evaluations discussed here. Nonetheless, neuropsychometric testing often provides useful supporting evidence and does provide a baseline against which changes after surgery can be measured.[34, 35]

Video-Electroencephalographic Monitoring

Video-EEG monitoring allows simultaneous recording using video and the EEG during the patient's seizures. EEG signals can be recorded from the scalp or from intracranial electrodes. Video-EEG monitoring is usually carried out in epilepsy monitoring units organized specifically for this purpose. This procedure is generally performed on an inpatient basis so that medications can be tapered to hasten the onset of seizures for recording. Trained personnel are available to examine the patient during and after the seizure. Because a permanent record is available, both clinical features of the seizure and ictal EEG studies can be repeatedly analyzed to obtain clues regarding the zone of seizure onset. Clinical features of recorded seizures can be reviewed with habitual observers of the patient's seizures to determine whether they are typical. At present, most centers require that at least three typical seizures be recorded in all patients before epilepsy surgery is considered. A few centers have recently questioned the need to record seizures in all patients referred for surgery.

The recording of an epileptic seizure is the only way to confirm that the patient suffers from epilepsy. Up to one-third of patients referred to epilepsy centers with intractable seizures experience nonepileptic events, as demonstrated with video-EEG monitoring.[36, 37] It is often difficult to distinguish epileptic seizures from nonepileptic events by history alone. Some patients with nonepileptic events have characteristic interictal epileptiform discharges recorded on routine EEG monitoring. Clearly, patients with nonepileptic events should not be referred for epilepsy surgery.

Review of clinical features of the seizure may help lateralize or localize area of seizure onset. Complex partial seizures arising in the frontal lobes are often short, with bizarre features such as shouting, thrashing, profane vocalizations, and sexual automatisms.[38–40] Patients may maintain some degree of awareness during the seizure, and there is often little postictal impairment. It is not surprising that these seizures are often misinterpreted as psychogenic events. Unlike psychogenic events, complex partial seizures arising in the frontal lobes are stereotyped, often occur at night, and are often associated with tonic-clonic seizures when anticonvulsants are tapered.[41] Seizures arising in the temporal lobes are usually longer (lasting more than 60 seconds); often start with arrest of ongoing activity or motionless stare; and classically exhibit oroalimentary automatisms, drooling, picking, or fumbling. Recent studies of temporal lobe seizures indicate that lateralized automatisms usually occur ipsilateral to the side of onset, and limb dystonia usually occurs contralateral to the side of seizure onset.[42] Postictal impairment is more profound than with frontal lobe seizures. Postictal aphasia is fairly common after seizures originating in the left temporal lobe and appears to be rare in seizures originating elsewhere.[43]

Scalp ictal EEG abnormalities lateralize to the side of seizure onset in 57–83% of temporal lobe seizures and in 12–65% of seizures originating in other regions of the brain;[44–46] in most of the remaining seizures, ictal EEG onset is diffuse, although the seizure is partial. Incorrect lateralization occurs in 3–7%, often in predictable circumstances.[45–47] Scalp ictal EEG monitoring is less useful in determining the lobe of seizure onset.[46] Sphenoidal and extra scalp electrodes are frequently used to improve yield of lateralization and localization, but the usefulness of these procedures has not been formally demonstrated. Computerized spike and seizure detection increases the amount of both interictal and ictal abnormalities recorded during video-EEG monitoring, with an acceptable degree of false positives.[17] In our experience, this procedure has increased the yield of video-EEG monitoring and addressed some of the sampling issues discussed in the section on interictal EEG monitoring.

There are several limitations to video-EEG monitoring. Clinical features during a seizure may reflect propagation of the seizure to areas outside the region of ictal onset rather than excitation of the region of onset. Although common pathways of propagation have been defined,[48] they are incompletely understood, and there are many exceptions. Similarly, seizure onset in the scalp EEG often occurs some time after clinical seizure onset, raising concerns that the EEG changes reflect regions to which the seizure has propagated rather than the area of seizure onset. Ictal EEG monitoring may show no change in 3–10% of complex partial seizures,[49, 50] and this may occur more frequently during complex partial seizures originating outside the temporal lobe. More frequently, artifact renders portions or all of the ictal EEG study uninterpretable. Given these limitations and the cost of video-EEG monitoring, a few authors have questioned the need for video-EEG monitoring in all cases evaluated for epilepsy surgery. Most believe, however, that epilepsy must be demonstrated unequivocally before elective resection of cortex; consequently, most centers require video-EEG monitoring to support the diagnosis of epilepsy before epilepsy surgery is performed.

Intracarotid Amobarbital Testing

With intracarotid amobarbital testing, amobarbital, a short-acting barbiturate, is injected into each carotid artery, resulting in anesthesia of one cerebral hemisphere. This allows for examination of language and memory function in the remaining unanesthetized hemisphere. Intracarotid amobarbital testing is used to confirm the hemisphere of language dominance. More than 90% of right hand–dominant patients have left-hemisphere language dominance; however, unusual localization of speech may be more common in patients with epilepsy.[51] Hemispheric anesthesia presumably inactivates the hippocampus, although the hippocampus does receive some perfusion from the posterior cerebral artery. Thus, in a rough way, hemispheric anesthesia reproduces the situation after temporal lobectomy, in which much of the hippocampus is usually removed. If a patient cannot learn new material with one hemisphere anesthetized, one can conclude that the anesthetized hippocampus is critical for learning and should not be removed. This procedure also allows one to determine whether the unanesthetized hippocampus is dysfunctional and can be removed without compromising memory. Thus, in theory, intracarotid amobarbital testing reveals whether a given hippocampus is critical for memory or whether it does not significantly assist memory. Intracarotid amobarbital testing is considered necessary to provide evidence that the hippocampus remaining after a proposed resection is sufficient to allow normal memory.[34, 35, 52]

Recent studies report that intracarotid amobarbital testing predicts the side of seizure onset,[53] distinguishes between temporal mesiobasal and temporal neocortical epilepsy,[54] and predicts outcome after temporal lobectomy.[55] Only one study[56] has correlated the results of this procedure with memory changes after temporal lobectomy. Although prevention of amnestic syndrome is considered to be the primary indication for performing the intracarotid amytal test, no study has demonstrated that the results of this procedure predict the occurrence of the amnestic sydrome. This would be a difficult study to conduct because amnestic syndrome is so rare.[52] Test-retest reliability has been low in some studies.[57, 58] Patients are often uncooperative during hemispheric anesthesia, making testing and interpretation difficult. Differing blood flow patterns probably result in somewhat different areas of induced anesthesia in different patients. In spite of these limitations, intracarotid amytal testing complements neuropsychometric testing and is required before temporal lobectomy or frontal lobectomy is performed in most centers.[34, 35, 52]

Advances in functional MRI and PET offer the promise of less invasive preoperative evaluation of language and perhaps eventually memory as well. It is not yet clear that these studies will be more reliable or practical than the intracarotid amobarbital test.

Integration of Noninvasive Data: Surgery or Invasive Studies?

After the above evaluation is completed, the epileptologists decide whether the available information has delineated the zone of seizure onset with sufficient precision that epilepsy surgery is likely to result in cure or whether further evaluation with invasive recordings is necessary. This decision is based on whether (1) an area of cortical hyperexcitability that appears to cause the patient's disabling seizures has been identified, (2) the presumed zone of seizure onset is confined enough that a resection is feasible, and (3) the presumed zone of onset can be resected without causing unacceptable deficits. Because individual situations are highly variable, no protocol or set of rules can include all cases of intractable epilepsy. Decisions are usually made by consensus and reflect the collective experience of the team. Some situations, however, occur relatively commonly and are approached similarly in many centers.

Although cortical hyperexcitability is often demonstrated with interictal or ictal scalp EEG monitoring, the relationship of the abnormal potentials to the underlying cerebral cortex is inexact, and the fields of these abnormal potentials may not allow localization to a discrete area of the cortex. If there is a lesion that is likely to be epileptogenic in the approximate region of cortical hyperexcitability, one can conclude that the lesion and the surrounding area are probably the region of seizure onset—that is, the lesion serves to provide implicit boundaries to regions of electrical abnormality, the boundaries of which may be indistinct with scalp EEG evaluations. Common epileptogenic lesions in this situation include low-grade gliomas, mesial temporal sclerosis, cavernous hemangiomas, arteriovenous malformations, and hamartomas. Consequently, many centers advise resection of the presumed epileptogenic lesion and surrounding tissue if scalp interictal or ictal epileptiform abnormalities are localized to this region and if the region can be safely resected.

Following similar reasoning, many centers advise anterior temporal lobectomy if mesial temporal sclerosis is demonstrated; if interictal abnormalities are, for the most part, confined to this region; if other noninvasive data support mesial temporal onset, at least in part; and if there is no strong evidence to suggest other areas of seizure onset. If mesial temporal sclerosis is present but interictal discharges are rare, most centers require that scalp ictal EEG monitoring demonstrate at least a high degree of lateralization and that other noninvasive data support mesial temporal onset to the seizure disorder. Occasionally, MRI does not demonstrate mesial temporal sclerosis, but EEG monitoring and other evidence suggest temporal onset. This situation is somewhat more problematic because of the possibility that the temporal neocortex rather than hippocampus constitutes the zone of seizure onset. Many centers proceed with temporal lobectomy if PET and all noninvasive data other than MRI support temporal lobe onset. Two arguments are raised in favor of this position: (1) Seizures originating in the temporal neocortex are said to be infrequent,[59] and (2) 4–5 cm of anterior temporal neocortex is routinely resected in anterior temporal lobectomy and may include the zone of seizure onset in these cases. Other centers are more cautious, especially if seizures arise from the dominant hemisphere and if prominent speech deficits occur early in the seizure. This approach requires that the zone of seizure onset be precisely defined with invasive recordings and that speech areas be mapped to allow a more definitive resection.

Approximately 25% of patients with seizures originating in the temporal lobes have epileptiform abnormalities occurring independently over the two temporal lobes,[10, 11, 60] suggesting two potential regions of seizure onset. It is not clear how many independent epileptiform abnormalities can be tolerated before another focus of seizure onset is strongly suspected. Concern is raised if 10–20% of the discharges are present contralateral to the "primary" focus.[61–63] Unless ictal EEG signals are consistently lateralizing and unless other noninvasive data strongly point to the "primary" focus, most centers require recording of seizures with intracranial electrodes covering at least both hippocampal regions. There is controversy whether epidural, subdural, or depth recording is the most useful in these situations.

Invasive recording is almost always indicated if seizures appear to arise from nontemporal regions and if a potentially epileptogenic lesion cannot be demonstrated. Areas of seizure onset in nonlesional neocortical epilepsy are often extensive, may change from seizure to seizure, and can rarely be defined with sufficient precision with noninvasive studies. Invasive recording can be contemplated if noninvasive evaluation suggests a potentially limited and resectable area of seizure onset. Even with invasive recordings, a localized zone of seizure onset is often difficult to define; consequently, seizure surgery is not as successful in these circumstances. Cure or significant palliation may result if a subtle lesion such as a limited area of cerebral dysgenesis is found after craniotomy that was not apparent with imaging.

Less frequently, invasive recording is considered necessary when noninvasive studies yield confusing or contradictory results. Occasionally, noninvasive studies strongly suggest that seizures arise from critical cortex, and precise definition of cortical regions that can be safely removed is necessary (see below). Finally, the patient may have multiple static central nervous system lesions that are potential areas of seizure onset, and EEG monitoring does not point to a single lesion as the clear source of seizures. If the patient has a single seizure type, intracranial recording from the regions surrounding the various lesions often determines the area of seizure onset.

Sperling and colleagues[63] devised and prospectively tested a protocol that included many of these ideas. This is the only explicit set of rules that has been prospectively tested, so it is described in detail. Patients were excluded if interictal EEG monitoring, MRI, or clinical features of seizures suggested a nontemporal seizure onset. If MRI demonstrated a temporal lobe lesion (not including mesial temporal sclerosis) and either interictal or ictal EEG findings supported temporal lobe onset, seizure surgery was recommended. If no temporal lobe lesion was found on MRI, one primary and two secondary criteria or two primary and one secondary criteria were required. The two primary criteria were lateralized-state independent interictal epileptiform discharges seen maximally in the sphenoidal electrode and initial seizure activity in the sphenoidal electrode within 30 seconds of seizure onset. Secondary criteria were lateralized sphenoidal interictal abnormalities only during sleep, lateralized sphenoidal slowing, and unilateral memory impairment with the intracarotid amobarbital test. Fifty-one of 103 patients evaluated for seizure surgery met the requirements for temporal lobectomy without invasive recordings; 80% of these were cured by seizure surgery, and all of these 51 patients had at least an 80% reduction in seizure frequency. Forty-seven of the patients not meeting requirements were evaluated with invasive recordings; 31 of 47 (66%) had seizures originating exclusively from one temporal lobe and were candidates for temporal lobectomy. This protocol appears to select most patients who can benefit from temporal lobectomy and to exclude most patients who do not have all seizures arising from one temporal lobe. Incorporating the presence of medial temporal sclerosis and temporal hypometabolism on PET may decrease the relatively large number of good candidates for temporal lobectomy who were thought to require invasive testing in this protocol. Clearly, further studies of this sort would be very useful.

Invasive Evaluation

In 20–50% of patients evaluated for temporal lobectomy, noninvasive testing does not define zone of seizure onset with sufficient precision. In these patients, invasive recording may serve to demonstrate a discrete zone of seizure onset that can be safely excised. Depth electrodes, subdural electrodes, and epidural electrodes are placed directly into or on the cortex to define a precise zone of seizure onset. Depth electrodes are usually used to record from medial cortical structures, especially the hippocampus, whereas subdural electrode grids or strips are used to record from larger areas of more superficial cortex. Intracranial electrodes allow direct recordings; thus, the relationship between the electrical abnormalities and the cortical structures is much more exact than with scalp recordings. Sampling is the major limitation of invasive recording. Because it is impossible to place electrodes over the entire brain, the interpreter is always concerned that the seizure started at a region removed from the intracranial electrode and then propagated to the electrode. The decision of where to place the intracranial electrodes is therefore very important. Intracranial electrodes are also associated with a 4% risk of infection and hemorrhage.[64]

Electrical stimulation of the cortex through the intracranial electrodes allows leisurely and precise definition of cortical function. Motor function, sensory function, and language can be defined relatively easily. Definition of higher cortical functions is much more difficult. Sensory-evoked potentials recorded from the cortex provide another means for defining primary motor and sensory areas before surgery. These procedures are invaluable when seizures appear to arise from critical areas of cortex. Comparison of electrodes involved in seizure onset with those in which stimulation causes neurologic deficits allows a relatively exact mapping of the cortical resection before exposure of the cortex.

Intracranial recordings provide sufficient information to allow seizure surgery in 30–60% of patients not thought to be candidates after noninvasive studies.[59–61, 65] Epilepsy surgery was generally less successful in these patients in earlier series because the seizure disorder was more complicated. Preliminary reports from some centers have recently reported nearly equal success in patients not requiring and in those requiring invasive study. This is probably because of the additional information provided by the ancillary studies discussed above.

Conclusion

New technology has increased the amount of information available in the selection of patients for seizure surgery. Nonetheless, the selection process for surgical treatment of partial seizures remains largely empirical. This situation should improve as multicenter studies evaluate and follow sufficient numbers of patients to demonstrate the usefulness of individual tests or combinations of tests. The current empirical nature of selection for seizure surgery is also the result of our poor understanding of how seizures start, how seizures propagate, and why epilepsy surgery works. For example, important concepts such as the *zone of seizure onset*, widely used in this literature, remain poorly defined. It is likely that the zone of seizure onset has different meanings in different situations. Clarification of such basic questions with further research will no doubt significantly change the selection process for surgical treatment of complex partial seizures.

References

1. Hauser WA. The Natural History of Drug Resistant Epilepsy: Epidemiologic Considerations. In WH Theodore (ed), Surgical Treatment of Epilepsy. New York: Elsevier, 1992;25.
2. Mattson RH, Cramer JA, Collins JF, et al. Comparison of carbamazepine, phenobarbital, phenytoin, and primidone in partial and secondarily generalized tonic-clonic seizures. N Engl J Med 1985;313:145.
3. Smith DB, Mattson RH, Cramer JA, et al. Results of a nationwide Veterans Administration cooperative study comparing efficacy and toxicity of carbamazepine, phenobarbital, phenytoin, and primidone. Epilepsia 1987;28(Suppl 3):S50.
4. Palmini A, Gloor P. The localizing value of auras in partial seizures: a prospective and retrospective study. Neurology 1992;42:801.

5. Boon PA, Williamson PD, Fried I, et al. Intracranial, intraxial, space-occupying lesions in patients with intractable partial seizures: an anatomo-clinical, neuropsychological, and surgical correlation. Epilepsia 1991;32:467.
6. Williamson PD, Thadani VM, Darcey TM, et al. Occipital lobe epilepsy: clinical characteristics, seizure spread patterns, and results of surgery. Ann Neurol 1992;31:3.
7. French JA, Saukin A, Pfeiffer L, et al. Early risk factor predicts successful epilepsy surgery [abstract]. Epilepsia 33(Suppl 3):27.
8. Marks DA, Kim J, Spencer DD, Spencer SS. Characteristics of intractable seizures following meningitis and encephalitis. Neurology 1992;42:1513.
9. Remillard GM, Anderman F, Rhi-Suasi A, Robbins NM. Facial asymmetry in patients with temporal lobe epilepsy. Neurology 1977;27:109.
10. Dodrill CB, Wilkus RJ, Ojemann GA, et al. Multidisciplinary prediction of seizure relief from cortical resection surgery. Ann Neurol 1986;20:2.
11. Walczak TS, Radtke R, Lewis DV, et al. Anterior temporal lobectomy for complex partial seizures: evaluation, results, and long term followup in 100 cases. Neurology 1990;40:413.
12. Zivin L, Ajmone-Marsan C. Incidence and prognostic significance of "epileptiform" activity in the EEG of non-epileptic subjects. Brain 1968;91:751.
13. Bennet DR. Spike-wave complexes in "normal" flying personnel. Aerospace Medicine 1967;38:1276.
14. Kellaway P. The Incidence, Significance, and Natural History of Spike Foci in Children. In CE Henry (ed), Current Clinical Neurophysiology. Update on EEG and Evoked Potentials. Amsterdam: Elsevier, 1980;151.
15. Cavazzuti GB, Cappella L, Nalin A. Longitudinal study of epileptiform EEG patterns in normal children. Epilepsia 1980;21:43.
16. Gotman J, Marciani MG. Electroencephalographic spiking activity, drug levels, and seizure occurrence in epileptic patients. Ann Neurol 1985;17:597.
17. Gotman J. Automatic seizure detection: improvements and evaluation. Electroencephalogr Clin Neurophysiol 1990;76:317.
18. Laster DW, Penry JK, Moody DM, et al. Chronic seizure disorders: contribution of MR imaging when CT is normal. AJNR 1985;6:177.
19. Theodore WH, Dorwart R, Holmes M, et al. Neuroimaging in refractory partial seizures: comparison of PET, CT, and MRI. Neurology 1986;36:750.
20. Heinz ER, Heinz TR, Radtke RA. Efficacy of MR vs CT in epilepsy. AJNR 1988;9:1123.
21. Jackson GD, Berkovic SF, Tress BM, et al. Hippocampal sclerosis can be reliably detected by magnetic resonance imaging. Neurology 1990;40:1869.
22. Cascino GD, Jack CR, Parisi JE, et al. Magnetic resonance imaging-based volume studies in temporal lobe epilepsy: pathological correlations. Ann Neurol 1991;30:31.
23. Jack CR, Sharbrough FW, Cascino GD, et al. Magnetic resonance image-based hippocampal volumetry: correlation with outcome after temporal lobectomy. Ann Neurol 1992;31:138.

24. Berkovic SF, McIntosh AM, Kalnins RM, et al. Preoperative MRI predicts outcome of temporal lobectomy: an actuarial analysis. Neurology 1995;45:1358.
25. Engel J, Kuhl DE, Phelps ME, Crandall PH. Comparative localization of the epileptic foci in partial epilepsy by PET and EEG. Ann Neurol 1982;12:529.
26. Abou Khalil BW, Siegal GJ, Sackellares JC, et al. Positron emission tomography studies of cerebral glucose metabolism in partial epilepsy. Ann Neurol 1987;22:480.
27. Radtke RA, Hanson MW, Hoffman JM, et al. Positron emission tomography predicts surgical outcome in temporal lobectomy. Neurology 1993;43:1088.
28. Radtke RA, Hanson MW, Hoffman JM, et al. Positron emission tomography: comparison of clinical utility in temporal lobe and extra-temporal epilepsy. J Epilepsy 1994;7:27.
29. Sperling M, Alavi A, Reivich M, et al. False lateralization of temporal lobe epilepsy with FDG positron emission tomography. Epilepsia 1995;36:722.
30. Homan RW, Paulman RG, Devous MD Sr, et al. Cognitive function and regional cerebral blood flow in partial seizures. Arch Neurol 1989;46:964.
31. Rowe CC, Berkovic SF, Sia STB, et al. Localization of epileptic foci with postictal single photon emission computed tomography. Ann Neurol 1989;26:660.
32. Markand ON, Shen W, Park HM, et al. Single Photon Imaging Computed Tomography for Localization of Epileptogenic Focus in Patients with Intractable Complex Partial Seizures. In WH Theodore (ed), Surgical Treatment of Epilepsy. Amsterdam: Elsevier, 1992;121.
33. Newton MR, Berkovic SF, Austin MC, et al. Dystonia, clinical lateralization, and regional blood flow changes in temporal lobe seizures. Neurology 1992;42:371.
34. Jones-Gotman M, Smith ML, Zatorre RJ. Neuropsychological Testing for Localizing and Lateralizing the Epileptogenic Region. In J Engel Jr (ed), Surgical Treatment of the Epilepsies (2nd ed). New York: Raven, 1993;245.
35. Rausch R. Role of the Neuropsychological Evaluation and the Intracarotid Sodium Amobarbital Procedure in the Surgical Treatment for Epilepsy. In WH Theodore (ed), Surgical Treatment of Epilepsy. Amsterdam: Elsevier, 1992;77.
36. Binnie CD, Rowan AJ, Overweg J, et al. Telemetric EEG and video monitoring in epilepsy. Neurology 1981;31:298.
37. Rowan AJ, Siegel M, Rosenbaum DH. Daytime intensive monitoring: comparison with prolonged intensive and ambulatory monitoring. Neurology 1987;37:481.
38. Geier S, Bancaud J, Talairach J, et al. Automatisms during frontal lobe epileptic seizures. Brain 1976;99:447.
39. Williamson PD, Spencer DD, Spencer SS, et al. Complex partial seizures of frontal lobe origin. Ann Neurol 1985;18:497.
40. Waterman K, Purves SJ, Kosaka B, et al. An epileptic syndrome caused by mesial frontal lobe seizure foci. Neurology 1987;37:577.

41. Saygi S, Katz A, Marks DA, Spencer SS. Frontal lobe partial seizures and psychogenic seizures: comparison of clinical and ictal characteristics. Neurology 1992;42:1274.
42. Chee MWL, Kotagal P, Van Ness PC, et al. Lateralizing signs in intractable partial epilepsy: blinded multiple observer analysis. Neurology 1993;43:2519.
43. Privitera MD, Morris GL, Gilliam F. Postictal language assessment and lateralization of complex partial seizures. Ann Neurol 1991;30:391.
44. Risinger MW, Engel J JR, Van Ness PC, et al. Ictal localization of temporal lobe seizures with scalp/sphenoidal recordings. Neurology 1989;39:1288.
45. Walczak TS, Radtke R, Lewis DV. Accuracy and interobserver reliability of scalp ictal EEG. Neurology 1992;42:2270.
46. Spencer SS, Williamson PD, Bridgers SL, et al. Reliability and accuracy of localization by scalp ictal EEG. Neurology 1985;35:1567.
47. Sammaritano M, Lotbinierre A, Andermann F, et al. False lateralization by surface EEG of seizure onset in patients with temporal lobe epilepsy and gross focal cerebral lesions. Ann Neurol 1987;21:361.
48. Ajmone-Marsan C, Ralston B. The Epileptic Seizure: Its Functional Morphology and Diagnostic Significance. Springfield, IL: Thomas, 1957.
49. Walczak TS, Lewis DV, Radtke R. Scalp EEG differs in temporal and extratemporal complex partial seizures. J Epilepsy 1991;4:25.
50. Quesney LF. Seizures of Frontal Lobe Origin. In BS Meldrum, TA Pedley (eds), Recent Advances in Epilepsy (Vol 3). Edinburgh: Churchill Livingstone, 1986;81.
51. Woods RP, Dodrill CB, Ojemann GA. Brain injury, handedness, and speech lateralization in a series of amobarbital studies. Ann Neurol 1988;23:510.
52. Hamberger M, Walczak TS. The Wada Test: A Critical Review. In T Pedley, B Meldrum (eds), Recent Advances in Epilepsy. London: Churchill Livingstone, 1995;57.
53. Loring DW, Meador KJ, Lee GP, et al. Wada memory performance predicts seizure outcome following anterior temporal lobectomy. Neurology 1994;44:2322.
54. Burgerman R, Sperling M, French J, et al. Comparison of mesial vs. neocortical onset temporal lobe seizures. Neurodiagnostic findings and surgical outcome. Epilepsia 1995;36:662.
55. Sperling MR, Saykin AJ, Glosser G, et al. Predictors of outcome after anterior temporal lobectomy: the intracarotid amytal test. Neurology 1994;44:2325.
56. Loring DW, Meador KJ, Lee GP, et al. Wada memory asymmetries predict verbal memory decline after anterior temporal lobectomy. Neurology 1995;45:1358.
57. Novelly RA. Relationship of intracarotid amytal procedure to clinical and neurosurgical variables in epilepsy surgery. [Abstract.] J Clin Exp Neuropsychol 1987;9:33.
58. Dinner DS, Luders H, Morris HH, et al. Validity of intracarotid sodium amobarbital (Wada test) for evaluation of memory function [abstract]. Neurology 1987;37(Suppl 1):142.

59. Spencer SS, Spencer DD, Williamson PD, Mattson R. Combined depth and subdural electrode investigation in uncontrolled epilepsy. Neurology 1990;40:74.
60. Van Buren JM, Ajmone-Marsan C, Matsuga N, Sadowsky D. Surgery of Temporal Lobe Epilepsy. In DP Purpura, HK Penry, RD Walter (eds), Neurosurgical Management of the Epilepsies (Advances in Neurology Vol 8). New York: Raven, 1975;155.
61. Chung MY, Walczak TS, Lewis DV, et al. Temporal lobectomy and independent bitemporal interictal activity: what degree of lateralization is sufficient? Epilepsia 1991;32:195.
62. Spencer SS, Spencer DD, Williamson PD, Mattson RH. The localizing value of depth electroencephalography in 32 patients with refractory epilepsy. Ann Neurol 1982;12:248.
63. Sperling MR, O'Connor MJ, Saykin AJ, et al. A noninvasive protocol for anterior temporal lobectomy. Neurology 1992;42:416.
64. Pilcher WH, Roberts DW, Flanigin HF, et al. Complications of Epilepsy Surgery. In J Engel Jr (ed), Surgical Treatment of the Epilepsies (2nd ed). New York: Raven, 1993.
65. Spencer SS, So NK, Engel J, et al. Depth Electrodes. In J Engel Jr (ed), Surgical Treatment of the Epilepsies (2nd ed). New York: Raven 1993.

16

Surgical Treatment of Epilepsy

Robert R. Goodman

Historical Review

The surgical treatment of epilepsy originated more than 100 years ago. Its origin is due in large measure to the work of J. Hughlings Jackson, whose observations and analysis of seizures led to the possibility of determining the localization of onset of certain seizures.[1] The experimental work of his colleague Ferrier[2] and of others confirmed his hypothesis regarding functional localization within the cerebral cortex. In 1884, Rickman J. Godlee used this information to perform an operation on a lesion in the right precentral gyrus of a patient with focal motor seizures and paralysis of the left arm and hand.[3] Victor Horsley, working with Hughlings-Jackson and having observed this operation, eventually became known as the father of the surgical treatment of epilepsy.[4] He made use of electrical stimulation to map the motor cortex in nonhuman primates and subsequently used similar electrical stimulation to guide areas of resection in an attempt to eliminate seizures. Beginning in 1886, Horsley applied the concept that a discrete epileptogenic area, or "focus," is responsible for the initiation of seizures, and its removal can eliminate them. In 1930, Foerster and Penfield reported the results of electrical stimulation of the brain in 100 patients operated on under local anesthesia in an attempt to control focal epileptic seizures resulting from focal brain injuries.[5] In 1934, Foerster and Altenburger reported the first use of electrocorticography (electrodes placed directly on or in the brain) to identify epileptic areas of the brain during surgery.[6] These approaches were greatly developed by Penfield and Jasper at the Montreal Neurological Institute during the next several decades.[7] These operations were guided by the presence of a structural abnormality or injury of the brain (e.g., a tumor, cyst, or traumatic injury). In the 1950s, Bailey and Gibbs reported operating on patients on the basis of electroencephalographic (EEG) evidence of partial complex seizures but of no known pathologic lesion.[8] This led to a great expansion of the application of surgery to the treatment of epilepsy, with the gradual development of various operations for the resection of portions of the temporal lobe and other cerebral cortical areas.

The major emphasis of epilepsy surgery and the focus of this chapter involve resection within the temporal lobe in patients who have intractable partial complex epilepsy who do not appear to harbor a neoplasm. Important related issues include the selection of appropriate patients for surgery, the evaluation and decision-making process to determine the region to be resected, and the various operations that are used. The first two of these issues are dealt with in more detail in Chapter 15 and are considered briefly in this chapter, whereas the latter issue is the main focus of this chapter. Some consideration is also given to other types of surgery used in the treatment of epilepsy, including the resection of mass lesions associated with intractable epilepsy, hemispherectomy, and cerebral commissurotomy.

Selection of Patients for Epilepsy Surgery

The selection of appropriate patients for surgery is the single most important factor in determining the success of surgery in the treatment of epilepsy.[9] Patients with focal, partial complex, or secondarily generalized seizures are considered potential candidates for surgery. Primary generalized epilepsy is not amenable to surgical intervention. Patients with seizures of focal origin who have failed to be adequately controlled despite thorough attempts (for at least 1 year) with antiepileptic medications can be considered for surgery.[9] Those whose seizures are found to originate in an area of brain that can be removed without producing an unacceptable neurologic deficit represent the group of patients that should be recommended for surgery.

The evaluation of these patients is a multifaceted procedure and continues to evolve with the application of new technologies. A careful history is helpful, both in determining pertinent risk factors for the development of focal epilepsy and in clinically characterizing the seizures to give clues as to the possible focality of the seizures' origin. Every patient is investigated with routine EEG studies, magnetic resonance imaging (MRI), neuropsychological testing, and usually also a positron emission tomography (PET) scan or a single photon emission computed tomography (SPECT) scan. In almost all centers, prolonged scalp EEG studies (usually with sphenoidal electrodes to sample the anteromedial temporal area) are carried out with video monitoring to record simultaneous video images and EEG tracings of patients' typical seizures.[10] In most centers, this video-EEG monitoring is believed to be an essential part of the evaluation, both to prove the diagnosis of epilepsy and to define the region of ictal onset (as it is this region that is generally believed to be the region that must be removed to eliminate the seizures).[11] Patients being seriously considered for surgical resection within the temporal lobe also will routinely undergo an intracarotid amytal (Wada) test to determine lateralization of language dominance and the ability of the contralateral temporal lobe to support important memory function.[12] These studies are generally considered part of a phase I evaluation and generally are analyzed together to determine whether a patient is an appropriate candidate for surgical resection.

When all of these data point to a single brain region as the source of the patient's seizures, surgical resection is often recommended. If these data are not fully concordant, often they will allow the clinicians to focus on a particular question with regard to the site of the patient's seizure onsets. This question often is an ambiguity between the two temporal lobes as the site of origin or regarding localization within a hemisphere that has been determined to be the hemisphere of seizure onset. When this is the case, patients are often recommended for a phase II evaluation, which involves placement of intracranial electrodes to better delineate the source of these seizures. The details of this type of intracranial investigation are discussed in Chapter 15 and are addressed only very briefly in this chapter.

The value of intracranial electrode investigation is completely dependent on the quality of the hypothesis that directs their implantation. The existing data must be analyzed and a hypothesis about the possible sites of origin of the patient's seizures developed. Electrodes are placed in such a way as to answer the particular question raised. Electrodes cannot cover all areas of the brain, and the answer that is arrived at by invasive monitoring is in many ways predetermined by the location of the electrodes implanted. Thus, if electrodes are implanted in both temporal lobes to assess the lateralization of a supposed temporal lobe seizure focus, it is important that an extratemporal onset has already been excluded as a realistic possibility.

The choice of the exact type of electrodes used is probably not nearly as important as the decision of where the electrodes should be placed in any particular patient. Some surgeons almost strictly use subdural strip electrodes for their invasive monitoring, others almost exclusively use intracerebral depth electrodes for monitoring, and many epilepsy centers use an approach that includes a combination of both. Also, in many centers, implanted subdural grid electrodes are used in many patients when the lateralization of the seizure onsets has been determined. These grid electrodes are often used for both localization of seizure onset and functional mapping through extraoperative stimulation studies. Although certainly it is important for the surgical team to apply the approach with which they are most comfortable, most likely there are certain patients for whom each of these different approaches would be most appropriate. Many centers use an individualized approach, in which each patient is discussed in detail and the best possible electrode implantation strategy is arrived at for each patient. It is certainly important to note that the risk of permanent morbidity or death with invasive electrode monitoring is quite low (less than 2%) and is similar for depth and subdural electrodes.[13]

The exactness with which the site of origin of a patient's seizures must be determined is in many ways influenced by the type of surgical resection that is contemplated. Thus, if a standardized temporal lobe resection is to be performed regardless of the site within the temporal lobe that a seizure focus is found, localization of seizure onsets to that temporal lobe is all that is needed. If resections are to be tailored for each individual patient based on their exact location of seizure onsets, a more exact localization of seizure onsets may be needed. Thus, it can be readily seen that the strategies for invasive electrode monitoring are intimately connected to the strategies for surgical resection, and both strategies vary widely among the various epilepsy centers.

The above exhaustive investigation is particularly relevant for patients with partial complex epilepsy without structural or mass lesions. The workup is much different for patients with mass lesions (particularly when the lesions are outside of the temporal lobe) and for patients with other seizure types (e.g., patients with secondarily generalized seizures and widespread hemispheric abnormalities), since they may be candidates for functional hemispherectomy or possibly disconnection surgery (e.g., corpus callosum sectioning). These latter patients generally do not require invasive monitoring.

Once the entire investigation of a patient has been accomplished, a team decision is generally reached with regard to the recommendation for surgery and, if surgery is recommended, the exact nature of the surgery to be performed. Criteria are generally established within each epilepsy center to choose patients who are considered to have medically intractable epilepsy; to be likely to obtain significant benefit from seizure control; and on the basis of the above diagnostic studies, to have their seizure origin adequately localized to a site amenable to resection (with acceptable risk of neurologic morbidity).

Focal Cortical Resection for Partial Epilepsy

The best candidates for surgical therapy of epilepsy are patients who have intractable partial complex (focal) seizures arising from a specific and removable area of the cerebral cortex. The temporal lobe is the area that has the greatest tendency to cause seizures and is the site of seizure origin in the vast majority of patients with partial complex seizures.

Temporal lobe resections generally fall into one of two approaches. Currently, the most widely applied of these two approaches is generally termed a *standardized resection;* the second approach is termed a *tailored resection.* Although several variations of the standard temporal lobe resection exist,[14–17] they have in common the objective of removing a specific portion of the temporal lobe defined by certain anatomic boundaries determined preoperatively. Various surgical teams have adopted different boundaries for the standard resection, but generally, the areas removed are quite similar. With this approach, preoperative evaluation is aimed at determining in which temporal lobe the partial complex seizures originate (and, further, whether they originate inferomesially or laterally). More precise localization is generally not required. For tailored resections, the boundaries of the temporal lobe tissue that is removed are determined by defining the epileptogenic brain tissue in each patient.[18] This generally requires performing intraoperative electrocorticography in an awake patient to define the areas of cortex to be removed. Frequently, electrical stimulation is carried out during these operations to define and spare eloquent cortex. These resections are obviously quite variable and individualized. The two approaches to temporal lobe resection are addressed separately.

Standard Temporal Lobe Resections

The resections carried out by Bailey and Gibbs in the early 1950s[8] involved resecting anterior temporal neocortex while sparing the medial structures (particularly the hippocampal formation). Their resections were carried back to the level of the central sulcus. Soon after this, Falconer and colleagues carried out a series of temporal lobe resections that purposefully included the en bloc removal of the hippocampus.[19, 20] This was done with the intent of obtaining important tissue for histologic study in this group of patients, in whom frequently no pathologic lesion had been found. This approach succeeded in identifying structural pathologic processes in the vast majority of their temporal lobectomy patients. Pathologic processes found included hippocampal sclerosis in 50% of patients and small hamartomas, tumors, or vascular lesions in 25%. The standardized en bloc anterior temporal lobectomy developed by Falconer was basically adopted and refined by Crandall at the University of California at Los Angeles Medical Center and used from 1960 to 1987.[15] The vast majority of these patients underwent a preoperative assessment that included prolonged EEG monitoring with a standard array of bilaterally implanted depth electrodes. Determining the area of ictal onset (particularly, determining in which temporal lobe the seizures originated) was accomplished by monitoring a number of seizures with this array of depth electrodes in place. In some patients, the temporal lobe to be operated on was determined by noninvasive EEG monitoring in conjunction with other studies (e.g., imaging with CT, MRI, or PET scan). Intracarotid amytal tests would be performed in these patients, both to lateralize language function and to assess memory reserve in the temporal lobe that was not resected.[21, 22] The boundaries of the temporal lobe resection in the nondominant and the dominant temporal lobe differed somewhat. The neocortical, or lateral temporal, resection extends 6 cm back from the anterior tip of the temporal lobe along the middle temporal gyrus on the nondominant side and 4.5 cm on the dominant side. The resection angles posteriorly along the inferior temporal gyrus to about 7–8 cm from the anterior tip (this can be done similarly on the dominant and nondominant sides) and angles anteriorly along the superior temporal gyrus to meet the sylvian fissure. Crandall's operation involved opening the sylvian fissure to provide access to the limen insulae, through which the medial incision is made to disconnect the anterior temporal stem (through the amygdala, uncinate fasciculus, and anterior commissure). At this point, attention is turned to the hippocampus and completing the resection. Coronal transection of the hippocampus is carried out 3.0–3.5 cm posteriorly to the anterior tip of the hippocampus. Dissection is then carried through the fimbria, and hippocampal arteries are carefully cauterized and cut. Then, inferior to this, the medial aspect of the parahippocampal gyrus is approached, and a subpial dissection is carried out until the edge of the tentorium is reached. The pia is then carefully cauterized and cut. This completes the en bloc resection and allows the hippocampus to be studied for pathologic changes.

The series of anterior temporal resections carried out in this manner provides an excellent experience for comparison with other approaches. Ultimately, when considering any alternative surgical approach, it is worthwhile to compare the outcome with seizure control and morbidity (including possible subtle changes in cognitive or language function). Modifications of this procedure have been developed for various reasons; some of these are mentioned here. One group recently reported a series of patients undergoing the original temporal lobectomy (Bailey and Gibb's procedure), which involved excision of temporal neocortex only, leaving the medial limbic structures (amygdala and hippocampus) intact.[23] The standard anterior temporal lobectomy performed for more than 30 years at the Montreal Neurological Institute (MNI) has evolved somewhat. The anterior temporal lobectomy practiced for many years by Rasmussen at the MNI involved a neocortical resection similar to that described by Crandall at the University of California at Los Angeles, but the decision about whether hippocampus would be resected and the extent of this resection was determined to a great extent by intraoperative electrocorticography.[24] The lateral neocortical resection stopped at the precentral sulcus (as defined by intraoperative stimulation) on the dominant side and at the central sulcus on the nondominant side. Also, on the dominant side, the speech areas would be localized with intraoperative stimulation. Thus, the patients were routinely operated on while they were awake, which was believed to provide more useful identification of interictal epileptiform discharges. During the past 20 years, Olivier (at the MNI) has modified this "tailored" approach (see the next section for further discussion) toward a more standard anterior temporal lobectomy procedure that now could be summarized as involving a resection of the anterior 5.5 cm of neocortex on the nondominant hemisphere and 4.5 cm on the dominant hemisphere, with extensive resection of the medial structures (amygdala and hippocampus).[14] Operations on the nondominant hemisphere are routinely performed with the patients under general anesthesia, whereas operations on the dominant side are performed with most patients awake for language mapping. Overall, the trend at the MNI has been to move from a tailored type of resection toward a standard anterior temporal lobectomy that is now quite similar from patient to patient and less affected by intraoperative electrocorticographic findings.

Spencer, at Yale University, developed a "standard" anteromedial temporal lobectomy with certain important differences from the previously developed standard resections.[16] Basically, this approach involves reducing the amount of lateral neocortex of the temporal lobe to be removed while maximizing the hippocampal resection, with the aim of minimizing visual field or other functional deficits. This approach developed as a consequence of a number of observations that included the early case reports of patients undergoing reoperation after having had lateral neocortex resection only.[8, 25] Many of these patients obtained seizure control by removal of the anterior hippocampus and other medial structures. Another observation has been with the extensive experience with intracranial recording (including depth electrodes in the medial temporal lobe), demonstrating that the vast majority of ictal events (in partial complex seizures) appear to originate in the medial temporal lobe (often documented in the hippocampus itself).[16] Furthermore, the vast majority of pathologic findings in resected temporal lobes occurred within the hippocampus, and the lateral neocortex rarely demonstrated a significant pathologic process.[26] The removal of the demonstrable pathologic process correlates very well with the success in obtaining seizure control. Thus, the approach at Yale[16] has been to identify patients who have evidence of seizure onset in the medial temporal lobe as supported by electrophysiologic studies (along with using all of the other data collected on each patient) and to carry out a standardized anteromedial temporal resection in these patients. The resection on the dominant hemisphere is the same as that on the nondominant hemisphere; both involve resection of the anterior 3.5 cm of the temporal neocortex (sparing the superior temporal gyrus) and a radical en bloc resection of the hippocampus that extends to the level of the superior colliculi (generally 3.5–4.0 cm of hippocampus). This approach obviates the need for operating on an awake patient with local anesthesia, since brain stimulation for language mapping and intraoperative electrocorticography for mapping of interictal epileptiform discharges are not needed. Also, the limited lateral resection nearly guarantees the avoidance of more than an upper quadrantic postoperative visual field deficit. It has been presumed that the limitation of neocortical resection will decrease the risk of cognitive impairment. The Yale experience seems to support this hypothesis, with visuospatial memory outcome in the nondominant hemisphere, but it is not clear whether a benefit is achieved with verbal memory on the dominant resections.[27]

An even more restrictive type of standard resection has been developed for a subset of patients characterized by Wieser as having a "mesiobasal limbic" subtype of complex partial seizures. In this subgroup of patients, a procedure of selective amygdalohippocampectomy has been recommended and performed by approaching the hippocampal formation through a transsylvian fissure approach.[17] The surgical technique for this procedure was developed by Yasargil. Basically, this surgical procedure allows for a direct approach through the sylvian fissure to reach the area of the amygdala and hippocampus without resecting lateral neocortex. The operation does involve significant disruption of white matter connections in the anterior medial temporal lobe and thus has effects on seizure spread beyond what might be expected by removal of the amygdala and hippocampal structures alone. The hippocampus is resected as an en bloc specimen, which generally includes 3–4 cm of hippocampal length. The objective with this operation is in many ways very similar to that of Spencer's anteromesial temporal resections. Operations are performed with the patients under general anesthesia, and intraoperative functional mapping and mapping of interictal epileptiform activity are not needed.

"Tailored" Temporal Lobectomy

The surgical approaches for temporal resection described in the previous section have in common the belief that the pathologic process underlying intractable temporal lobe epilepsy is similar from patient to patient and generally localizable to medial temporal structures (especially the hippocampus). An alternative and quite different approach to this same problem is to assume that there is great variability from patient to patient, both in the area of the pathologic process causing the seizures and in the location of important functional areas of neocortex. This latter approach was originally developed by Penfield and Jasper[7] and has been most fully applied recently by Ojemann.[18, 28] With this approach, the pathologically affected cortex to be removed (the "epileptogenic zone") is to a large extent defined by interictal epileptiform activity monitored by the direct electrocorticogram, performed intraoperatively. Using this approach, quite differing regions of the temporal neocortex and hippocampus are found to be "epileptogenic" from patient to patient. Furthermore, intraoperative stimulation of the temporal neocortex in awake patients allows for the precise mapping of functional areas. This is particularly important in the tailored approach, since the localization of important functions has been found to be quite variable and often reaches into or close to areas believed to be epileptogenic. In some patients, areas of language function have been mapped into the anterior temporal lobe in areas believed to be "safe" for resection in many of the standard temporal lobectomy procedures. This may explain the occurrence of anomic aphasia, which has been reported with standard anterior temporal resection,[29] although many large series of standard resections have been reported without the occurrence of severe dysphasia.[7, 30–32] One of the most important aspects of this tailored approach is that a less extensive preoperative assessment is needed compared with the approach for standard temporal resections. The area of seizure onset needs only to be lateralized to the appropriate temporal lobe, and precise localization of the ictal onset within that temporal lobe is not needed. Thus, intracranial prolonged EEG monitoring is frequently avoided, and in some patients, scalp ictal monitoring is believed to be unnecessary. In many cases, interictal routine EEG studies in combination with imaging studies, neuropsychologic testing, and the intracarotid sodium amytal test represent the only information needed before proceeding with surgery. One great advantage of this approach, emphasized by Ojemann, is the ability to reduce the hospital stay and the cost of the evaluation for these patients. Also, the risks associated with invasive monitoring can be avoided in certain patients. Mapping of both the epileptogenic zone and the critical functional cortical areas can be accomplished either by the implantation of grids of subdural electrodes or intraoperatively with an awake patient. Implantation of chronic grids of electrodes allows for the monitoring of both interictal and ictal epileptiform activity.[33] Also, this allows for much more time to carry out stimulation studies to map areas of critical function. This approach is certainly needed in patients who cannot cooperate for craniotomies performed under local anesthesia (e.g., children). This approach, however, requires two successive craniotomies and certainly increases the risk of infection. There is some reason to think that intraoperative stimulation mapping may be more accurate in certain circumstances. In many cases, some surgeons believe that the proper resection can be guided by the intraoperative recording of interictal epileptiform activity and thus avoids the need for grid implantation and two craniotomies. If this is true, this approach would reduce somewhat the risk to the patient and greatly reduce the cost, time, resources, and money required for performing this surgery.

The success of this approach to temporal resection depends on the degree to which interictal epileptiform discharges identify the critical tissue that must be removed to control seizures. Ojemann has summarized the several lines of evidence that suggest that excision of tissue identified as epileptogenic by the interictal epileptiform discharges or spikes is quite successful in obtaining seizure control.[18] Although Ojemann acknowledges examples of cases in which scalp ictal onsets were localized to the opposite side of the interictal discharges, it is not clear which is the better guide to the tissue that must be excised to obtain seizure control.[34] In general, the temporal resections carried out by Ojemann using this approach involve excision of the anterior 1.0–1.5 cm of hippocampus and the anterior pole of the temporal lobe (of course, after excluding the existence of functional cortex in this region). Further extension of more posterior basal and medial temporal lobe structures, including posterior hippocampus, relies on the identification of epileptiform discharges in these regions and the absence of critical functions. The extent of resection of the inferior temporal gyrus and fusiform gyrus with this approach is generally more than that accomplished with many of the standard resections. This may be beneficial, because larger basal/medial resections (as determined by postoperative MRI) correlate with better seizure control.[35] Of course, not all interictal epileptiform discharges need be eliminated at the end of the resection. Activation of cortex adjacent to a resection is a well-known phenomenon[7] but may not correlate with an area of epileptogenic cortex.[32] The failure of temporal resections to control seizures generally occurs when epileptiform abnormalities persist in the adjacent cortex, however.[36] Also, interictal discharges in important functional areas have been left in many patients who have subsequently proven to be seizure-free.[37] The primary objective is to remove areas of epileptiform discharge that are identified before the resection is carried out. These areas are believed to be the areas responsible for the patient's spontaneous seizures.

The approach of "tailoring" temporal resection obviously requires a great deal of intraoperative decision-making. Also, the ability to successfully perform such operations on awake patients (the recent introduction of a new anesthetic agent, propofol, has greatly improved this approach, because it allows readily reversible deep sedation without endotracheal intubation) and to obtain the desired information require extensive knowledge on the part of the operative team. One drawback of this approach is that the variability with which this approach is applied by different surgical teams makes it difficult to compare results with those obtained with standard resections.

Cortical Resection with Mass Lesions

Cortical resections in patients with medically intractable partial complex seizures and space-occupying lesions (primarily benign intra-axial neoplasms, hamartomas, and cavernous or arteriovenous vascular malformations) represent a distinct group. Although varying approaches are used in these patients, generally good results with seizure control are obtained.[7, 32, 35, 38, 39]

A large number of these lesions have been discovered in patients who have been treated for seizures for many years with previously unremarkable imaging only because they appear on MRI scans. Recently, this type of patient has become less common, because most newly diagnosed seizure patients undergo MRI before they are treated long enough to be considered medically intractable. Most centers approach these latter patients as they would patients with lesions alone (without seizures), attempting to achieve resection of the mass lesion only. Some centers use the same approach with these patients as they do with patients with mass lesions and intractable seizures: extending resections beyond the margins of the lesion to resect tissue defined as epileptogenic. Epileptogenic tissue is defined either with chronically implanted subdural electrodes[33] to detect seizure onsets or with intraoperative measures to detect interictal epileptogenic abnormalities.[40] Another approach used in these patients is to aggressively ensure complete lesion resection (as defined by negative margins on frozen sections) without defining epileptogenic tissue.[41] In general, the preoperative evaluation in these patients is much less extensive than in patients without mass lesions. There is an excellent correlation between the site of mass lesions and the region of seizure onset.[42] Some studies suggest that removal of apparent epileptogenic cortex is less important than removal of the mass lesion as far as seizure outcome is concerned.[7]

It seems that the approach in patients with mass lesions and intractable seizures should be influenced by the location of the lesion. Lesions located in the medial temporal lobe might best be treated by prompt radical resection of medial temporal structures along with the mass lesion, as this would increase the chance of seizure control without a significantly increased risk of producing cognitive or neurologic deficits.[43] Mass lesions in the frontal or temporal poles might best be approached by including a significant surrounding margin and by localizing the epileptogenic cortex (either with prolonged ictal recording or intraoperative interictal mapping). Mass lesions localized in, beneath, or adjacent to exquisite cortex might be best approached by removal of the mass lesion (abnormal tissue) only to see if this will provide seizure control before considering an operation that would carry more risk of producing a neurologic deficit. One option to consider in these areas is the use of multiple subpial transections, since this appears to allow for the reduction or elimination of epileptogenicity without affecting cortical function.[44] The effectiveness of this approach has not yet been clearly demonstrated, since in many cases it has been applied in conjunction with a cortical resection. I have had limited experience with this technique and have found that it very effectively eliminates active epileptiform activity without producing functional deficits (unpublished observations). The usefulness of this technique can be demonstrated only by its application alone (i.e., without resection) in clearly important functional areas and with adequate long-term follow-up. It is hoped that this type of experience will be acquired.

Extratemporal Resections

Patients with an extratemporal seizure origin and without a structural abnormality on imaging studies represent a difficult challenge for surgical treatment. Precise localization of epileptogenic cortex is often unnecessary because even radical resections are less successful than temporal resections. Thus, resections should be limited only by the avoidance of exquisite cortex. If seizure onsets are localized to the frontal lobe (either with noninvasive or intracranial electrodes), a maximal frontal resection (defined anatomically) should be performed.[45] This would extend to the precentral sulcus and in the dominant hemisphere would spare the 2.5 cm of inferior frontal gyrus anterior to this sulcus. Parietal and occipital origins are encountered less often. Resections in these areas generally warrant more precise localization of epileptogenic cortex (often with chronically implanted subdural electrodes) and must include identification and avoidance of critical sensory cortex.[45]

The most radical resective surgical procedures for epilepsy are multilobar resections and hemispherectomies. Multilobar resections have generally yielded relatively poor seizure control. This is understandable because frequently these are performed in patients whose epileptogenic zone is diffuse and difficult to define. Success is often limited because of the proximity of this zone to critically functional areas. Preresection evaluation generally requires monitoring with subdural electrodes as described previously. In patients with preservation of cortical function on the resected side, critical areas are avoided during resective surgery. If intractable or disabling seizures persist afterward, reoperation using subpial transections can be considered. Patients with intractable partial complex, focal motor or sensory, or secondarily generalized seizures originating in a hemisphere with contralateral hemiparesis (with loss of useful hand function) are excellent candidates for hemispherectomy. These patients most frequently have congenital hemiplegia syndrome, unilateral dysplastic syndrome (e.g., hemimegalencephaly), or Rasmussen's chronic encephalitis. Initially, anatomic hemispherectomies were performed. Although these had a relatively high success rate for seizure control without unacceptable early morbidity, the late complication of progressive deterioration (attributed to cerebral hemosiderosis) led to a sharp decline in the number of these operations performed. Rasmussen's procedure of an "anatomically incomplete, but physiologically complete, hemispherectomy," or "functional hemispherectomy," was developed in the 1970s and provided similar results without the late complication of cerebral hemosiderosis.[46] In recent years, the number of functional hemispherectomies has been increasing, but it probably remains a significantly underused procedure.

Cerebral Commissurotomy

Disconnection of the cerebral hemispheres (partial or complete) is another option available as a surgical intervention for medically intractable secondarily generalized seizures. Patients with atonic ("drop attack") seizures are considered to be the best candidates for this surgery, and it is also quite appropriate to consider cerebral commissurotomy for patients with generalized motor or tonic seizures when a resectable seizure focus cannot be identified.[47, 48] Generally, these patients have no focal structural abnormality on MRI studies and no focal epileptiform abnormalities on interictal or ictal EEG studies. Neuropsychological studies and Wada (intracarotid amytal) testing are often helpful in evaluating these patients. Concern has been raised that commissurotomy (particularly when complete) may lead to significant cognitive impairment in patients with mixed cerebral dominance.[48] Currently, most centers perform a partial corpus callosotomy in these patients (anterior four-fifths, unless evaluation suggests a posterior onset). Most patients obtain good results with this approach, while reoperation to complete the sectioning is considered only in those patients without adequate response to the first operation.

The objective of cerebral commissurotomy is not the complete elimination of seizures, but rather the elimination or marked reduction of the seizure type(s) for which the operation was performed. A very high success rate (80–90%) is generally achieved in this regard;[49] however, partial seizures persist and are not infrequently increased in frequency. In some patients, callosal sectioning allows the subsequent identification of a resectable seizure focus that will lead to focal resection and the possibility of complete seizure elimination. Overall, this procedure has yielded very satisfactory outcomes and is being performed increasingly in recent years.

Outcome

The primary objective of epilepsy surgery is the elimination, or "cure," of chronic, medically intractable seizures. The fraction of patients permanently seizure-free after surgery is one important indicator of epilepsy surgery outcome. The assessment of the overall, or "true," outcome is a very complex and, as yet, poorly accomplished goal, however. Assessment of the overall outcome would require determination of possible improvements of behavioral patterns (e.g., increased independence and improved social skills), cognition, employment, and other factors. In essence, this would involve determining the effect of epilepsy surgery on patients' quality of life. It is hoped that data addressing these issues will be forthcoming in the foreseeable future, but this will most likely require a coordinated multicenter database. Also, it is generally believed that the impact of epilepsy surgery is more positive when it is carried out in younger patients, who are less disabled by this chronic disease. For now, seizure control data are the most readily available tool for the assessment of epilepsy surgery outcome and are briefly considered here.

Seizure outcome is generally classified as excellent improvement (e.g., no seizures, aura only, or possibly rare seizures), good or "worthwhile" improvement (precise definition varies among studies), and poor or "not worthwhile" improvement. Long-term follow-up is necessary for reliable results and should last at least 2 years. Different centers have reported quite variable results for the various resection procedures.[50] The averages of results of studies reported in 1987[51, 52] for seizure-free outcome with at least 1-year follow-up were 55% for temporal lobectomy, 43% for extratemporal resection, and 77% for hemispherectomy. Similar results for temporal lobectomy were reported by review of the literature from 1928 to 1973.[53] Studies reported up to 80% of patients being seizure-free, with an average of 68% in the 1986–1990 survey.[50] It is not clear whether this percentage represents a truly improved outcome for this operation. It is also unclear what the explanations might be if it does represent a truly improved outcome. Patient selection factors and more aggressive resections may be responsible for this apparent improvement. Also, the ability to identify structural abnormalities with MRI has probably increased the likelihood that pathologic tissue will be resected. Resection of pathologic tissue correlates well with successful seizure control.[54] Improved imaging techniques (i.e., MRI, PET, SPECT) and more aggressive intracranial monitoring may also improve the outcome with extratemporal resections. The relatively new technique of multiple subpial transections has been reported to yield long-term seizure control in 55% of patients.[44] Patients undergoing corpus callosum sectioning often have multiple seizure types and almost never obtain elimination of all seizures. Outcome is best assessed with regard to the specific seizure type or types for which the surgery was performed. Complete callosal section eliminates or markedly reduces secondarily generalized seizures in 80–90% of patients.[49] Partial sectioning is less successful. Callosal section markedly reduces partial complex seizures in less than 50% and worsens partial seizures in about 25% of patients. Some behavioral changes have been reported to occur, both worsening (35%) and improvement (15%).[52] Some (generally not disabling) neurologic impairments (e.g., apraxias, language disturbances, memory decline, or disconnection syndromes) are seen in about 20% of patients.

Resective procedures have other effects in addition to seizure control.[52] Some studies report improvement of personality traits and behavior in some patients. Psychosis is reported in some (5–15%) resective patients pre- and postoperatively, with possibly 10% of patients developing psychosis only after surgery. Relatively little information is available with regard to the functional outcome from resective surgery. Some improvement of work or school status and social situation has been reported. Further studies of these variables are needed for a better understanding of the value of resective surgery.

The serious complication rate for epilepsy surgery, including invasive evaluation, resective surgery, and callosal sectioning, is quite low.[55] The intracarotid amytal (Wada) test carries the small risk (less than 0.5%) of a cerebrovascular accident. Depth electrodes cause intracerebral hemorrhages in about 1% of patients (with a minority of these resulting in death or permanent neurologic deficit) and infection (meningitis or abscess) in about 1% (usually without permanent sequelae). Subdural strip and grid electrodes have been used and reported on less extensively but seem to carry about the same 1–2% risk of bleeding or infection (usually with full recovery). Complications with temporal lobe resections include about a 2% occurrence of permanent hemiparesis (thought to be caused by manipulation of the anterior choroidal or middle cerebral arteries), about a 2% occurrence of significant (more than a full quadrant) visual field defect, and about a 1% incidence of global memory impairment. Mild language deficits occur in less than 5%; severe language deficits are rare. Verbal memory impairments are frequent but usually are only very significant if preoperative verbal memory was good or important for the patient's occupation. Other rare complications include infections, venous infarctions, and epidural hematomas. Neurologic complications occurring with extratemporal lobe resections depend on the functional cortex in the resected region (e.g., motor, sensory, speech, and visual deficits). Physiologic identification of functional cortex and avoidance of injury to subcortical white matter and passing arteries minimize complication occurrence. Anatomic hemispherectomy has been reported to have a mortality rate of 6.6% and a 33% risk of delayed cerebral hemosiderosis (with progressive deterioration). Functional hemispherectomy has been reported to have a lower mortality rate and to avoid the late complication of hemosiderosis. Corpus callosotomy frequently causes transient mutism and an increase of focal seizures. Rarely, permanent neurologic deficits may occur, including the "split-brain syndrome," which has been attributed to bilateral significant language representations.

Conclusions

The value of surgery for the elimination of medically intractable seizures has become progressively better recognized by physicians and patients during the past 20 years. The generally high success rate and relatively low risk of serious morbidity and mortality have been the most important factors underlying this change. The appreciation that medically intractable partial complex and secondarily generalized seizures (generally in young patients) have a very adverse effect on a person's quality of life has also been a key factor in this process. One future challenge will be to begin to recognize and intervene in these conditions earlier, which will allow us to have the greatest positive impact on the quality of life of these patients.

References

1. Jackson JH. A Study of Convulsions. Transactions of the St. Andrews Medical Graduate Association (Vol. 3, pp 1–45). In J Taylor (ed), Selected Writings of John Hughlings Jackson. London: Hadder & Stoughton, 1931;8.
2. Ferrier D. Experimental researches in cerebral physiology and pathology. West Riding Lunatic Asylum Medical Reports 1873;3:30.
3. Kirkpatrick DB. The first primary brain-tumor operation. J Neurosurg 1984;61:809.
4. Horsley V. Brain surgery. BMJ 1886;2:670.
5. Foerster O, Penfield W. The structural basis of traumatic epilepsy and results of radical operation. Brain 1930;53:99.
6. Foerster O, Altenburger H. Electrobiological Process in the Human Cortex. Proceedings of the Association of German Neurologists, 22nd Anniversary. Munich, Berlin: Vogel Press, 1934;93.
7. Penfield W, Jasper H. Epilepsy and the Functional Anatomy of the Human Brain. Boston: Little, Brown, 1954.
8. Bailey P, Gibbs FA. The surgical treatment of psychomotor epilepsy. JAMA 1951;145:365.
9. McNaughton FL, Rasmussen T. Criteria for Selection of Patients for Neurosurgical Treatment. In DP Purpura, JR Penry, RD Walter (eds), Advances in Neurology (Vol. 8). New York: Raven, 1975;37.
10. Darcey TM, Williamson PD. Computer System for Automated Seizure Detection, Recording, and Reformatting. In P Wolf, M Dam, D Janz, FE Dreifuss (eds), Advances in Epileptology (Vol. 16). New York: Raven, 1987;269.
11. Gumnit RA (ed). Advances in Neurology: Intensive Neurodiagnostic Monitoring. New York: Raven, 1980.
12. Milner B. Hemispheric Specialization: Scope and Limits. In FO Schmidt, FG Worden (eds), The Neurosciences: Third Study Program. Boston: MIT Press, 1974.
13. Spencer SS. Controversies in epileptology: depth vs. subdural electrodes. J Epilepsy 1989;2:123.
14. Olivier A. Commentary: Cortical Resections. In J Engel Jr (ed), Surgical Treatment of the Epilepsies. New York: Raven, 1987;405.
15. Crandall PH. Standard "En Bloc" Anterior Temporal Lobectomy. In SS Spencer, DD Spencer (eds), Surgery for Epilepsy. Boston: Blackwell, 1991;118.
16. Spencer DD, Spencer SS, Mattson RH, et al. Access to the posterior medial temporal lobe structures in the surgical treatment of temporal lobe epilepsy. Neurosurgery 1984;15:667.
17. Yasargil M, Wieser HG. Selective Amygdalohippocampectomy at the University Hospital, Zurich. In J Engel Jr. (ed), Surgical Treatment of the Epilepsies. New York: Raven, 1987;653.
18. Ojemann GA. Temporal Lobectomy Tailored to Electrocorticography and Functional Mapping. In SS Spencer, DD Spencer (eds), Surgery for Epilepsy. Boston: Blackwell, 1991;137.
19. Hill D, Falconer M, Pampliglione G, Liddell DW. Discussion on the surgery of temporal lobe epilepsy. Proc R Soc Med 1953;46:965.

20. Falconer MA, Hill D, Meyer A, et al. Treatment of temporal lobe epilepsy by temporal lobectomy—a survey of findings and results. Lancet 1995;1:827.
21. Wada J, Rasmussen T. Intracarotid injection of sodium amytal for the lateralization of cerebral speech dominance: experimental and clinical observations. J Neurosurg 1960;17:266.
22. Woods R, Dodrill C, Ojemann G. Brain injury, handedness and speech lateralization in a series of amobarbital studies. Ann Neurol 1988;23:510.
23. Keogan M, McMackin D, Peng S, et al. Temporal neocorticectomy in the management of intractable epilepsy: long term outcome and predictive factors. Epilepsia 1992;33:852.
24. Rasmussen T. Neurosurgical treatment of focal epilepsy. Mod Probl Pharmacopsychiatry 1970;4:306.
25. Penfield W, Paine K. Results of surgical therapy for focal epileptic seizures. Can Med Assoc J 1955;73:515.
26. Babb TL, Brown WJ, Petorius J, et al. Temporal lobe volumetric densities in temporal lobe epilepsy. Epilepsia 1984;25:729.
27. Spencer DD. Anteromedial Temporal Lobectomy: Directing the Surgical Approach to the Pathologic Substrate. In SS Spencer, DD Spencer (eds), Surgery for Epilepsy. Boston: Blackwell, 1991;129.
28. Ojemann G, Dodrill C. Intraoperative techniques for reducing language and memory deficits with left temporal lobectomy. Adv Epileptol 1987;16:327.
29. Heilman K, Wilder B, Malzone W. Anomic aphasia following anterior temporal lobectomy. Trans Am Neurol Assoc 1972;97:291.
30. Van Buren JM. Focal Epilepsy. In CM Long (ed), Current Therapy in Neurological Surgery. Toronto: Decker & Mosby, 1985;49.
31. Crandall PH. Post-Operative Management and Criteria for Evaluation. In DP Purpura, JR Penry, RD Walter (eds), Advances in Neurology: Neurosurgical Management of the Epilepsies (Vol. 8). New York: Raven, 1975;265.
32. Rasmussen T. Surgical treatment of patients with complex partial seizures. Adv Neurol 1975;11:415.
33. Luders H, Lesser R, Dinner D, et al. Commentary: Chronic Intracranial Recording and Stimulation with Subdural Electrodes. In J Engel Jr (ed), Surgical Treatment of the Epilepsies. New York: Raven, 1987;297.
34. Dodrill C, Wilkus R, Ojemann G, et al. Multidisciplinary prediction of seizure relief from cortical resection surgery. Ann Neurol 1986;20;2.
35. Nayel MH, Awad IA, Luders H. Extent of mesiobasal resection determines outcome after temporal lobectomy for intractable complex partial seizures. Neurosurgery 1991;29:55.
36. Ajmone-Marsan C. Depth Electrography and Electrocorticography. In M Aminoff (ed), Electrodiagnosis in Clinical Neurology. New York: Churchill Livingstone, 1980;167.
37. Bengzon A, Rasmussen T, Gloor P, et al. Prognostic factors in the surgical treatment of temporal lobe epileptics. Neurology 1968;18:717.
38. Kelly PJ, Cascino GD. Stereotactic Methods in Surgery of Epilepsy. In H Luders (ed), Epilepsy Surgery. New York: Raven, 1991;579.
39. Boon PA, Williamson PD, Fried I, et al. Intracranial, intraaxial space-occupying lesions in patients with intractable partial seizures: anatomoclinical, neuropsychological, and surgical correlations. Epilepsia 1991;32:467.

40. Berger MS, Ojemann GA, Lettich E. Neurophysiological monitoring during astrocytomy surgery. Neurosurg Clin North Am 1990;1:65.
41. Fried I, Kim JH, Spencer DD. Hippocampal pathology in patients with intractable seizures and temporal lobe masses. J Neurosurg 1992;76:735.
42. Sperling MR, Sutherling WW, Nuwer MR. New Techniques for Evaluating Patients for Epilepsy Surgery. In J Engel Jr (ed), Surgical Treatment of the Epilepsies. New York: Raven, 1987;235.
43. Spencer DD, Ingerni J. Temporal Lobectomy. In H Luders (ed), Epilepsy Surgery. New York: Raven, 1991;533.
44. Morrell F, Whisler WW, Bleck TP. Multiple subpial transection: a new approach to the surgical treatment of focal epilepsy. J Neurosurg 1989;70:231.
45. Olivier A. Extratemporal Cortical Resections: Principles and Methods. In H Luders (ed), Epilepsy Surgery. New York: Raven, 1991;559.
46. Tinuper P, Andermann F, Villemure J-G, et al. Functional hemispherectomy for the treatment of epilepsy associated with hemiplegia: rationale, indications, results and comparison with callosotomy. Ann Neurol 1988;24:27.
47. Spencer SS, Spencer DD, Williamson PD, et al. Corpus callosotomy for epilepsy. I. Seizure effects. Neurology 1988;38:19.
48. Sass KJ, Spencer DD, Spencer SS, et al. Corpus callosotomy for epilepsy. II. Neurologic and neuropsychological outcome. Neurology 1988;38:24.
49. Spencer SS. Corpus callosum section and other disconnection procedures for medically intractable epilepsy. Epilepsia 1988;19(Suppl 2):S85.
50. Engel J Jr, Van Ness PC, Rasmussen TB, Ojemann LM Outcome with Respect to Epileptic Seizures. In J Engel Jr (ed), Surgical Treatment of the Epilepsies (2nd ed). New York: Raven, 1993;609.
51. Engel J Jr. Outcome with Respect to Epileptic Seizures. In J Engel Jr (ed), Surgical Treatment of the Epilepsies. New York: Raven, 1987;553.
52. Spencer SS, Spencer DD. Dogma, Data, and Directions. In SS Spencer, DD Spencer (eds), Surgery for Epilepsy (Contemporary Issues in Neurological Surgery). Boston: Blackwell, 1991;181.
53. Jensen I. Temporal lobe surgery around the world. Acta Neurol Scand 1975;52:354.
54. Babb TL, Brown WJ. Pathological Findings in Epilepsy. In J Engel Jr (ed), Surgical Treatment of the Epilepsies. New York: Raven, 1987;511.
55. Pilcher W, Roberts DW, Flanigin HF, et al. Complications of Epilepsy Surgery. In J Engel Jr (ed), Surgical Treatment of the Epilepsies (2nd ed). New York: Raven, 1993;565.

17

Psychosocial and Rehabilitative Treatment of Epilepsy

Venkat Ramani

Introduction

Epilepsy is a chronic disorder characterized by recurrent seizures. Like other chronic illnesses, it is a major psychosocial stressor. The protracted nature of the disorder taxes the resources of affected individuals and interferes with their successful adaptation to life. The unpredictability of seizure occurrence often engenders in them a state of vigilant anxiety and inhibition of behavior that leads to progressive social withdrawal. The social stigma associated with epilepsy persists even today despite evidence from recent surveys indicating increased awareness about the illness among those in the general public.[1] Individuals with epilepsy face a number of problems in their everyday life related to emotional, social, vocational, financial, and legal matters. These diverse issues are often collectively lumped together, perhaps without justification, under the convenient label "psychosocial problems."[2] In a study by Dodrill and his colleagues, 55% of epileptic patients showed evidence of significant psychosocial problems on the Washington Psychosocial Seizure Inventory.[3] Poor seizure control, multiple seizure types, and associated neurologic deficits seem to render patients more vulnerable to psychosocial difficulties.

Psychosocial problems associated with epilepsy are often more disabling than seizures themselves. Epilepsy cannot be managed with drugs alone; in fact, effective seizure control is often difficult to achieve without a reasonable degree of psychosocial stability. A comprehensive approach to seizure management with attention to psychological and social problems is therefore essential for lasting benefit. For the sake of convenience, psychosocial problems of epilepsy may be discussed under three headings: (1) psychological and psychiatric issues, (2) social and vocational issues, and (3) legal issues.

Psychological and Psychiatric Issues

The prevalence of psychiatric disorders in epilepsy is difficult to estimate because of methodologic problems. Nevertheless, there is good evidence to indicate a higher incidence of psychiatric problems in people with epilepsy than in the general population.[4] Furthermore, controlled studies suggest that emotional symptoms may be more common in epileptic patients than in medical or nonepileptic neurologic patients.[5] Although psychiatric manifestations may be directly related to seizure activity in some patients, in the vast majority of cases they are interictal in nature, resulting from complex interaction of biological and environmental factors.[6] The specificity of these mental syndromes and their relationship to various types of epilepsies remain controversial. For example, the existence of a unique temporal lobe personality or syndrome has been questioned by many investigators.[4] Such controversies notwithstanding, from a practical point of view, early recognition and vigorous treatment of emotional disorders are very important in epilepsy management. Lack of attention to a patient's psychological needs invariably leads to a strained patient–physician relationship, noncompliance with treatment, unsatisfactory seizure control, and perpetuation of the patient's psychosocial problems.

Recognition of personality disorders is usually not difficult in clinical practice. A broad psychosocial history obtained at the time of initial seizure evaluation is usually adequate for identifying a major psychopathologic process. This initial survey should include information about the patient's current life situation (marital status, employment, living conditions, etc.), past and present emotional problems, and attitudes about illness and treatment. Sometimes the existence of psychological problems is revealed by subtle signs such as missed appointments, frequent telephone calls to the physician, irregular compliance with treatment, and inexplicable variations in seizure control. A sympathetic attitude on the part of the physician and sensitive exploration of patient's emotional life in a supportive milieu often result in psychological improvement, obviating the need for formal psychiatric intervention. Patient education is an important aspect of this strategy. An excellent review of comprehensive patient and family education in epilepsy care can be found in a recent article by Shope.[7]

The major psychiatric disorders encountered in patients with epilepsy are depression, anxiety, aggression, psychosis, and pseudoseizures (PSs). The diagnosis and management of these specific syndromes is discussed below.

Depression

Depression is fairly common among patients with epilepsy. The magnitude of this problem, however, is not reliably known. There is agreement in the literature that depression is the most frequently encountered emotional disorder in people with epilepsy.[8] Ictal depression is rare. It tends to be brief, lasting only a few seconds to minutes, and often represents the initial aura of complex partial seizures. Prolonged ictal depression lasting days to weeks and resembling psychogenic depressive episodes has not been convincingly documented, and for all practical purposes, clinically significant depression in epilepsy is an interictal phenomenon. Transient depression may occur as a prodromal symptom before seizures or as a postictal event. A clearly defined alternating relationship between depression and seizures appears to be relatively rare in clinical practice. The topic of depression in epilepsy has been comprehensively reviewed by Robertson and Trimble.[8]

Diagnosis

The full-blown syndrome of depression is characterized by the presence of specific emotional, cognitive, behavioral, and somatic symptoms. The patient feels sad and is preoccupied with depressive thoughts. Thought process is slow, and the patient experiences difficulties in memory and concentration. There is a lack of initiative, and psychomotor retardation is prominent. Sleep and appetite are disturbed, and sexual drive is diminished. The diagnosis of depression is obvious in the presence of the above signs and symptoms; however, it can be difficult because of certain problems unique to epilepsy. Many patients have varying degrees of cognitive impairment and may lack social and communication skills. They are often withdrawn and inhibited as a consequence of chronic psychosocial stresses, and low self-esteem is very common in this group. Some of these features can mimic clinical depression and create diagnostic difficulties. Often clinicians fail to make the distinction between transient feelings of depression and more enduring depressive illness. Although depressive symptoms are fairly common among people with epilepsy, there is no convincing evidence to indicate that depressive illness is more common in this group than in the general population. The diagnostic difficulty is compounded by the fact that antiepileptic drugs (AEDs) often induce sedation and sometimes even frank depression of mood. This is particularly the case with phenobarbital and primidone.

Management

Early diagnosis of depression in epileptic patients may be difficult, and a high index of suspicion is important. AED toxicity should be ruled out and multiple drug therapy reduced. Carbamazepine and valproate seem to cause the least amount of cognitive and mood impairment, and monotherapy with these agents should be instituted whenever possible. Sedative drugs such as phenobarbital and primidone should be gradually discontinued. Emotional support, encouragement, and tangible assistance to the patient to cope with the problems of daily living are generally sufficient to overcome depression in most cases. Antidepressant drug (ADD) treatment is only occasionally indicated. The risk of seizure precipitation by ADDs, although real, is not a major concern in clinical practice. Also, pharmacokinetic interactions between AEDs and ADDs are not clinically significant. High-dose therapy and the use of certain ADDs such as maprotiline appear to increase the risk of seizures and therefore should be avoided.

Electroconvulsive therapy (ECT) may be required in rare cases of intractable depression, particularly when there is a risk of suicide. There is an increased risk of suicide in patients with epilepsy,[9] and prompt psychiatric consultation should be obtained whenever such a possibility is suspected. ECT is not contraindicated in epilepsy; in fact, ECT has been used as adjunct therapy for intractable seizures because of its presumed gamma-aminobutyric acid system–mediated anticonvulsant properties.[10] The theoretic risk of aggravating seizures by kindling does not appear to be clinically significant in short-term ECT for epilepsy-depression syndromes.

Anxiety

Anxiety symptoms are common in seizure patients. A state of chronic anxiety is generated by the ever present risk of unpredictable seizures, and patients often dread the consequences of having a seizure, such as social embarrassment, public exposure of their illness, physical injury, and potential loss of a job. In most cases, anxiety is vague and generalized but at times may evolve into discrete phobic syndromes or manifest itself as PSs. Transient fear or anxiety symptoms frequently occur as initial auras in complex partial seizures. Persistent or chronic anxiety, however, is almost always an interictal disturbance. As in depression, supportive psychotherapy is usually adequate for managing mild anxiety symptoms. Benzodiazepines may be used in more severe cases. Biofeedback and relaxation therapy can be very effective in reducing anxiety symptoms in selected patients.

Aggression

There is no evidence to support the popular belief that aggression is more common in epileptics than in nonepileptics.[11] Ictal aggression is very rare. Criminal acts involving well coordinated directed aggression are never the result of seizures. Some patients may exhibit aggressive behavior in postictal confusional states, particularly when subjected to forcible restraint. Most often, interictal aggression is related to environmental triggers and is generally encountered in institutionalized mentally retarded patients. AEDs such as phenobarbital, primidone, and benzodiazepines may precipitate hyperactivity and aggressive behavior in some patients, particularly children.

When the aggressive behavior is medication-induced, the offending drug should be discontinued. Environmental manipulation and behavior modification can be very effective in reducing aggressive behavior in the institutionalized population.[12] A number of drugs are potentially useful in the symptomatic control of aggression. They include neuroleptics such as chlorpromazine and haloperidol, propranolol, methylphenidate, and lithium. Valproate and carbamazepine have been reported to be useful in some cases.[13]

Psychosis

Psychosis occurs in about 5% of patients with epilepsy. Usually, these patients have a long history of seizures. Complex partial seizure type and bilateral mesial temporal or frontal epileptogenic foci seem to increase the risk for psychosis. The pathogenesis and specificity of epileptic psychoses are largely unknown. Clinically, they represent a heterogeneous group, and some bear a superficial resemblance to schizophrenia.[14, 15] Sometimes, there is an alternating relationship between seizures and psychosis, and the electroencephalogram (EEG) in such cases may show the phenomenon of "forced normalization" during the phase of psychosis.[16] Prolonged nonconvulsive status epilepticus may be misdiagnosed as psychosis. Patients in this condition show clouding of sensorium, mental confusion, and behavioral automatisms, and the EEG shows diagnostically specific ictal changes. Savard et al. recently described a syndrome of postictal psychosis after complex partial seizures in nine patients.[17] Management of interictal psychosis is essentially symptomatic and is no different from that of the so-called functional psychoses. Antipsychotic medications are quite effective and may be used safely without undue concern about aggravation of seizures.

Pseudoseizures

About 10–15% of patients admitted to specialized epilepsy centers are found to have PSs with or without coexisting epilepsy. The incidence of PSs in the general population is unknown. According to Roy, the typical PS patient is female with a personal and family history of psychiatric disorders, history of sexual maladjustment, attempted suicide, and current depression.[18] PSs may occur in both sexes and in all age groups. History of incest appears to be common at least in a subgroup of PS patients.[19] PSs do not represent a unitary disorder; rather, they are a symptom of diverse psychiatric conditions such as conversion disorder, anxiety, depression, and psychosis.[20] Reports of frequent "seizures" by the patient despite vigorous treatment with major AEDs should raise the suspicion of PSs, particularly when the EEG repeatedly fails to reveal any abnormalities. Simultaneous video-EEG documentation is usually required for definitive diagnosis. Treatment should be individualized and directed toward underlying conditions.[21] A detailed discussion of the diagnosis and management of PSs is beyond the scope of this chapter and may be found elsewhere.[22]

Social and Vocational Issues

People with epilepsy face a number of social problems. Many are unemployed or underemployed. They experience difficulty in obtaining life, health, and automobile insurances. Lack of secure employment, inadequate insurance, and the high cost of medical treatments impose a heavy financial burden on these individuals and their families. Financial limitations prevent access to high-quality medical care, resulting in inadequate seizure control. Poor seizure control in turn leads to deterioration in the patient's psychosocial status and further downward drift in society.

Employment

The economic cost of caring for epilepsy was estimated at more than $3 billion by the Epilepsy Foundation of America (EFA) in 1975. This figure is undoubtedly many times higher today. Two-thirds of epileptic patients have additional neurologic or cognitive deficits, and the unemployment rate is high in this group.[23] In one study, the unemployment rate for persons with epilepsy was estimated to be about twice that of the general population (7.6% vs. 3.6%).[24] There is no doubt that there has been an increased awareness about epilepsy and a concomitant decline in prejudicial attitudes toward people with seizures among those in the general population in recent years. Nevertheless, employers continue to show reluctance to hire individuals with epilepsy, even when they are qualified for the job. Deeply ingrained prejudices, doubts about the applicant's competence, image considerations, liability, and insurance issues are some of the usual reasons for employer resistance. Although it may seem that some of these concerns are justified, closer scrutiny does not support that position. The job performance of people with epilepsy compares well with that of their peers without epilepsy, and their rate of absenteeism is not higher.[24] Epileptics do seem to have a slightly higher rate of job-related injuries, but it has not been proved that these injuries are caused by seizures. People with epilepsy must contend with a number of realistic problems that may interfere with their ability to secure and retain employment. Many have some degree of additional neurologic handicaps and may be deficient in their communication and job-seeking skills. Lacking driving privileges, they often depend on public transportation and are therefore limited in their mobility.

The physician's primary role, of course, is to aim for good seizure control and minimize undesirable side effects; however, good seizure control alone is not sufficient to guarantee employment in many cases, particularly in cases of individuals with various neurologic and cognitive deficits. A systematic program of vocational rehabilitation is necessary in such cases, and it is important for the physician to be aware of the various resources available in the community that provide such services. There are a number of vocational rehabilitation agencies, some of which are federally sponsored and others funded at the state or local levels. The best known program is the Training and Placement Services (TAPS), which is sponsored by the EFA with federal funding. These programs offer a variety of services, including comprehensive assessment of the client's job potential, psychological counseling, training in job-seeking skills, referrals to potential employers, and postplacement followups. TAPS has a 76% success rate in placement and 70% success rate in job retention by clients.[24] The local epilepsy association can assist clients with information on a variety of issues such as financial matters, insurance, education, housing, transportation, and legal assistance.

Physicians are frequently asked to submit medical reports to various rehabilitation agencies and employers on behalf of their patients regarding their seizure control and disability status. A comprehensive and meaningful report will greatly help these agencies and facilitate the process of successful job placement. The best predictors for successful outcome in vocational rehabilitation are high patient motivation, normal intelligence, good seizure control, and absence of significant neurologic deficits. The physician's report should contain the following information: (1) a concise description of neurologic and psychiatric deficits; (2) reports of neuropsychological assessments, if available; (3) summary of seizure-related disability, incorporating information on seizure type, frequency, presence of aura, loss of consciousness, degree of impairment in awareness, specific precipitants, time, circumstances of seizure occurrence, and medication effects; (4) realistic appraisal of the patient's suitability for the job in question from a medical perspective, based on knowledge of the job requirements; and (5) special problem areas and specific activities to be avoided in the work situation. As a general rule, patients should avoid working at heights and operating power tools or heavy machinery.

Two sensitive issues concern patients with respect to employment. First is the question of whether to divulge the history of epilepsy in job applications; the second is about mandatory drug testing of employees and job applicants by the employer in many job sectors. The EFA advises clients to divulge their condition to the employer, not at the time of application, but after the job has been offered and before accepting it. The foundation has also taken a strong stand on the issue of drug testing and has issued a position statement aimed at protecting the rights of clients in such situations. This publication can be obtained by contacting the EFA (1-800-EFA-1000).

Education

There are a number of important issues regarding the educational needs of people with epilepsy. Most educational programs are not sensitive to the special needs of children with epilepsy, and considerable ignorance about the disease still prevails in the school system. Children may be subjected to unnecessary restriction of various school activities based on unfounded fears. Absence seizures may be misinterpreted by the teacher as a sign of inattentiveness or dullness. To complicate matters further, children with epilepsy often have a number of realistic handicaps that may interfere with learning. The treating physician can provide a valuable service to these children by providing comprehensive information to the school staff about the nature and extent of their neurologic deficits and the functional consequences of the seizures. Federal and state laws provide important protection from discrimination in education based on disabilities; this point is discussed further in the section on legal issues.

Lifestyle Concerns

Patients frequently ask a number of questions concerning adjustments to daily living. These relate to seizure precautions, factors that may aggravate seizures such as sleep loss, excess caffeine or alcohol consumption, restrictions in sports and recreational activities, and so forth. Patients should be encouraged to exercise moderation and use common sense in these matters. A balanced and nutritious diet, adequate rest, and regular physical activities should be prescribed. Sleep deprivation is to be avoided. Moderate intake of caffeine and occasional use of alcohol may be permitted. Patients should not be allowed to swim alone. There is no justification to restrict contact sports, but high-risk activities such as rock climbing, scuba diving, sky diving, and hang gliding are strictly prohibited.

Legal Issues

Historically, people with epilepsy have had to face a number of legal restrictions. In many states, they were prohibited from marrying and were denied the right to adoption and child custody. Compulsory sterilization of individuals with epilepsy was legally permitted in some states. Immigration into the United States was denied on the basis of epilepsy. In some states, such restrictions existed until the 1980s. Such archaic laws have largely been repealed and are only of historical interest now. In recent years, a number of laws have been enacted to protect the rights of individuals with mental and physical disabilities and to prevent discrimination in employment, education, public facilities, housing, and transportation. The Rehabilitation Act of 1973 prohibits discrimination on the basis of handicaps in educational programs by recipients of federal financial assistance. The Education for All Handicapped Children Act guarantees every handicapped child the right to free and appropriate education in the least restrictive setting. Another important series of legislative acts is the Developmentally Disabled Assistance and Bill of Rights Act. The landmark piece of legislation, Americans with Disabilities Act, which was signed into law by President George Bush in 1990, gives civil rights protection to individuals with disabilities in several important areas.

Despite such major reforms, social prejudices and negative perceptions about epilepsy linger in the public mind. For epileptic patients, obtaining legal redress in cases of discrimination is often a lengthy and expensive process that cannot be achieved without the concerted efforts of legal and medical professions.[25] Patients who experience seizures in public places face the risk of being unjustly arrested for disorderly conduct or for possibly being under the influence of drugs or alcohol. To avert such mistakes, law enforcement officials in many states are required to search for medical information on all individuals who are unconscious or appear impaired before arresting an individual. Patients should be advised to wear Medic Alert bracelets and carry their medications in labeled containers.

Driver's Licensing

Perhaps the single most important legal issue that concerns both patients and physicians alike is the problem of an epileptic patient having a driver's license. Driving is a social and economic necessity in our society. Restriction of driving privileges not only leads to limitation of employment opportunities and financial hardship, but also to social isolation and low self-esteem. On the other hand, seizures can and do cause automobile accidents and thus endanger public safety. Physicians treating epileptic patients are frequently caught in the dilemma of conflicting interests—between their obligation to assist the patient on the one hand and safeguarding the broader interests of society on the other. Regulations concerning drivers licensing vary considerably from state to state and are often quite arbitrary. The requirements for seizure-free period, mandatory physician reporting to the state's department of motor vehicles (DMV), and periodic medical reviews are far from uniform in the various states. Mandatory physician reporting is required in six states. It does not appear that such a regulation has had any effect in reducing seizure-related accidents in these states. Concern has been expressed that mandatory physician reporting to the authorities may actually discourage patients from seeking medical help and thus prove counterproductive to the patient's welfare. Ten states have no minimum seizure-free period requirement before relicensing, whereas 25 states require a 12-month period, and most others between 6 and 9 months. Freedom from seizures for 2 years is required only in one state. The regulations for interstate trucking are quite stringent and prohibit anyone suffering from epilepsy or on AED therapy from operating commercial vehicles on national highways.

Physicians treating patients with epilepsy have the responsibility to submit periodic medical statements to the state DMV in support of their application for the renewal of driver's license. This seemingly routine function often involves a complex decision-making process to determine the risk the applicant poses to incur a seizure-related accident while driving. Unfortunately, reliable information necessary to make such a complex decision is not available. The key questions in this respect are:

1.   What is the incidence of seizure-related accidents in people with epilepsy, and how different is it from the general population?

2.   Do epileptics pose a greater risk for traffic accidents than people with other chronic medical conditions?

3.   What is the nature of seizure-related accidents, and what are the important factors that determine accident proneness?

4.   What are the predictors of seizure recurrence, remission, and relapse?

The answers to these questions are not clear, and data available in the literature are limited.

It appears that people with epilepsy have a slightly greater risk for traffic accidents than the population at large. The magnitude of this risk, however, is unclear. One study found the risk to be twice as high.[26] Other studies have found that although the risk for epileptic drivers is higher than that for the general population, it is not significantly different from that for other chronic medical conditions such as diabetes and cardiovascular disease.[27, 28] In a study of 82 epileptic patients who had definite seizures while driving, Gastaut and Zifkin found that 55% of the seizures resulted in an accident.[29] On the other hand, van der Lugt found that only 11% of accidents caused by epileptic drivers were actually the result of a seizure and that, in general, the accidents were less severe than average, involving single vehicles and occurring more often in rural areas.[30] Fatalities are significantly fewer in seizure-related accidents compared with those caused by alcohol intoxication.[31]

The risk of seizure recurrence after the first unprovoked seizure ranges from 16% to 61%.[24] Remote symptomatic causes, partial seizures, and abnormal EEG findings appear to increase the likelihood of recurrent seizures. In the study by Gastaut and Zifkin, complex partial seizures accounted for 88% of seizure-related accidents.[29] On the other hand, simple partial seizures without impairment of awareness and exclusively nocturnal seizures seem to be associated with lowest risk for traffic accidents. It is important to keep in mind, however, that 30% of patients with only nocturnal seizures may develop additional daytime seizures on long-term follow-up.[32] Brief myoclonic seizures without impairment of consciousness or motor control do not pose a major risk for driving. The presence of a reliable aura before seizures allows the patient sufficient time to take protective measures to avoid traffic accidents. It is reasonable to assume that the likelihood of a seizure occurring while driving is related to the degree of seizure control in general. In this respect, the number of seizures in the last 2 years and the longest seizure-free interval during this period are useful clinical indicators of the state of seizure control.[32] Patients with idiopathic generalized seizures and normal neurologic examinations are most likely to enter seizure remission and are least likely to be involved in accidents caused by seizures. The rate of relapse is also low in such patients. Even in this group, there is a small risk of relapse during AED withdrawal, and ideally patients should refrain from driving during periods of physician-directed reductions in medication. Seizures precipitated by planned AED reduction or other specific provocative factors such as hypoglycemia are relatively benign with respect to the probability of recurrence, and a certain measure of leniency is justified in such cases during DMV evaluations. On the other hand, frequent seizures, multiple seizure types, history of noncompliance with treatment, repeated alcohol intoxications, and prior accidents are reasons for caution or even denial of a driver's license.

Practical recommendations for DMV evaluations include:

1. Establish the diagnosis of epilepsy.

2.   Formulate a comprehensive assessment of the seizure disorder, including seizure cause, seizure type, frequency, and specific seizure precipitants.

3.   Determine if there are mitigating or complicating factors that may affect seizure control.

4.   Estimate the likelihood of seizure occurrence and the potential for traffic accidents based on seizure-related data, the patient's lifestyle, and his or her driving habits.

5.   Know your state laws regarding epilepsy and driving.

In states where reporting to DMV is not mandatory, advise patients about their obligation to inform the authorities and document such action. The physician's divulgence of the diagnosis of epilepsy to the DMV when it is not mandatory can be construed as a breach of patient–physician confidentiality and may result in legal action against the physician. When there is a substantial foreseeable public risk or danger, however, physicians may and perhaps are even required to report patients with seizures to the authorities at the risk of breaking the ethics of patient confidentiality.

Resources for People with Epilepsy

Physicians should be aware of the various resources available in the community for people with disabilities. Only a brief overview of the major resources is given here; detailed information may be obtained by contacting local epilepsy associations or other social agencies.

Health Care

Medicare is a federal health insurance program that serves individuals older than 65 years of age and disabled people younger than 65 years of age if they are eligible for Social Security benefits. Medicaid is a joint state and federal program that provides health care services to people with low income. Crippled Children's Services provides medical services to handicapped children from birth to 21 years of age. Aid to Families with Dependent Children provides care to families in which one or both parents are disabled. Veterans Affairs benefits are available to people who have served in the armed forces.

Financial Assistance

Supplemental Security Income is available for individuals with disabilities who cannot obtain gainful employment, even if they have not contributed to the Social Security system. Social Security Disability Insurance, on the other hand, is designed for people with disabilities who have made Social Security contributions. The Workmen's Compensation Fund compensates for disabilities resulting from work-related injuries.

Insurance

People with epilepsy can obtain term group life insurance through the EFA underwritten by the Government Employees Life Insurance Company. State-sponsored second injury funds encourage employers to hire people with disabilities by protecting employers from additional financial liabilities. Automobile insurance may be available to qualified individuals with epilepsy through state-sponsored assigned risk plans, although at a higher premium.

Legal Assistance

People with epilepsy and other handicaps may contact a number of agencies for information on legal matters pertaining to their disabilities. These resources include state and local legal aid programs as well as the local bar and epilepsy associations. The Legal Advocacy Department of the EFA is another important resource for legal advice and referral services.

The Epilepsy Foundation of America

The EFA is a national volunteer health organization dedicated to the comprehensive care of individuals with epilepsy. It has a large number of state and local affiliates and seeks to accomplish its goals and mission through support of research, education, advocacy, and service. Detailed information about the various activities and services provided by the EFA may be obtained by contacting the foundation's office, which is located in Landover, Maryland. Their toll-free telephone number is 1-800-EFA-1000.

Conclusion

There has been significant progress in the field of epileptology during the last two decades. Major advances have taken place in AED treatment, intensive seizure monitoring techniques, and epilepsy surgery. The long-ignored psychosocial predicament of people with epilepsy is only now beginning to receive the attention it deserves. Specialized epilepsy centers were first established in the mid 1970s; and in the years that followed, comprehensive medical and psychosocial treatment of epilepsy has become the standard of care. Funding for research into the psychosocial problems of epilepsy is more readily available from sources such as the EFA. Research in this area has suffered in the past because of a general lack of interest in the subject, methodologic problems, and flawed study designs. The importance of well designed, controlled studies is being increasingly recognized. These developments in the profession are paralleled by an equally impressive, enlightened progress in the social and legal environment. It is hoped that comprehensive care of epilepsy will increasingly become a reality rather than remain an idealized concept.

References

1. Caveness WF, Gallup GH Jr. A survey of public attitudes towards epilepsy in 1979 with an indication of trends over the past thirty years. Epilepsia 1980;21:509.
2. Trostle JA. Social Aspects of Epilepsy. In WA Hauser (ed), Current Trends in Epilepsy: A Self-Study Course for Physicians, Unit I. Landover, MD: Epilepsy Foundation of America, 1988;39.
3. Dodrill CB, Breyer DN, Diamond MB, et al. Psychosocial problems among adults with epilepsy. Epilepsia 1984;25:168.
4. Dodrill CB, Batzel LW. Interictal behavioral features of patients with epilepsy. Epilepsia 1986;27(Suppl 2):64.
5. Kogeorgos J, Fonagay P, Scott DF. Psychiatric symptom patterns of chronic epileptics attending a neurological clinic: a controlled investigation. Br J Psychiatry 1982;140:236.
6. Hermann BP. Interictal Psychopathology in Patients with Epilepsy. In WA Hauser (ed), Current Trends in Epilepsy: A Self-Study Course for Physicians, Unit I. Landover, MD: Epilepsy Foundation of America, 1988;29.
7. Shope JT. Educating Patients and Families to Successfully Manage a Seizure Disorder. In WA Hauser (ed), Current Trends in Epilepsy: A Self-Study Course for Physicians, Unit II. Landover, MD: Epilepsy Foundation of America, 1988;40.
8. Robertson MM, Trimble MR. Depressive illness in epilepsy. A review. Epilepsia 1983;24(Suppl 2):109.

9. Mathews WS, Barabas G. Suicide and epilepsy: a review of the literature. Psychosomatics 1981;22:515.
10. Sackeim HA, Prohovnik I, Decina P, et al. Anticonvulsant Properties of Electroconvulsive Therapy: Theory and Case Report. In M Baldy-Moulinier, DH Ingvar, BS Meldrum (eds), Current Problems in Epilepsy. London: John Libbey, 1983;370.
11. Treiman DM. Epilepsy and violence: medical and legal issues. Epilepsia 1986;27(Suppl 2):77.
12. Gardner WI, Cole CE. Aggression and Related Conduct Difficulties. In JL Matson (ed), Handbook of Behavior Modification with the Mentally Retarded (2nd ed). New York: Plenum, 1990;225.
13. Post RM, Trimble MR, Pippenger CE (eds). Clinical Use of Anticonvulsants in Psychiatric Disorders. New York: Demos, 1989.
14. Trimble MR. Interictal psychoses of epilepsy. Adv Neurol 1991;55:143.
15. Ramani V, Gumnit RJ. Intensive monitoring of interictal psychosis in epilepsy. Ann Neurol 1982;11:613.
16. Pakalnis A, Drake ME, John K, Kellum JB. Forced normalization. Acute psychosis after seizure control in 7 patients. Arch Neurol 1987;44:289.
17. Savard G, Andermann F, Olivier A, Remillard GM. Postictal psychosis after partial complex seizures: a multiple case study. Epilepsia 1991;32:225.
18. Roy A. Hysterical seizures. Arch Neurol 1979;36:447.
19. Goodwin J, Simms M, Bergman R. Hysterical seizures: a sequel to incest. Am J Orthopsychiatry 1979;49:698.
20. Ramani V, Quesney LF, Olson D, Gumnit RJ. Diagnosis of hysterical seizures in epileptic patients. Am J Psychiatry 1980;137:705.
21. Ramani V, Gumnit RJ. Management of hysterical patients in epileptic patients. Arch Neurol 1982;39:78.
22. Riley TL, Roy A (eds). Pseudoseizures. Baltimore: Williams & Wilkins, 1982.
23. Rodin EA, Shapiro HL, Lennox M. Epilepsy and life performance. Rehab Lit 1977;38:34.
24. Hauser WA, Hersdorffer DC. Epilepsy. Frequency, Causes and Consequences. New York: Demos, 1990.
25. Golinker LA, Lehman C. Legal Aspects of Epilepsy. In WA Hauser (ed), Current Trends in Epilepsy: A Self-Study Course for Physicians, Unit III. Landover, MD: Epilepsy Foundation of America, 1988:24.
26. Waller JA. Chronic medical conditions and traffic safety. N Engl J Med 1965;273:1413.
27. Crancer A, McMurray L. Accident and violation rates of Washington's medically restricted drivers. JAMA 1968;205:272.
28. Hansotia P, Broste SK. The effect of epilepsy or diabetes mellitus on the risk of automobile accidents. N Engl J Med 1991;324:22.
29. Gastaut H, Zifkin BG. The risk of automobile accidents with seizures occurring while driving: relationship to seizure type. Neurology 1987;37:1613.
30. van der Lugt PJM. Traffic accidents caused by epilepsy. Epilepsia 1975;16:747.
31. Engel J Jr. Seizures and Epilepsy. Philadelphia: FA Davis, 1989;475.
32. Spudis EV, Penry JK, Gibson P. Driving impairment caused by episodic brain dysfunction. Arch Neurol 1986;43:558.

18

Recent Advances in the Management of Epilepsy: A Synopsis

Sudhansu Chokroverty

Introduction

Epilepsy is by definition a condition of recurrent unprovoked seizures. An overall prevalence of 5–8 per 1,000 population has been determined based on studies in the United States, Europe, Japan, China, and India.[1] The cause of seizures in approximately 70% of all cases remains unknown.[1] In the remaining 30%, the causes of seizures include developmental disorders (5.5%); cerebral vascular disease (13.2%); head trauma, including birth injuries (4.1%); brain tumors (3.6%); central nervous system infection (2.6%); degenerative central nervous system diseases (1.8%); and miscellaneous other causes (0.5%).[1] The incidence of epilepsy is slightly higher in males than in females for most seizure types except absence seizure, which has an incidence that is twice as high in females as in males. Epilepsy can begin at any age, but the highest incidences are reported in the very young and in the elderly.

In this chapter, recent advances in the management of epilepsy are summarized, and the general principles of practical treatment are highlighted. There is considerable individual variation in response to drug treatment, and each patient must be managed on an individual basis. The details of modern management have been described in various chapters in this volume. In the last two decades, several developments have led to recent advancements and improvements in the management of epilepsy.[2, 3] Such developments include a better understanding of the mechanism of epileptogenesis; an improved classification of epilepsy and epileptic syndromes; technical advances and improved diagnostic precision by use of magnetic resonance imaging (MRI) and long-term video-electroencephalographic (EEG) monitoring, including subdural and depth EEG recordings; a better understanding of the pharmacokinetic and the pharmacodynamic interactions of the antiepileptic drugs (AEDs); the concept of monotherapy being superior to the long-standing practice of multiple drug therapy in the management of most epileptic patients, including patients with seizures that are thought to be intractable or refractory; the availability of several new promising AEDs developed on the basis of neuronal cellular and neurotransmitter mechanisms; and, finally, a better method of localization of an epileptic focus for surgical treatment in a small percentage of patients with medically refractory epilepsy.

Does the Patient Have Epilepsy?

Before treating a patient for epilepsy, the diagnosis of epilepsy must be unequivocally confirmed. This is accomplished by obtaining a detailed history and physical examination and by differentiating the recurrent seizures from conditions that may mimic epilepsy (see Chapters 3 and 5). The role of EEG is crucial and has been described in detail in Chapter 5. An attempt should be made in suspected secondary cases of epilepsy to determine the cause by obtaining imaging studies (e.g., a computed tomographic [CT] scan of the brain and MRI) and other laboratory tests to diagnose systemic metabolic or toxic causes.

What Type of Epilepsy Does the Patient Have?

The next step is to determine what type of epilepsy (e.g., partial or localization-related and generalized) the patient has based on an electroclinical correlation and the International Classification of Epileptic Seizures and Epileptic Syndromes (see Chapter 2).

Which Patients Should be Treated and When?

Next, a decision must be made whether to treat a patient with a single unprovoked seizure (see Chapter 9) or to wait until the patient has a second or more seizures. A single seizure by definition does not constitute epilepsy. The benefit of treating a single seizure must be weighed against the possibility of adverse effects associated with AED treatment. Recurrence rate after a first unprovoked seizure ranges widely, from 23% to 71%, based on both retrospective and prospective studies.[4] However, two important prospective studies by Hauser et al.[5] and Shinnar et al.[6] have determined that a second episode of seizure within the next 3 years occurs in only 26–29% of cases. Predictors of seizure recurrence after first seizure include a history of prior neurologic illness (the most important factor); an abnormal EEG finding; a family history of epilepsy; prior history of acute seizures, including febrile seizures, status epilepticus, or multiple seizures at the onset, and Todd's paralysis (i.e., partial seizure).[7] Most epileptologists therefore would elect not to treat a patient with a single unprovoked seizure and thus avoid the unnecessary use of AEDs, which are often associated with adverse reactions in the majority of the subjects. An exception can be made for an adult whose livelihood depends on driving, in whom a second seizure may be hazardous to his or her driving, and whose driver's license may therefore be suspended. Another exception for treating patients experiencing a single seizure can be made in cases where the factors predicting recurrence suggest a strong possibility of seizure recurrence, and hence the benefit of AEDs outweigh their potential disadvantages.[8]

Recurrent seizures (epilepsy) may cause damage or loss of cerebral neurons, degeneration of the neuronal and dendritic spines ("seizure begets seizure"),[9] as well as psychosocial and vocational disturbances.[8] Therefore, patients with epilepsy should be adequately treated with AEDs. Additional reasons for treating epilepsy with AEDs are the controversial question of kindling and genesis of a mirror focus. Most investigators, however, do not believe in the existence of human kindling.

Selection of Antiepileptic Drugs

Once a decision to treat has been made, the most appropriate AEDs for the particular type of epilepsy or epilepsy syndromes must be selected.

The AEDs in current use may be divided into three categories according to their efficacy and toxicity;[10] a new class of promising AEDs[11, 12] should also be considered (see Chapters 4 and 19).

The first-line drugs (highest efficacy and least toxicity) include phenytoin (PHT), carbamazepine (CBZ), valproic acid (VPA), and ethosuximide (ETS). Second-line drugs (high efficacy but may cause excessive sedation and other side effects) include phenobarbital (PB), and primidone (PR). Clonazepam (Klonopin) also may be considered a second-line drug for certain seizure types. The third-line drugs (useful to only a few patients but with troublesome adverse effects) include clorazepate, mephobarbital, methsuximide, mephenytoin, ethotoin, phenacemide, and acetazolamide. The serious side effects of third-line drugs outweigh their efficacy; therefore, they are rarely used with some exception. The fourth category of promising new AEDs[11, 12] includes felbamate (Felbatol), gabapentin (Neurontin), lamotrigine (Lamictal), and vigabatrin (GVG). All of these drugs have been used in several thousand patients in Europe for several years. Felbamate, gabapentin, and lamotrigine are now available in the United States for general use; vigabatrin may be available in the future. Felbamate was restricted several months after its availability, however, because of an increasing incidence of aplastic anemia and liver failure causing deaths in a few patients.

Two multicenter Veterans Affairs double-blind, controlled cooperative studies compared several of the first- and second-line AEDs. The first study[13] compared PHT, CBZ, PB, and PR in 622 patients with simple and complex partial seizures and with secondary generalized tonic-clonic seizures. There was no statistically significant difference in efficacy between these drugs in treating secondarily generalized tonic-clonic seizures. The second study[14] compared CBZ and VPA in 480 patients with complex partial seizure and secondarily generalized tonic-clonic seizures. CBZ was statistically superior to VPA in patients with complex partial seizures, but no significant difference was noted between the two drugs in treating secondarily generalized tonic-clonic seizures. In four well-controlled, double-blind studies,[15–18] VPA and PHT showed equal efficacy as monotherapy for primary generalized tonic-clonic seizures. Approximately 60–75% of these patients became seizure-free. Even in children, a double-blind, multicenter, controlled study showed that PHT, CBZ, PB, and VPA had equal efficacy as monotherapy, but patients taking PB had to drop out of the study because of its adverse effects (sedation and behavioral effects).[19]

Specific Recommendations

Specific recommendations for the first choice for AED are summarized as follows[3, 8, 20–22] (see also Chapters 6, 7, and 10):

For simple or complex partial seizures with or without secondary generalization, CBZ is the initial drug of choice. The cosmetic or possible behavioral side effects of PHT preclude its initial use, particularly in women, children, and young adults, although it is as effective as CBZ in seizure control.

For classic absence seizures, ETS is the first drug of choice; however, those with atypical absence seizures, especially when associated with myoclonic, tonic, or tonic-clonic seizures, should be treated with VPA unless pre-existing hepatic dysfunction contraindicates its use.

VPA is the first drug of choice for primary tonic-clonic generalized seizures. This is also the first drug of choice for juvenile myoclonic epilepsy or other primary generalized epilepsies or epileptic syndrome, such as generalized tonic-clonic seizures on awakening, generalized tonic-clonic seizures with associated myoclonus, and generalized tonic-clonic seizures with photoconvulsive EEG responses. VPA is also the first drug of choice for Lennox-Gastaut syndrome, which may be associated with tonic, atonic, akinetic, myoclonic, or atypical absence or mixed seizures. When a patient is having frequent recurrent seizures that interfere with day-to-day functioning, a drug must then be chosen that can be given as a loading dose either parenterally or orally to achieve rapid therapeutic effects.[21] Therefore, PHT or PB has an advantage in these cases over VPA. Table 18-1 lists the recommended drugs (as first, second or third choice) for particular seizure types.[3]

Initiation of Antiepileptic Drug Therapy

Before initiating therapy, the following baseline laboratory tests must be performed: hematologic tests (e.g., measurements of total and differential white blood cell count, hemoglobin levels, platelet count, and prothrombin time), liver function tests (e.g., measurements of plasma protein levels including those of albumin and globulin, aspartate aminotransferase, alanine aminotransferase, gamma-glutamyl transferase, bilirubin, and alkaline phosphatase), blood urea nitrogen and creatinine measurements, and urinalysis. These baseline measurements are important because any alteration of these test results after AED treatment is begun may be an early indication of adverse effects. Also,

Table 18-1. Selection of Antiepileptic Drugs

Seizure Type	First Choice	Second Choice	Third Choice
Partial seizure (simple, complex, with or without secondary generalization)	CBZ	VPA	PHT, newer AEDs
Generalized seizure			
Classic absence	ESM	VPA	—
Atypical absence	VPA	VPA + ESM	—
Tonic-clonic	VPA	CBZ	PHT, newer AEDs
Myoclonic	VPA	CLN	PB, newer AEDs
Tonic, atonic, akinetic, clonic or mixed	VPA	CLN	PHT, newer AEDs
Infantile spasms	ACTH	Prednisone	CLN

AED = antiepileptic drug; CBZ = carbamazepine; VPA = valproic acid; PHT = phenytoin; ESM = ethosuximide; CLN = clonazepam; PB = phenobarbital; ACTH = adrenocorticotropic hormone.
Source: Modified from JK Penry. Epilepsy: Diagnosis, Management, Quality of Life. New York: Raven, 1986.

contraindications to certain AEDs (e.g., VPA treatment in a patient with abnormal liver function test results) may be determined before initiating treatment.

The basic principle of AED therapy is to start with a low dose and then increase the dose slowly, except in the case of PHT, where an initial loading dose should be given.[8, 20–23] Before initiating AED therapy, the physician must have a basic understanding of the pharmacology of the drugs, including knowing the plasma half-life and steady state of the drugs, drug interactions, drug dosages, the drugs' therapeutic plasma levels, and possible toxicities. See the section on pharmacologic data in this chapter; anticonvulsant toxicity has been discussed in Chapter 13.

Table 18-2 lists the essential pharmacologic data of the first- and second-line AEDs and the four new AEDs. Plasma half-life and steady state are listed in Table 18-3. It is important to know drug plasma half-lives, as any dose change in an AED should be made when a steady state is achieved (this usually occurs at every five plasma half-lives of the drug).

Table 18-2. Pharmacologic Data of First- and Second-Line Antiepileptic Drugs and Four Newer Antiepileptic Drugs

Drug	Initial Dose	Maintenance Dose (mg/kg/day)	Plasma Level (µg/ml)	Protein-Bound (%)
Phenytoin (after a loading dose)	100 mg bid	200–600 (5–8/kg)	10–20	90
Carbamazepine	100 mg bid	400–1,800 (15–20/kg)	4–12	70–80
Valproate	125 mg bid	1,000–3,000 (20–40/kg)	50–100	90–100
Phenobarbital	30 mg nocte	30–240 (2–4/kg)	15–40	45
Primidone	125 mg nocte	500–1,500 (20/kg)	5–15	<20
Ethosuximide	250 mg bid	500–1,500 (15–20/kg)	50–100	0
Clonazepam	0.5 mg bid	1–10 (0.025–0.25/kg)	0.02–0.08	50–80
Felbamate	600 mg bid	2,400–3,600	20–80	20–25
Gabapentin	100 mg tid	900–1,800	2–3	0
Lamotrigine	50 mg qid	200–500	2–4	55
Vigabatrin	500 mg bid	1,500–3,000	Not relevant	0

Table 18-3. Plasma Half-Life and Steady State

Drugs	Half-Life	Steady State (Five Half-Lives) (Days)
Carbamazepine	0.5 day	3
Valproic acid	0.5 day	3
Primidone	0.5 day	3
Phenytoin	1 day	5
Ethosuximide	2 days	10
Phenobarbital	4 days	21
Felbamate	1 day	5
Gabapentin	5–7 hours	1.0–1.5
Lamotrigine	0.5–2.0 days	3–10
Vigabatrin	5 days	25

After AED therapy is initiated, a stable dose and a reduction of the initial side effects (e.g., mild gastrointestinal disturbances, sedation, and dizziness) is achieved generally within the first 4–8 weeks.[8, 20] A follow-up visit is necessary 4–8 weeks after initiation of drug therapy to emphasize compliance and monitor clinical efficacy and side effects. Occurrence of seizures during dosage adjustment should not necessitate further adjustment of medication unless the seizures are frequent or severe. Sixty percent to 70% of patients will have almost complete control of seizures after 1 or 2 years. Some patients may have breakthrough seizures.

Pharmacologic Data

The essential pharmacologic data for the first- and second-line AEDs and the four newer AEDs are summarized here (see also Chapters 4 and 19).[2, 11, 12, 24, 25]

Carbamazepine

CBZ is available as 100-mg and 200-mg tablets and 100 mg/5 ml (teaspoon) suspension. Peak absorption occurs 3–8 hours after ingestion (the average amount of time it takes for peak absorption is 4 hours). Seventy percent to 80% of CBZ is bound to plasma protein. The half-life of CBZ is about 12 hours; hence at least twice daily dosing is required. The starting dose is 200 mg/day (100 mg bid) in most adults. The dose should be increased by 200 mg every 3 days (5 × half-life) until a dose of 10–20 mg/kg/day is achieved. The suggested maximum dose is 1,200 mg/day, but in difficult cases and in those with multidrug regimens, a higher dosage may be needed. The daily maintenance dose may vary from 400 mg to 1,800 mg.

In children, treatment should be started with 5 mg/kg/day in two divided doses. Every 3–4 days, the dose should be increased by half of the starting dose up to a total of 10–15 mg/kg/day.

After 2–4 weeks, CBZ induces its own metabolism; hence, the dosage may need to be increased after several weeks. The full effect of CBZ occurs after 2–3 months.

The therapeutic range of CBZ is 4–12 µg/ml. The plasma level should be obtained 5–7 days after a stable dosage is achieved. Determination of the level should be repeated at 1-month intervals for the next 2 months to diagnose any fall in the level caused by autoinduction. Once the patient is on a stable regimen, a plasma level should be determined.

Most AEDs (e.g., PHT, PR, PB, ETS) increase (stimulate) CBZ metabolism and lower its plasma level; hence, in a multidrug regimen, the CBZ dose may need to be increased. VPA displaces CBZ from protein-binding sites, resulting in an increase of free levels of CBZ and possible clinical toxicity. Certain drugs (e.g., cimetidine, erythromycin, isoniazid, propoxyphene, fluoxetine, and calcium channel blockers) inhibit CBZ metabolism and increase its plasma concentration, causing toxicity. CBZ may increase the metabolism of certain drugs, such as warfarin, thus reducing its anticoagulant effect, and of VPA, PHT, ETS, and clonazepam, lowering their plasma levels.

Phenytoin

PHT is available as 100-mg and 30-mg capsules, 50-mg tablets, and 125 mg/5 ml suspension. PHT is also available as 2-ml ampules of 50 mg/ml for parenteral use. Dilantin is absorbed in 6–12 hours, but most generic formulations are absorbed within 2 hours after ingestion. Approximately 90% of PHT is bound to serum albumin, and the drug has a half-life of approximately 24 hours.

Treatment may be begun with a loading dose on the first day (which should be three to four times the predicted daily dose). The usual range of maintenance dose is 150–600 mg/day. The usual dose of PHT is 5–8 mg/kg/day. A single daily dose may be given in adults. In children, the half-life of PHT is short; hence, a twice or thrice daily dose is given. PHT should be given every 4–6 hours in infants.

The therapeutic range of PHT is 10–20 µg/ml. Steady state is achieved in 5–7 days if the plasma level is below 10 µg/ml. An early morning trough plasma level should be obtained at this time. The half-life increases as the plasma level rises, and the drug may need 2–3 weeks to reach steady state.

Certain drugs stimulate PHT metabolism and lower PHT plasma levels, such as AEDs (CBZ, PB, PR, clonazepam), non-AEDs (e.g., theophylline, salicylates, ethanol [chronic abuse], antacids, phenothiazine, and phenylbutazone). The interaction between VPA and PHT is complex. Most reports indicate a decrease of total plasma PHT concentration, but by displacing the protein-bound fraction,valproate may cause an increase of free PHT concentration. Certain drugs inhibit PHT metabolism and increase plasma levels, causing toxicity; they include cimetidine, chloramphenicol, chlordiazepoxide, diazepam, isoniazid, propoxyphene, and some AEDs such as ETS.

PHT may stimulate the metabolism of certain drugs (e.g., contraceptive pills, cortisone, theophylline, haloperidol, bishydroxycoumarin), decreasing their plasma levels and efficacy.

Valproate

Depakene is available as 250-mg capsules. Depakote (divalproex sodium) is available as 125-mg capsules or 125-mg, 250-mg, and 500-mg tablets. Valproate sodium is rapidly absorbed, and peak concentration occurs within 3–4 hours of ingestion in the fasting state or if given before meals; however, absorption is slower if given after meals. More than 90% of valproate is protein-bound. Its half-life is about 12 hours.

The usual dose is 20–30 mg/kg/day, but adults with resistant seizures may need up to 40 mg/kg/day and sometimes 60–80 mg/kg/day. In children, higher dosage may be needed. The usual range of maintenance dose is 600–3,000 mg/day. During multiple drug therapy with enzyme-inducing AEDs, larger doses may be needed in both adults and children. Treatment should be started with small dose, such as 10 mg/kg/day, and gradually increased to 20 mg/kg/day within 2 weeks. The dose is then increased further if necessary at 1- to 2-week intervals. In very unusual cases, more than 40 mg/kg/day may be needed. Valproate is given twice daily. During polytherapy when the clearance is rapid, it may be given three to four times a day. To reduce gastrointestinal irritation, the drug can be taken after meals.

The therapeutic range is 50–100 µg/ml. In monotherapy, plasma levels are not absolutely necessary but useful. During multiple drug therapy, if valproate is added to the existing AED (e.g., PHT or CB2), blood levels of both AEDs should be monitored; likewise, if another AED (e.g., PHT or CB2) is added to the existing regimen of valproate therapy, blood levels of both AEDs should be monitored.

Enzyme-inducing AEDs (e.g., CBZ, PHT, PB, PR) stimulate the metabolism of valproate and lower its plasma level. Valproate may increase blood levels of PB as a result of inhibition of metabolism. It may increase free PHT levels as a result of competition with protein-binding sites but later, because of redistribution, may lead to lower total PHT concentration. Valproate may also increase ETS levels.

Phenobarbital

PB is available as 15-mg, 30-mg, 60-mg, and 100-mg tablets. Peak serum absorption occurs 1–6 hours after ingestion, and 45% is bound to plasma proteins. The half-life of PB is 4 days.

A single daily dosage is usually given in the evening. The maintenance dose in adults is 1–3 mg/kg/day; in children 1–15 years of age, the dose is 1–4 mg/kg/day; and in infants younger than 1 year of age, the dose is 3–4 mg/kg/day. The usual range of maintenance dose is 30–240 mg/day. Therapeutic range is 15–40 µg/ml.

VPA inhibits PB metabolism and raises its level in plasma. PB may stimulate the metabolism (enzyme-inducing effect) of PHT and VPA and hence may decrease their plasma levels. PB, because of its enzyme-inducing effect, may stimulate the metabolism of many non-AEDs (e.g., oral contraceptives, digoxin, steroids, bishydroxycoumarin, quinidine, antidepressants, rifampin) and decrease their levels and effectiveness.

Primidone

PR is available as 50-mg and 250-mg tablets, and its time to peak absorption is about 2–5 hours after ingestion. Less than 20% of PR is protein-bound, and its half-life is approximately 12 hours.

The dosage must be initiated very slowly because of PR's acute toxicity. The starting dose may be 50 mg/day in children and 125 mg/day in adults. The dose is then gradually increased every 5–7 days (about 5 × half-life). The maintenance dose in children is 10–20 mg/kg/day and 8–15 mg/kg/day in adults. The dose is generally in the range of 500–1,000 mg. The dose is given twice or thrice daily in divided doses. PB levels should be monitored for all patients on PR.

Clonazepam

Clonazepam (Klonopin) is available as 0.5-mg, 1-mg, and 2-mg tablets. Its peak absorption occurs 1–3 hours after ingestion, and 50–80% is bound to plasma protein. The half-life of clonazepam is 20–40 hours.

Adults generally require 8–10 mg/day. In children, doses should be begun with 0.01–0.03 mg/kg/day and should be increased gradually to 0.2 mg/kg/day; increments should be at the rate of 0.25–0.50 mg/week.

The effective therapeutic range has not been determined but may be in the range of 0.02–0.08 µg/ml.

Ethosuximide

ETS is available as 250-mg capsules. Its peak serum level occurs 3–7 hours after ingestion; ETS does not bind with protein, and its half-life is 2 days.

ETS treatment should be begun by giving 250 mg after lunch and should be gradually increased to the full dosage of 15–20 mg/kg/day. In resistant cases, higher dosages may be needed (e.g., 30 mg/kg/day in adults and 40 mg/kg/day in children). The drug can be given twice daily after meals to lessen gastrointestinal irritation. The usual maintenance dose is 500–1,500 mg/day. The therapeutic range is 50–100 µg/ml. Trough sampling of the plasma level should be obtained. If the response is poor and the patient continues to have seizures and if noncompliance is suspected, regular monitoring of the plasma level is needed.

Valproate may increase the half-life of serum ETS levels, causing ETS toxicity.

Felbamate

Felbamate (Felbatol) is available as 400-mg and 600-mg tablets and 600 mg/5 ml oral suspension. More than 90% of felbamate is absorbed, and peak absorption occurs in 1–3 hours. Twenty percent to 25% of felbamate is bound to proteins, and its half-life is 13–23 hours.

The dosage of felbamate is 600 mg bid. The dosage is then increased by 600–1,200 mg/week to an effective clinical level, up to its maximum dose of 3,600 mg/day, or up to the level when toxicity appears. The therapeutic range is 20–80 µg/ml.

The drug has hepatic enzyme–inducing action and major interactions with other AEDs. It is best used as monotherapy. The following drug interactions have been noted:

1.   Felbamate increases serum PHT and valproate levels.

2.   Felbamate decreases CBZ levels but increases the CBZ-10,11-epoxide metabolite level.

3.   CBZ and PHT decrease felbamate levels, but VPA does not significantly alter felbamate levels.

Felbamate causes nausea, dizziness, headache, insomnia, and ataxia. However, serious side effects, such as aplastic anemia and hepatotoxicity in several patients, with fatalities in some, forced its manufacturer, Carter Wallace, to restrict its use.

Felbamate's exact mechanism of action is not known. Most likely it blocks sodium channels, thus preventing seizure spread. Felbamate has been found to be useful in the treatment of uncontrolled partial seizures with or without secondarily generalized tonic-clonic seizures and of Lennox-Gastaut syndrome.

Gabapentin

Gabapentin (Neurontin) is available as 100-mg, 300-mg, and 400-mg capsules. It is rapidly absorbed and reaches peak level in 2–4 hours. Gabapentin does not bind to serum proteins, and its half-life is 5–7 hours.

Gabapentin is recommended as an add-on therapy. The full dosage is 900–1,800 mg/day, which is reached in the course of a few days. Gabapentin is given three times a day (e.g., the initial dose is 100 mg tid and increased to 300 mg tid on the third or fourth day). The therapeutic range is 2–3 µg/ml.

Gabapentin has no hepatic microsomal enzyme–inducing action and no major interactions with other AEDs. It is safe and has mild side effects, including somnolence, dizziness, fatigue, and ataxia. Pancreatic carcinomas found in toxicologic studies in rodents have not been noted in human studies.

Gabapentin's mechanism of action remains unknown. It does not act by interacting with the gamma-aminobutyric acid (GABA) system. The drug is indicated as an add-on treatment in refractory simple and complex partial seizures with and without secondary generalization in individuals older than 12 years of age.

Lamotrigine

Lamotrigine (Lamictal) is available as 50-mg, 100-mg, and 250-mg tablets. It is rapidly absorbed and widely distributed after oral administration. Fifty-five percent of the drug is bound to serum proteins, and its half-life is 12–48 hours. If used alone, lamotrigine's half-life is 24 hours. If used with AEDs with hepatic enzyme inductions, its half-life is then 12 hours. If used with valproate, which is an enzyme inhibitor (metabolic inhibitor), its half-life is 48 hours.

The total daily dosage is 200–500 mg. A single daily dose is given in monotherapy. The dose is increased gradually over the course of several weeks to reduce the toxic effects. A therapeutic range of 2–4 μg/ml has been quoted in the literature, but this is of uncertain significance for monitoring the clinical improvement or toxicity.

Generally, lamotrigine does not interact significantly with other AEDs except for elevation of CBZ-10,11-epoxide metabolite serum levels, causing possible CBZ toxicity. There is one report of valproate acutely inhibiting lamotrigine metabolism. Its half-life may be reduced if used with enzyme-inhibiting AEDs.

Lamotrigine is a relatively safe drug; this safety has been established after its widespread use in more than 10,000 epileptics in 15 countries. Mild side effects include incoordination, dizziness, double vision, somnolence, and skin rash. It is indicated for refractory partial seizures and Lennox-Gastaut syndrome.

Lamotrigine's mechanism of action is to decrease presynaptic release of glutamate and aspartate, two excitatory neurotransmitters in the central nervous system. It also acts on the voltage-dependent sodium channels and blocks influx of sodium ions into rapidly firing neurons.

Vigabatrin

Vigabatrin (GVG) is available as 500-mg tablets. Its peak absorption occurs within 2 hours of oral ingestion. No significant binding to serum proteins has been noted. Vigabatrin has a half-life of 5–7 hours, but its pharmacodynamic effect is much longer, in the range of days.

The total daily dose is 1,500–3,000 mg/day. Vigabatrin should be started with 500 mg bid to reduce side effects and then increased weekly by 500–1,000 mg/day. In children, the daily dosage may be increased to 50 mg/kg/day or, in some difficult cases up, to 100 mg/kg/day. Serum level determination is of uncertain value for monitoring the clinical effects.

Vigabatrin has minimal interactions with other AEDs and minimal hepatic enzyme induction. A slight decrease in serum PHT level has been reported. The drug has relatively mild side effects, including somnolence, fatigue, gastrointestinal irritation, confusion, and weight gain. A low incidence of severe behavioral problems has been reported in some studies. Myelin vacuoles found in earlier animal toxicologic studies have not been found in monkeys or humans.

Vigabatrin decreases GABA catabolism by inhibiting the rate-limiting enzyme, GABA-transaminase. It is useful as an add-on therapy in patients with intractable partial seizures. The drug is also useful in intractable pediatric seizures, such as Lennox-Gastaut syndrome and infantile spasms.

Role of Antiepileptic Drug Plasma Level Monitoring

When monitoring AED serum levels, physicians should use serum levels as guidelines rather than strictly adjusting the dose according to the level. The goal is to use the medicine in a dosage high enough to stop seizures irrespective of the recommended upper limit of the drug dose or the serum drug level. The toxic side effects are, of course, limiting factors. It should be remembered that the therapeutic blood levels are just statistical values. Some patients may cross the highest level without showing adverse effects, whereas some may show adverse effects in the lowest level. Furthermore, some patients may require higher than the maximum recommended therapeutic level for seizure control without showing side effects, whereas others may have seizure control with the lowest level of the therapeutic level. The most important thing to remember is that clinical monitoring is much more important than AED blood level monitoring.[26] Drug level determinations are, of course, important in cases of suspected drug interactions, noncompliance or poor compliance, and other coexisting diseases.[26, 27]

Monotherapy Versus Multiple Drug Therapy

Multiple drug therapy was practiced in the past on the mistaken belief that AEDs are additive or synergistic in efficacy in controlling seizures. On the contrary, recent pharmacokinetic investigations have clearly shown that this practice decreases the efficacy because of drug interactions (metabolic induction causing acceleration of metabolism, metabolic inhibition, displacement of protein-bound fractions by competing with the binding sites and other complex interactions) and increases the toxicity of each drug even though both drugs are within their accepted therapeutic ranges.[2, 3, 8, 20–23] In fact, recent investigations have documented an improvement of seizure control when multiple drug therapy is changed to monotherapy.[28–32]

In patients with severe prolonged epilepsy and in those with brain damage and progressive central nervous system structural lesions, monotherapy is less likely to succeed. Even in these cases, however, there is no clear evidence that a multiple drug regimen would be more effective.

Advantages of Monotherapy

The advantages of monotherapy can be summarized as follows:

Improved Seizure Control

Schmidt[29] in his study has clearly shown an improvement in seizure control in more than 36% of patients on changing from multiple drug therapy to monotherapy. Similarly, Shorvon and Reynolds[31] reported a reduction in seizure frequency by at least 50% in just over half of the patients with intractable seizures when multiple drugs were changed to a single drug regimen. Albright and Bruni[28] also noted improvement in seizure frequency on changing from multiple drug therapy to monotherapy in 39 patients followed for 16 months.

Management of Dose-Related Toxicity

It may be difficult to decide which drug is responsible for toxicity during multiple drug therapy.[21, 22] The serum levels of the drugs may be within the therapeutic range, and toxicity results from additive effects. Efficacy does not necessarily have an additive effect in multiple drug therapy. Beghi et al.[33] in a multicenter survey of 500 patients on long-term AEDs documented adverse reactions in 44% of those taking three or more AEDs, in 34% taking two AEDs, and in only 22% on monotherapy. Dose-related adverse reactions in monotherapy are easy to recognize and manage by simple dose reductions. Such side effects can be correlated with serum drug levels and can be easily maintained and treated.

Ability to Control Idiosyncratic Reactions

Hypersensitivity reactions are unpredictable and may occur at the initiation of therapy or months later.[21, 22] It is easy to monitor and control idiosyncratic reactions when only a single drug is used. With multiple drug therapy it is not possible to know which drug is causing such reactions. Sometimes, there is a cross-hypersensitivity reaction because of similar chemical configurations of the drugs (e.g., between PHT and PB). In multiple drug therapy, it may be necessary to discontinue both drugs even though only one drug is responsible for such hypersensitivity reactions. Risk of idiosyncratic reaction also decreases with monotherapy.[21, 22] For example, the incidence of VPA-related fetal hepatoxicity decreased from 1 in 500–1,000 to 1 in more than 10,000 patients.[34]

Reduced Chances of Chronic Toxicity

Chronic toxicity increases with multiple drug therapy and is not necessarily dose-related.[21, 22] Monotherapy decreases the chance of developing chronic toxicity, particularly long-term behavioral effects and impairment of memory, cognition, attention, and learning. An improvement in neuropsychological test scores has been noted on conversion from multiple drug therapy to monotherapy.[28, 29, 31, 35] PHT and PB are particularly associated with cognitive and behavioral dysfunction.

Reduced Drug Interactions

Multidrug treatment can cause complex drug interactions.[21, 22] These interactions can manifest in several ways:

1.   Dose-related side effects are additive when two drugs are used even though each drug is within the therapeutic plasma level.

2.   The enzyme-inducing drugs (e.g., CBZ, PHT, PB, PR) may accelerate the metabolism of one drug, resulting in a subtherapeutic concentration of the initial drug and loss of seizure control. For example, if PB is added to PHT, serum PHT levels fall, causing breakthrough seizures. When enzyme-inducing AEDs are added to VPA, VPA blood levels may fall, and an increased dose of VPA is needed to maintain therapeutic level. When the same enzyme-inducing AEDs are reduced or withdrawn, however, the VPA dose must be decreased, or VPA toxicity will develop.

3.   Some drugs may inhibit the metabolism of others, causing toxic concentrations—for example, VPA inhibits the metabolism of PB.

4.   Some drugs may compete for the protein-binding sites and displace the other drugs—for example, VPA may displace PHT from the protein-binding site, causing a rise of free PHT levels, although the total serum PHT level remains unchanged and toxicity may result from an excessive amount of free PHT.

Compliance

Noncompliance is the single most important cause of AED failure.[36] Monotherapy improves compliance. Patients on multidrug regimens often forget and may suffer drug-related memory and cognitive impairment; therefore, it may be difficult to remember complex drug schedules.

Reduced Teratogenicity

A multi-institutional study by Nakane et al.[37] has shown a reduction of teratogenic risk by two- to threefold in the babies of mothers taking only one AED instead of two AEDs.

Cost Benefit

Monotherapy is obviously less costly for the patients than multiple drug therapy. Furthermore, drug interactions may require some drug doses to be increased, thus raising the cost of the drugs.

Disadvantages of Multiple Drug Therapy

The disadvantages of multiple drug therapy can be summarized as follows: loss of seizure control, an increase of dose-related side effects, an increased risk of chronic toxicity, an increased risk of idiosyncratic reactions, effects of drug interactions, an increase of noncompliance, an increased risk of teratogenicity, and an increase in the cost of the drugs.

In a recent pilot study Lammers et al.[38] re-examined the question of the incidence and severity of the adverse effects after monotherapy versus multiple drug therapy to control seizures. They quantitated the adverse effects by using clinimetric indices (rating scales) and found no statistically significant difference between monotherapy and multiple drug therapy groups. These authors are planning an experimental prospective study to verify or refute this conclusion.

How to Begin Monotherapy

Monotherapy can control seizure disorders in 70–75% of patients.[20–22] The first basic principle in monotherapy is to diagnose the type of seizure or epilepsy syndrome. The next step is to choose the drug with the highest level of efficacy for the particular seizure type and the lowest toxicity. The final step is to initiate the drug with an average dose and then gradually increase the dose while monitoring the patient clinically and if necessary by measuring drug levels.

Monotherapeutic treatment can be determined by following the steps below:

- Step 1. Determine whether the patient has epilepsy.

- Step 2. Determine the patient's type of seizure or epilepsy syndrome (based on clinical and EEG findings).

- Step 3. Select the appropriate drug for the particular seizure type.

- Step 4. Discuss with the patient and the family members the plan of action. For monitoring seizures, the patient should keep a seizure diary. Various adverse reactions of the drug should be explained to the patient and the family members so that the toxicity of the drug can be monitored. It should be remembered that some effects (e.g., mild nausea, dizziness, sleepiness) are transient at the onset and will disappear on continuing the medication after a week or so.

- Step 5. Obtain baseline blood tests for hepatic and hematopoietic functions.

- Step 6. Begin drug therapy with an average initiating dose (see Tables 18-1 and 18-2 and section on pharmacological data).

- Step 7. After waiting for five half-lives to pass (i.e., when steady state is reached), monitor seizure control, and increase the dose by the same amount as the initial dose every five half-lives. Monitor the patient's serum drug level. Usually in 1 to 2 months a stable dose is reached.

- Step 8. If the seizures are controlled at an "average" maintenance dose without significant side effects, continue follow-up with the patient, monitoring clinical effects and attending to the psychosocial, vocational, and educational problems of the patient.

- Step 9. If seizures are not controlled and the patient does not have significant side effects, the dose can be increased irrespective of the serum levels (it should be remembered that the therapeutic range is a statistical average and that there is considerable individual variation) until seizures are under control or the patient experiences unacceptable side effects.

- Step 10. If seizures are not controlled despite administering the highest recommended dose (make certain about compliance) and the highest recommended therapeutic range (serum drug level should be obtained) or the patient has severe and unacceptable adverse reactions, try a second first-line drug as monotherapy.

• Step 11. Begin monotherapy with a second AED. Two AEDs must be temporarily continued. The original AED should be reduced, and the new AED added using the average initiating dose (see Table 18-2 and section on pharmacological data). The reduction of the original drug and the increment of the new AED by an amount equivalent to the initiating dose should be at an interval of five elimination half-lives until the original drug is totally discontinued and the new AED is pushed to the maximal tolerable dose without significant side effects.

• Step 12. If seizures are controlled with the new AED, continue follow-up as in Step 8. If the second drug fails, a third first-line drug may be tried as a monotherapy using the above scheme.

• Step 13. In a small percentage of patients (less than 20% in primary generalized seizures and about 25–30% in partial seizures), monotherapy fails and a two-drug or, rarely, a three-drug regimen or one of the new promising AEDs may be tried before labeling the seizures as medically refractory and before consideration for surgical treatment in a small percentage of cases (about 5–10%).

Indications for Multiple Drug Therapy

Approximately 70% of patients will achieve adequate seizure control with a single drug (monotherapy) using either the initial AED or an alternative choice of AED as discussed above. Hence, in the remaining 30% of patients, multiple drug therapy is justified. Furthermore, 10–15% will be controlled by a two-drug regimen or rarely, a three-drug regimen.[20] There is no evidence to suggest that any further improvement will occur by the addition of another AED. Usually there is not much improvement after a two-drug regimen, and an improvement in multidrug regimen means partial rather than complete remission. Thus, about 15% of patients are left with unsatisfactory control and may be considered to have intractable seizures. Some of these patients may control their seizures using one of the newer AEDs (e.g., lamotrigine monotherapy or add-on with gabapentin or vigabatrin). Finally, surgical treatment is indicated and needed in many of these remaining cases of medically refractory seizures.[20, 21]

Despite the many disadvantages of multiple drug therapy and the reduced control of seizures that characterizes multidrug regimens, there are indications for this approach. Multiple drug therapy is indicated when a patient has multiple seizure types (e.g., seizures of different pathophysiologic types), for the treatment of status epilepticus, and when adequate monotherapy fails (in a small percentage of cases).

How to Change from Multiple Drug Therapy to Monotherapy

When a patient on a multidrug regimen whose seizures are not controlled or who has unacceptable drug-induced side effects is seen for the first time, an attempt should be made to change from multiple drug therapy to monotherapy. There is ample evidence in the literature that such a change may improve seizure control.[29, 30] Schmidt[29] found an improvement in at least 36% of patients. Reynolds and Shorvon[30] noted that 70–75% of patients could be completely controlled with one drug. A change from multiple drug therapy to monotherapy is a difficult undertaking and needs the commitment of the physician, patient, and family members. The steps should be individualized, but a general outline based on the recommendations[22, 39] in the literature is given here:

- Step 1. Re-evaluate the patient. Obtain history, physical examination, and EEG studies. If a structural lesion is suspected, appropriate imaging studies should be performed.

- Step 2. If no cause or precipitating or aggravating factors (e.g., sleep deprivation, intercurrent infection, other medical or surgical disorders, alcohol abuse) are found, establish the type of seizure or epileptic syndrome based on the clinical evaluation and EEG findings.

- Step 3. Measure morning trough levels of all AEDs the patient has been taking.

- Step 4. Discuss the plan of action for changing from multiple drugs to monotherapy with the patient and family members.

- Step 5. Obtain baseline blood tests for hepatic and hematopoietic functions.

- Step 6. Initiate withdrawal of drugs one at a time. Begin withdrawal of the drug that is least likely to cause withdrawal seizures (e.g., acetazolamide). Also, gradually withdraw any drug that has a subtherapeutic level or that is suspected to be causing major toxicity.

• Step 7. After the initial withdrawal, introduce the desired AED using an initial average dose, or if this agent is already part of the multiple drug regimen, increase its dose by an amount used in the beginning. Continue to increase the drug dosage every five elimination half-lives until the maximum recommended dose and the therapeutic serum level of this agent are attained.

• Step 8. As the dose of the desired AED is increased every five elimination half-lives, continue at the same time the process of withdrawal of the other agents every five half-lives. CBZ, PR, or valproate can be decreased by 15–25% of the maximal dose at weekly intervals, and PB doses can be halved every 3 weeks.[22] PHT, however, must be withdrawn more cautiously than the other agents because of its zero kinetics at the higher end of the therapeutic serum level. Therefore, for PHT, a smaller amount is withdrawn every 10–14 days.[22] The withdrawal of these agents may require 1–3 months.

• Step 9. Throughout the process of withdrawal of the undesirable AEDs and the increment of the desirable AED, continue to monitor the patient clinically (look for toxicity, control of seizure, and compliance), and obtain periodic AED serum levels.

• Step 10. If the seizures are controlled with the desirable AED and all the other agents have been successfully withdrawn, monotherapy is established. The patient should have periodic follow-up so that the physician may monitor the clinical effects and attend to the patient's psychosocial, vocational, and educational problems.

• Step 11. If seizures are not controlled by a new agent or by the already existing desirable agent despite using the highest recommended dose (make certain about compliance) and attaining the therapeutic serum level (monitor the drug levels regularly during conversion from multiple drug therapy to monotherapy) or if the patient experiences an unacceptable adverse reaction, try another conventional AED or one of the newer promising AEDs (e.g., lamotrigine as monotherapy) and withdraw the previous agent following the steps outlined above.

• Step 12. In a small percentage of patients, monotherapy fails. A two-drug and, rarely, a three-drug regimen of the first- and second-line drugs or one of the newer promising drugs (e.g., gabapentin, lamotrigine or vigabatrin) as add-on therapy may be tried before labeling the seizures as medically refractory and considering surgical treatment in a small number of cases (about 5–10%).

Treatment Considerations in Special Situations

Epilepsy in Children

Seizure classification is critical in childhood seizures (see also Chapter 10). It is important to correctly classify the seizure type and choose the right AED based on the seizure classification, as certain AEDs may exacerbate some childhood seizures. For example, CBZ or PHT often worsens atonic, typical, or atypical absence or myoclonic seizures. ETS may increase the frequency of myoclonus. Clonazepam may occasionally aggravate myoclonus. The new AED vigabatrin may exacerbate nonprogressive myoclonic epilepsy.

Some childhood seizures have distinguishing features. Knowing these characteristics helps to correctly classify the seizure type and to choose the AED that will best control the seizures. Certain childhood seizures are self-limiting (e.g., febrile seizures, rolandic seizures). Several epileptic syndromes are age-dependent, such as febrile seizures, rolandic epilepsy, absence seizures, West's syndrome, Lennox-Gastaut syndrome, and juvenile myoclonic epilepsy of Janz. There is a higher incidence of neurologic handicap, mental retardation, or learning disorders in children with epilepsy.

Pregnancy and Epilepsy

Special consideration should be paid to an epileptic woman who wants to become or who has become pregnant (see also Chapter 11). The incidence of seizures increases in approximately 25% of epileptic women who become pregnant, in 25% the seizures improve, and in 50% there is no change in the frequency of seizure.[40] The increased incidence of seizures during pregnancy may be detrimental not only to the mother, but also to the fetus because seizures in the mother can cause intracranial bleeding. There is clear evidence of an increased incidence of pregnancy-related complications, such as abruptio placentae, hydramnios, and premature birth.

During pregnancy, the metabolism of AEDs is altered because of changes in their absorption or changes in compliance. Often, the dosage of AEDs must be increased during pregnancy, but it must be decreased when the pregnancy ends to avoid toxicity.

Despite considerable controversy, there is clear evidence of an increased incidence of AED embryopathy and teratogenicity. Intrauterine development of the fetus is often delayed in epileptic mothers on AEDs. There is a two- to threefold increase of teratogenicity (congenital malformation) in epileptic mothers taking AEDs. The following recommendations are suggested for pregnant epileptic women taking AEDs:

1.   AED withdrawal should be considered before conception.

2.   Monotherapy is preferable to multiple drug therapy because drug toxicity is avoided and the chances of teratogenicity are reduced.

3.   If seizures are controlled, the AED should not be changed. It should be noted that more than 90% of pregnancies in epileptic women are uncomplicated.

4.   Frequent clinical and serum AED level monitoring, including free drug level monitoring, should be performed to avoid toxicity.

5.   The drug dosage should be adjusted during pregnancy and adjusted again in the postpartum period.

6.   If the patient is taking valproate or CBZ, serum alpha-fetoprotein should be measured and ultrasonography studies performed to detect spina bifida. This malformation has been noted in 1% of patients taking valproate; there also have been some reports of similar neural tube defects in the children born to epileptic mothers on CBZ treatment.

7.   If the patient is taking PHT or barbiturates, vitamin K therapy should be administered to the mother during the last week before the expected delivery date. The newborn should receive vitamin K and, if necessary, fresh plasma if bleeding tendencies are noted.

Epilepsy in the Elderly

The highest incidence of epilepsy is in the very young and in the elderly. The most common type of seizure is partial seizure with or without secondary generalization; the most common cause of epilepsy in the elderly is cerebrovascular disease. Because of slowing of the hepatic metabolism as a result of reduced hepatic blood flow and hepatocellular mass and because of reduced plasma protein levels related to decreased protein synthesis, the drug dosage in elderly patients should be lowered.[41, 42] Generally, a reduction by a factor of one-third to one-fourth of the recommended younger adult dose is required.[41] Elderly patients are also very sensitive to the neurotoxic effects of AEDs;[41, 42] in particular, the drugs affect coordination, cognition, behavior, and alertness in elderly patients. Hence, frequent AED plasma level monitoring may be required. Particular attention should be paid to free-drug levels in patients receiving highly protein-bound drugs such as PHT and VPA. Elderly patients are also susceptible to certain other AEDs side effects, such as osteoporosis and osteomalacia (in those receiving PHT, PB, and PR) and cardiac conduction defects (in those receiving CBZ and PHT).

Intractable Seizures

Intractable seizures should be differentiated from refractory seizures.[43] Intractable means "difficult to treat," whereas refractory means "not responsive to treatment" (in the case of seizures, not responsive to AED treatment).[43] Approximately 5–10% of cases of epilepsy prove to be refractory; seizures continue to occur severely and frequently despite optimal medical treatment in this group. Such cases may comprise up to 3,000 patients with newly diagnosed epilepsy annually in the United States, and these patients may require surgical treatment.[43]

Causes of intractable seizures include:[43]

1. Incorrect diagnosis of nonepileptiform spells (e.g., alcohol withdrawal seizures, pseudoseizures) as epilepsy.

2. Incorrect classification of the seizure type and consequent incorrect drug therapy.

3. Inadequate or faulty medications.

    a. Incorrect medication given because of an incorrect diagnosis.

    b. Administration of excessive medication.

    c. Undermedication. The therapeutic drug levels in the blood have not been reached; therefore, it is advisable to increase the dose (rather than switch to a second drug) until toxic signs appear and then reduce it to the optimum level.

d. Faulty combinations in a multiple drug therapy. Multiple drug therapy may have been with multiple AEDs or AEDs with other medications, causing cancellation effects. Thus, drug interactions or other pharmacokinetic factors may have been responsible for intractability.

4.   Noncompliance or poor compliance (the single most important cause of drug failure in epilepsy treatment).

5.   Complications of drug abuse or alcoholism.

6.   Unrecognized precipitating factors for seizures (e.g., unrecognized sleep disturbances, psychological stress, or intercurrent infections).

7.   Incorrect association of the seizures with a variety of medical and surgical conditions.

8.   The presence of a static or progressive neurologic lesion that may need surgical treatment.

Approach a patient with intractable seizures according to the following steps:[43, 44]

• Step 1. Re-evaluate the patient by clinical means and by obtaining laboratory tests, including EEG studies.

• Step 2. The patient should be hospitalized, and, if necessary, long-term video-EEG monitoring should be performed.

• Step 3. Serum AED levels should be monitored.

• Step 4. If the patient is on multiple drug therapy, convert him or her to monotherapy as described previously.

• Step 5. If monotherapy fails, try a newer AED (e.g., gabapentin or lamotrigine).

• Step 6. If monotherapy with the above regimen fails, a combination of two and, rarely, three appropriate drugs, including the newer AEDs as add-ons, may improve seizure control in a small number of patients.

• Step 7. In a small subset of medically refractory patients, a surgical option should be considered.

Presurgical Evaluation and Surgical Procedures

Details of surgical treatment preceded by presurgical evaluation have been described in Chapters 15 and 16. Briefly, the presurgical evaluation should include a history and physical examination; standard EEG recording; prolonged noninvasive video-EEG monitoring; invasive EEG recording (if necessary), including depth EEG or subdural grid EEG recording; neuropsychological assessment; Wada test (intracarotid amytal test); and imaging studies, including MRI, SPECT, and PET.

Surgical procedures that are available include temporal lobectomy for refractory partial complex seizures; nontemporal resection for partial complex seizures of extratemporal origin; hemispherectomy for refractory unilateral seizures with hemiparesis; and corpus callosotomy for "drop attacks" and tonic, atonic, and secondarily generalized seizures that have been refractory to medical treatment.

Epilepsy is not a life-long condition, contrary to the general perception of the past. Approximately 70–75% of all patients will eventually become seizure-free (5-year remission) on medication, and 40–90% of those entering remission will remain seizure-free after withdrawal of AEDs.[7]

Factors favoring remission after medical treatment[7, 45, 46] include young age at onset, diagnosis of generalized seizures at onset, normal findings on neurologic examination, and idiopathic seizure cause. Unfavorable factors for remission after medical treatment[7, 45–47] include symptomatic epilepsy (known cause), partial seizure or complex partial seizure types, abnormal EEG findings (especially a generalized spike and wave pattern), increased number and duration of seizures before diagnosis and initiation of treatment, and mental retardation or cerebral palsy. Only 60% of patients will have remission if seizures are not controlled within the first year, and only 10% of patients will enter remission after medical treatment if control is not achieved by 4 years.

The favorable and unfavorable predictors for recurrence and nonrecurrence of seizure after AED withdrawal and the method of withdrawal have been described in Chapter 14. An overall recurrence rate of 30% both in adults and in children has been quoted in the literature.

Briefly, the favorable predictors for nonrecurrence after AED withdrawal include normal EEG findings, primary generalized tonic-clonic or absence seizure type, normal findings on neurologic examination, and improvement on monotherapy. The unfavorable predictors for recurrence after withdrawal are age of onset of seizure before age 3 years or after age 30 years, abnormal findings on neurologic examination, partial complex seizure type, frequent seizures before improvement on AEDs, an abnormal EEG finding at the time of withdrawal, a long duration of epilepsy before control, mixed seizures, and juvenile myoclonic epilepsy.

Conclusion

In 1881, Sir William Gowers said, after the discovery of bromides in 1857 as the first pharmacotherapy for epilepsy, that "although the condition of many sufferers is still gloomy enough, it is not without hope and we must surely trust that the progress of the recent past is the dawn of a brighter day."[48] Today we are leaping into the twenty-first century with a new understanding in the management of epilepsy and with the developments of promising new drugs to control and possibly to cure the suffering of the unfortunate victims of epilepsy.

References

1. Annegers JF. The Epidemiology of Epilepsy. In E Wyllie (ed), The Treatment of Epilepsy: Principles and Practice. Philadelphia: Lea & Febiger, 1993;157.
2. Wyllie E. The Treatment of Epilepsy: Principles and Practice. Philadelphia: Lea & Febiger, 1993.
3. Penry JK. Epilepsy: Diagnosis, Management, Quality of Life. New York: Raven, 1986.
4. Berg AT, Shinnar S. The risk of seizure recurrence following a first unprovoked seizure: a quantitative review. Neurology 1991;41:965.
5. Hauser WA, Anderson VE, Loewenson RB, McRoberts SM. Seizure recurrence after a first unprovoked seizure. N Engl J Med 1982;307:522.
6. Shinnar S, Berg AT, Moshe SL, et al. Risk of seizure recurrence following a first unprovoked seizure in childhood: a prospective study. Pediatrics 1990;85:1076.
7. Hauser WA. The Natural History of Seizure. In E Wyllie (ed), The Treatment of Epilepsy: Principles and Practice. Philadelphia: Lea & Febiger, 1993;165.
8. Camfield CS, Camfield PR. Initiating Drug Therapy. In E Wyllie (ed), The Treatment of Epilepsy: Principles and Practice. Philadelphia: Lea & Febiger, 1993;791.
9. Reynolds EH. The prevention of chronic epilepsy. Epilepsia 1988; 29(Suppl):S25.
10. Ferrendelli JA. Clinical Uses of Current Antiepileptic Drugs. Gainesville, FL: Epilepsy Research Foundation of Florida, 1993.
11. Fisher RS. Emerging antiepileptic drugs. Neurology 1993;43(Suppl 5):S12.

12. Leppik IE, Graves N, Devinsky O. New antiepileptic medications. Neurol Clin 1993;11:923.
13. Mattson RH, Cramer JA, Collins JF, et al. Comparison of carbamazepine, phenobarbital, phenytoin, and primidone in partial and secondarily generalized tonic-clonic seizures. N Engl J Med 1985;313:145.
14. Mattson RH, Cramer JA, Collins JF, et al. Valproate in the treatment of partial and secondarily generalized tonic-clonic seizures in adults: a comparison with carbamazepine. N Engl J Med 1992;327:765.
15. Ramsay RE, Wilder BJ, Murphy JV, et al. The efficacy and safety of valproic acid vs phenytoin as sole therapy for newly diagnosed primary generalized tonic-clonic seizures. J Epilepsy 1992;5:55.
16. Wilder BJ, Ramsay RE, Murphy JV, et al. Comparison of valproate and phenytoin in newly diagnosed tonic-clonic seizures. Neurology 1983;33:1474.
17. Turnbull DM, Rawlins MD, Weightman D, et al. A comparison of valproic acid and phenytoin in previously untreated adult epileptic patients. J Neurol Neurosurg Psychiatry 1982;45:55.
18. Callaghan N, Kenny RA, O'Neill B, et al. A prospective study between carbamazepine, phenytoin and sodium valproate as monotherapy in previously untreated and recently diagnosed patients with epilepsy. J Neurol Neurosurg Psychiatry 1985;48:639.
19. DeSilva M, McArdle B, McGowan L, et al. Monotherapy for newly diagnosed childhood epilepsy: a comparative trial and prognostic evaluation [abstract]. Epilepsia 1989;30:622.
20. Mattson RH, Cramer JA. The Choice of Antiepileptic Drugs in Focal Epilepsy. In E Wyllie (ed), The Treatment of Epilepsy: Principles and Practice. Philadelphia: Lea & Febiger, 1993;817.
21. Smith DB. Antiepileptic Drug Selection in Adults. In DB Smith (ed), Epilepsy: Current Approaches to Diagnosis and Treatment. New York: Raven, 1990;111.
22. Wilder BJ. Treatment considerations in anticonvulsant monotherapy. Epilepsia 1987;28(Suppl 2):S1.
23. Porter RJ. General Principles: How to Use Antiepileptic Drugs. In R Levy, R Mattson, B Meldrum, et al. (eds), Antiepileptic Drugs. New York: Raven, 1989;117.
24. Levy R, Mattson R, Meldrum B, et al. Antiepileptic Drugs (3rd ed). New York: Raven, 1989.
25. Physicians' Desk Reference (49th ed). Montvale, NJ: Medical Economics Data, 1995.
26. Schmidt D, Jacob R. Clinical and Laboratory Monitoring of Antiepileptic Medication. In E Wyllie (ed), The Treatment of Epilepsy: Principles and Practice. Philadelphia: Lea & Febiger, 1993;798.
27. Pellock JM, Willmore LJ. A rational guide to routine blood monitoring in patients receiving antiepileptic drugs. Neurology 1991;41:961.
28. Albright P, Bruni J. Reduction of polypharmacy in epileptic patients. Arch Neurol 1985;42:797.
29. Schmidt D. Reduction of two drug therapies in intractable epilepsy. Epilepsia 1983;24:368.
30. Reynolds EH, Shorvon SD. Monotherapy or polytherapy for epilepsy? Epilepsia 1981;22:1.

31. Shorvon SD, Reynolds EH. Reduction in polypharmacy for epilepsy. BMJ 1979;2:1023.
32. Shorvon SD, Reynolds EH. Unnecessary polypharmacy for epilepsy. BMJ 1977;1:1635.
33. Beghi E, DeMascio R, Sasanelli F, et al. Adverse reactions to antiepileptic drugs: a multicenter survey of clinical practice. Epilepsia 1986;27:323.
34. Dreifuss FE, Santilli N, Longer DH, et al. Valproic acid hepatic fatalities: a retrospective review. Neurology 1987;37:379.
35. Thompson PJ, Trimble MR. Anticonvulsant and cognitive functions. Epilepsia 1982;23:531.
36. Pippenger CE, Lesser RP. An overview of therapeutic drug monitoring principles. Cleve Clin Q 1984;51:241.
37. Nakane Y, Oltum T, Takahashi L, et al. Multi-institutional study on the teratogenicity and fetal toxicity of anticonvulsants: report of a collaborative study group in Japan. Epilepsia 1988;21:663.
38. Lammers MW, Hekster YA, Keyser A, et al. Monotherapy or polytherapy for epilepsy revisited: a quantitative assessment. Epilepsia 1995;36:440.
39. Dean JC, Penry JK. Valproate monotherapy in 30 patients with partial seizures. Epilepsia 1988;29:140.
40. Schmidt D. The Effect of Pregnancy on the Natural History of Epilepsy: Review of the Literature. In D Janz, M Dam, A Richen, et al. (eds), Epilepsy, Pregnancy and the Child. New York: Raven, 1982;3.
41. Troupin AS. Antiepileptic Drug Therapy: A Clinical Overview. In E Wyllie (ed), The Treatment of Epilepsy: Principles and Practice. Philadelphia: Lea & Febiger, 1993;785.
42. Scheuer ML, Cohen J. Seizures and epilepsy in the elderly. Neurol Clin 1993;11:787.
43. Pedley TA. The Challenge of Intractable Epilepsy. In D Chadwick (ed), New Trends in Epilepsy Management: The Role of Gabapentin. Royal Society of Medicine Series No. 198. London: Royal Society of Medicine, 1993;3.
44. Morris HH, Lesser RP, Luders H, Dinner DS. Medical therapy for intractable complex partial seizure. Cleve Clin Q 1984;51:255.
45. Gross-Tsur V, Shinnar S. In E Wyllie (ed), The Treatment of Epilepsy: Principles and Practice. Philadelphia: Lea & Febiger, 1993;858.
46. Shinnar S, Berg AT, Moshe SL, et al. Discontinuing antiepileptic drugs in children with epilepsy: a prospective study. Ann Neurol 1994;35:534.
47. Tennison M, Greenwood R, Lewis D, Thorn M. Discontinuing antiepileptic drugs in children with epilepsy. N Engl J Med 1994;330:1407.
48. Thrush DC. Epilepsy: clinical management. Proc R Coll Physicians Edinb 1993;23:455.

19

Newer Antiepileptic Medications

Rajesh C. Sachdeo

Introduction

The history of the treatment of epilepsy has encompassed a host of therapeutic modalities and dates back centuries. Initially, nonmedicinal therapies that included rituals, potions, and special diets were the mainstays. The modern era of antiepileptic drugs (AEDs) began with Merritt and Putnam,[1] who demonstrated, through the use of animal models of epilepsy, screening procedures with which to select potential AEDs. Since that time, there has been an increase in AED development. Despite the availability of numerous AEDs, between 25% and 40% of patients continue to have breakthrough seizures or undesirable side effects. It is therefore important to continue developing new AEDs to allow better control of seizures.

There have been several long hiatuses during which no new AEDs were marketed. Since the introduction of carbamazepine (CBZ) in 1974 and valproic acid (VPA) in 1978, no new AEDs were marketed in the United States until 1993, when felbamate (FBM) was approved by the Food and Drug Administration (FDA). Since 1993, a number of new AEDs, many of which were born from the program developed by the National Institutes of Health/National Institute of Neurological Disorders and Stroke (NINDS) Epilepsy Branch, have been introduced on the market. In addition, formulation alterations with specific therapeutic advances have occurred, and several new AEDs are expected in the next 3 years. These new AEDs include FBM, fosphenytoin, gabapentin (GBP), lamotrigine (LTG), oxcarbazepine (OXC), an extended-release formula of CBZ called Tegretol-XR, tiagabine, topiramate, and vigabatrin (VGB). Three of these agents (FBM, GBP, and LTG) recently received approval for use in United States, and several other products are expected to be approved by the FDA in the next 3 years. All have been in use in some countries outside the United States. These agents are discussed in an alphabetical order in this chapter. Table 19-1 lists drug interactions when combinations of these newer and the standard AEDs are used.

Felbamate

FBM is 2-phenyl-1,3-propanediol dicarbamate. FBM inhibits seizure activity in maximal electroshock and pentylenetetrazol models as well as seizures induced by N-methyl-D-aspartate (NMDA), suggesting potential effects in a broad range of epilepsy types.[2, 3] FBM appears to have multiple mechanisms of action, including effects at the sodium voltage–gated channels,[4] NMDA receptor complexes, and gamma-aminobutyric acid (GABA) receptor complexes.[5]

When given orally, FBM is well absorbed (approximately 90%),[6] with peak plasma concentrations being reached after 2–6 hours.[7, 8] Terminal elimination half-life ranges from 15 hours to 23 hours,[7] with dose-related increases in the area under the curve (AUC) and maximal plasma concentration (Cmax). Food does not affect the rate or extent of absorption.[9] FBM is 22–25% reversibly bound to human plasma proteins.[10] FBM is relatively lipid-soluble and readily crosses the blood–brain barrier.[11] Approximately 40–50% of the absorbed dose appears unchanged in urine. None of the metabolites identified in human urine has significant anticonvulsant activity.

FBM is predominantly metabolized by the cytochrome P-450 system (CYP450), which probably accounts for its interactions with other AEDs.[12] Through induction of CYP450, FBM reduces CBZ levels by approximately 20%, whereas levels of the active metabolite CBZ-10,11-epoxide increase by 30–50%.[13] FBM increases plasma phenytoin (PHT) levels in a dose-dependent manner, probably through a competitive inhibition of CYP450 isozyme responsible for phenytoin hydroxylation.[14] Similarly, FBM at a dose of 2,400 mg/day increases phenobarbital plasma concentration by approximately 25%.[15] At doses of 1,200 and 2,400 mg/day, FBM increases VPA serum levels by 28% and 54%,[16] respec-

Table 19-1. Antiepileptic Drug-Drug Interactions

Added Drug	Effect on Plasma Concentration of:										
	Carbamazepine	Felbamate	Gabapentin	Lamotrigine	Oxcarbazepine	Phenobarbital	Phenytoin	Tiagabine	Topiramate	Valproic Acid	Vigabatrin
Carbamazepine	—	↑	nc	↓	nc	uk	↑↓	↓	↓	↓	nc
Valproic acid	↑ CBZ epoxide	↑	nc	↑	nc	↑	↑*	nc	nc	—	nc
Phenobarbital	↓	↓	nc	↓	↓	—	↑↓	↓	↓	↓	nc
Phenytoin	↓	↓	nc	↓	nc	↑↓	—	↓	↓	↑↓	nc
Felbamate	↓ CBZ ↑ epoxide	—	uk	nc	nc	↑	↑	↑	uk	↑	nc
Gabapentin	nc	uk	—	uk	uk	nc	nc	uk	uk	nc	uk
Lamotrigine	↑ CBZ epoxide	uk	uk	—	uk	nc	nc	uk	uk	↓	uk
Oxcarbazepine	nc	nc	uk	uk	—	uk	uk	uk	uk	↑	nc
Tiagabine	nc	uk	uk	uk	uk	uk	nc	—	uk	↓	uk
Topiramate	nc	uk	uk	uk	uk	nc	nc	uk	—	nc	uk
Vigabatrin	nc	nc	uk	uk	uk	↓	↓	uk	uk	nc	—

nc = no change; uk = unknown; ↑ = increased concentration of the initial drug; ↓ = decreased concentration of the initial drug; ↑↓ = variable results.

*Free fraction.

tively, probably through an inhibition of β-oxidation of valproate.[17] In studies in healthy volunteers, FBM at a dose of 2,400 mg/day had no clinically significant effect on the pharmacokinetics of clonazepam,[18] the active monohydroxy metabolite of OXC,[19] VGB,[20] or LTG.[21]

The enzyme-inducing AEDs PHT, CBZ, and phenobarbital increase clearance of FBM, leading to reduced plasma concentrations.[13, 15, 22] VGB does not affect the pharmacokinetics of FBM.[20] To minimize toxicity of other AEDs during their concomitant administration, doses of CBZ, PHT, valproate, and phenobarbital should be reduced by 10–30% initially, depending on the dosing increment of FBM.

The efficacy claim for FBM in patients with partial onset seizures with and without secondary generalization is based on the results of five controlled studies (three in multiple drug therapy and two in monotherapy) with patients with therapy-resistant seizures despite optimal plasma concentrations of one or two AEDs.[23–27]

FBM is unusual among new AEDs in that it is effective in secondary generalized as well as localization-related epilepsy. In a double-blind, add-on, parallel study involving 73 mostly pediatric patients with Lennox-Gastaut syndrome, FBM at a dose of up to 45 mg/kg/day reduced the frequency of atonic seizures by 34% (p = .01) and all seizures by 19% (p = .002). A quality of life measure, the global evaluation score, was significantly better in the FBM group than in the placebo group.[28]

The historical adverse events profile of FBM during the clinical trial program of about 1,700 patients was favorable, with the most common events being gastrointestinal and nonspecific central nervous system symptoms. In July 1993, FBM was approved in the United States by the FDA for the treatment of patients with partial onset seizures or Lennox-Gastaut syndrome. Since then, an estimated 150,000 patients have been exposed to the compound. With this wide postmarketing exposure, some idiosyncratic adverse events were reported.[29] The increased risk of aplastic anemia (e.g., about 30 cases have been reported) and hepatotoxicity in some cases led to a restriction in the clinical use of FBM to include only patients who have failed to respond to available relevant AEDs.

Fosphenytoin

Fosphenytoin is a disodium phosphate ester prodrug of PHT. Fosphenytoin is formulated in a TRIS buffer aqueous solution at a pH of

8.8 provided as a sterile solution containing 50 mg/ml (all fosphenytoin doses, IV rates, and solution concentrations are expressed as the amount of phenytoin provided after conversion in the body). The increased water solubility allows fosphenytoin to be formulated without organic solvents (e.g., propylene glycol and ethanol) and the caustic pH (e.g., pH 12) required for parenteral PHT (Dilantin).

Fosphenytoin is rapidly and completely converted to PHT in the body, and its pharmacologic activity is the result of its conversion to PHT, as fosphenytoin has no known activity of its own. PHT derived from fosphenytoin has the same pharmacokinetics and adverse events as PHT, and therapeutic plasma concentrations are monitored similarly as with PHT.[30] The half-life of conversion is approximately 15 minutes. Fosphenytoin is completely converted to phenytoin independent of dose, rate of intravenous (IV) administration, and route of administration.[31] Therapeutic plasma concentrations of PHT (more than 10 μg/ml of total PHT or more than 1 μg/ml of free PHT) are rapidly achieved after IV or intramuscular (IM) fosphenytoin loading doses, generally within approximately 10 minutes of the start of IV infusion or within 30 minutes after IM injection. It has been shown that a significant crossreactivity of fosphenytoin occurs with the TDx/TDxFLx and Emit 2000 PHT immunoassays, resulting in an overestimation of the PHT concentration. When it is necessary to measure PHT concentrations shortly after administration, it is recommended that a blood sample be obtained at least 2 hours after IV dosing and 4 hours after IM dosing when using an immunoassay. Blood samples obtained earlier must be analyzed by a method specific to measure phenytoin in the presence of fosphenytoin (e.g., an HPLC assay).

The types and incidence of adverse events reported with fosphenytoin are similar to those with PHT (see Chapter 13). The most common side effects are nystagmus, dizziness, ataxia, and somnolence. Transient skin sensations characterized by perineal itching and tingling (pruritus or paresthesia) have been reported with IV fosphenytoin and appear to be dose- and rate-related. The itching and tingling sensation is self-limiting and generally disappears within 1 or 2 minutes of completing the IV infusion. In some patients, the infusion has been temporarily interrupted to alleviate the symptoms, and, rarely, the IV infusion has been discontinued before completing the prescribed dose. IV or IM fosphenytoin is very well tolerated in contrast to IM PHT, which causes severe pain and burning at the injection site in addition to causing muscle abscesses.[32] Safety and pharmacokinetics in children younger than 5 years of age have not been studied.

Fosphenytoin may be used to load and maintain plasma PHT in patients requiring parenteral PHT. Fosphenytoin may be admixed with normal saline or dextrose 5% IV solutions. A concentration range of 1.5–25 mg/ml of diluted solution is recommended. IV admixtures may be stored at room temperature for up to 8 hours and under refrigeration for up to 24 hours before use.[33] Fosphenytoin has been studied in clinical situations, with maintenance dosing of up to 14 days' duration.[34]

For status epilepticus the recommended dose is 20–30 mg/kg IV at a rate of 100–150 mg/minute (2–3 mg/kg/minute for children weighing less than 50 kg). The dose may be reduced to 15 mg/kg in elderly patients. Possible additional treatment would include IV lorazepam or diazepam. The desired trough PHT plasma concentration should be maintained by initially administering 4–6 mg/kg/day, IM or IV either once or divided into two doses. IM fosphenytoin is injected undiluted in the gluteal, deltoid, or other suitable muscle. Two-site injections may be required for large volumes as with loading doses. Single-site injection volumes of 10–20 ml have been well tolerated. The IV infusion rate will be adjusted according to clinical circumstances (e.g., whether seizures stop or are continuing). Monitoring of blood pressure and electroencephalographic findings is recommended during infusion of IV loading doses.

For patients temporarily unable to take their current oral PHT, equimolar dose of fosphenytoin IM or IV may be administered at the same daily frequency. The free levels of both fosphenytoin and PHT reach peak plasma concentration at the same time. Plasma concentrations are maintained with IM fosphenytoin after equimolar dose substitution for a patient's oral PHT when the oral route is temporarily not feasible. IM fosphenytoin is completely and reliably absorbed (essentially 100% bioavailable).

In summary, the advantages of fosphenytoin over PHT include greater water solubility, lower pH (i.e., pH of 8.8 versus 12), faster rate of administration, shorter period for infusion and monitoring, fewer IV rate and site changes, and fewer problems with infiltration. Other advantages are absence of precipitation, stability of IV mixture, compatibility with normal saline or dextrose water, and complete and reliable absorption from the IM site. Finally, fosphenytoin does not require solvents such as propylene glycol or ethanol.

Gabapentin

GBP is a carboxylated amino acid that was designed to transport GABA across the blood–brain barrier without affecting GABA uptake by the nerve terminals.[35] It does not appear to act as a GABA agonist or antagonist and has no effects on the sodium channel, GABA A receptors, or GABA B receptors. The anticonvulsant action of GBP is probably mediated by altering the concentration or metabolism of brain amino acids.[36–38] The oral bioavailability of GBP is 56%. It is absorbed by the gastrointestinal tract by a mucosal L amino acid transport mechanism that is saturable.[39]

The plasma half-life of GBP is 5–8 hours, but its effect on the brain may last longer than this. Because of its half-life, tid dosing is recommended. Because of the saturable transport mechanisms, however, absorption is nonlinear above 3,600 mg/day. Therefore, patients who are taking more than 3,600 mg/day may need to take the drug four times a day. It has no active metabolites. GBP is excreted unchanged by the kidneys, and the renal clearance of GBP equals the total glomerular filtration. In patients with impairment of renal function, the dose needs to be reduced.[40] GBP is not protein-bound and is not a hepatic enzyme inducer. There appears to be no drug interaction.

Several double-blind, placebo-controlled studies[41–43] have been conducted using doses of GBP ranging from 900 mg to 1,800 mg/day. The results show that 26% of patients treated with 1,800 mg of GBP have at least a 50% reduction in their seizure frequency. Some patients can tolerate a higher dosage of up to 4,800 mg with improved efficacy, however. Trials comparing the results of gradually incrementing GBP from 300 to 900 mg/day in 3 days with the results of administering an initial loading dose of 900 mg on the first day and then 300 mg tid showed no difference between the two regimens. The most common side effects reported are somnolence (24%), dizziness (20%), ataxia (17.4%), and fatigue (11%). Most of the side effects are mild, with development of tolerance to the side effects in 4 weeks. GBP is the drug of choice in patients with acute intermittent porphyria, since it has no effect on the liver. In elderly epileptics, who are usually on multiple drugs, GBP becomes the drug of choice because of its lack of drug interactions.

Lamotrigine

LTG is a recently approved AED that has a unique mode of action involving inhibition of the release of excitatory neurotransmitters, primarily glutamate.[44, 45] LTG is almost completely absorbed, with no effect of food on its absorption. It is extensively metabolized and is excreted predominantly by the kidneys, with 8% of the dose being recovered unchanged in urine.[46] It induces its own metabolism, resulting in a 25% decrease in the elimination half-life at steady state. It has linear pharmacokinetics.[47] LTG's half-life is about 29.6 hours.[48] LTG has no significant drug interactions, as it does not have enzyme-inducing properties; however, the effect of other AEDs on the kinetics of LTG are clinically significant. In the presence of enzyme-inducing drugs such as PHT and CBZ, its half-life is reduced to 12.5 hours. With valproate, LTG's half-life is increased to 69.6 ± 14.8 hours.[49] LTG has no effect on PHT but decreases VPA levels slightly. Although it has no effect on CBZ levels, CBZ epoxide levels increase by 10–50%, resulting in clinical manifestations of toxicity. Acetaminophen enhances the metabolism of LTG and decreases the serum level by approximately 20%.[50] Two parallel studies; seven crossover, double-blind, placebo-controlled studies; and several open-label studies have been undertaken. To date, more than 120,000 patients have been exposed to the drug. In crossover studies, Messenheimer et al.,[51] Schapel et al.,[52] and Matsuo et al.[53] found that 25% of patients had at least a 50% reduction in seizures. These studies clearly show that LTG is efficacious in patients with partial seizures with or without secondary generalization. Several open-label studies[54, 55] have also claimed efficacy in patients with primarily generalized tonic-clonic seizures, although in patients with severe primary juvenile myoclonic epilepsy and other primary generalized seizures, it was difficult to convert patients to LTG monotherapy. As adjunctive therapy, the dosage of VPA was reduced by 90%.

The most common side effects of LTG were dizziness, headache, diplopia, ataxia, and somnolence. Diplopia was more frequent when combined with CBZ, whereas ataxia and somnolence were more frequently seen when combined with PHT. Skin rash was seen in approximately 10% of patients. The incidence is lower with enzyme-inducing AEDs but higher in patients taking VPA. The rash is usually self-limited but can progress to Stevens-Johnson syndrome. Rash in the beginning of therapy does not predict severity. Generally, the incidence of rash can be reduced by initiating LTG on a lower dosage than that indicated in the drug insert. LTG may be started at 25 mg/day for 1 week, and then the daily dosage may be increased by 25 mg every week until a dose of 100 mg/day is reached. At this point, the daily dose of LTG can be increased by 50 mg every week until the daily maximum dose of 500 mg is reached. Occasionally, patients may need a slightly higher dosage. In patients taking VPA, the daily dosage increment should be undertaken at a slower speed than this.

LTG is 55% protein-bound, and therapeutic blood levels have not been established. Levels of 0.5–10.0 µg/ml have been reported in patients taking therapeutic doses. Although enzyme-inducing AEDs reduce the half-life of LTG and VPA increases the half-life of LTG, the combination of enzyme-inducing AEDs and VPA appear to cancel their effects. Monotherapy trials in Europe for newly diagnosed patients have been found to be efficacious.

Oxcarbazepine

OXC (Trileptal) is the 10-keto-analogue of CBZ. The compound is currently marketed in some 25 countries worldwide and is under development for registration in North America and Europe. The presence of a keto moiety confers a radically different metabolic profile in comparison with CBZ and most other AEDs. OXC is reduced to a long-acting metabolite (half-life of 9–13 hours), 10-mono-hydroxy-CBZ (MHD). Based on its half-life and preclinical profile, MHD is considered the primary mediator of OXC's therapeutic effects. The absence of an oxidative step in OXC metabolism eliminates the occurrence of an epoxide intermediate and minimizes the likelihood of induction of cytochrome P450 enzymes.[56] At present, the only known drug interaction of clinical significance is with oral contraceptives.[57] In a Scandinavian double-blind multicenter study,[58] 235 patients suffering from newly diagnosed epilepsy were randomly allocated to treatment with either OXC or CBZ. There was no difference in the number of seizures between the two treatment groups (mean 0.4 ± 3.0 for OXC; mean 0.3 ± 1.4 for CBZ). A global evaluation of efficacy was made by the physicians at the end of the treatment. Efficacy was judged as either excellent or good in 96% of the patients receiving OXC and in 97% of those treated with CBZ. In both groups, at least 80% of patients experienced a 50% or higher reduction in seizures compared with baseline. The number of patients with adverse experience (68% for OXC versus 74% for CBZ) and the mean number of side effects per patient (2.8 for OXC versus 3.5 for CBZ) tended to be lower with OXC than with CBZ. Particularly with respect to adverse events leading to discontinuation, this difference was statistically significant in favor of OXC ($p = .04$). The most commonly reported side effects were fatigue, headache, dizziness, and ataxia.[59] This suggests a profile of equivalent efficacy and better tolerability than CBZ.

A randomized, double-blind, crossover, add-on polytherapy trial[60] in 42 refractory patients with mixed seizure types comparing CBZ and OXC demonstrated significantly reduced frequencies of tonic and tonic-clonic seizures in patients taking OXC compared with those taking CBZ. Partial seizures also were somewhat reduced in patients taking OXC. With respect to tolerability, OXC was rated superior to CBZ in terms of patient and physician willingness to continue therapy.

A recent review[61] of OXC treatment further supports a favorable safety profile. Allergic skin reactions were rare, and cross-reactivity in CBZ-sensitive patients was only 25%. The only noteworthy clinical laboratory abnormality, hyponatremia, was generally benign, provided that water intoxication was managed. An analysis of 350 Danish patients on chronic OXC therapy indicated that hyponatremia necessitated discontinuation in about 1% of patients.[61] Van Amelsvoort et al.,[62] in a review of 128 papers dealing with hyponatremia that was associated with OXC treatment, found that no baseline values of sodium were obtained in many cases. Thus, some of the reported incidence may reflect a pre-existing condition. They also confirmed that most cases of hyponatremia were asymptomatic.

Overall, OXC has been shown to be at least as effective as CBZ for the treatment of generalized tonic-clonic seizures and partial seizures, with and without secondary generalization, in both monotherapy and polytherapy. The equivalent dose is about 50% higher than that of CBZ. A simplification of the dose regimen (from tid to bid) may be possible in some patients.

Tegretol-XR

Tegretol-XR is an extended-release formulation of CBZ recently approved by the FDA. It makes use of a novel osmotically driven mechanism for delivery of the drug that ensures a constant release of CBZ over an extended period. Practically, this allows twice daily dosing.

Two randomized clinical trials using this formulation have been published.[63, 64] A randomized crossover kinetic trial[64] of Tegretol-XR and CBZ, each administered for 21 days, indicated bioequivalence of the two dosage forms based on 24-hour AUC, Cmax, and time to maximal plasma level for the parent compound and epoxide. Both treatments were tolerated well, and no changes in seizure frequency were noted between treatments on crossover. The kinetic trial included a sizable cohort of pediatric patients, and general labeling of CBZ recently was extended to include pediatric patients of all ages. A larger multicenter double-blind, crossover trial[63] compared the safety, efficacy, and kinetics of Tegretol-XR and Tegretol monotherapy administered serially for 56 days. Ninety-eight percent of Tegretol-XR patients had trough plasma levels in a therapeutic range, compared with 97% of Tegretol patients. No statistically reliable differences in overall seizure rate were noted across compartments, and the authors concluded that physicians could switch to a twice daily dosage with no loss of control but with compliance advantages.

Tiagabine

Tiagabine is a novel anticonvulsant that acts by inhibiting GABA uptake by presynaptic neurons and glial cells.[65] Tiagabine hydrochloride crosses the blood–brain barrier and has no effect on other neurotransmitters. Tiagabine is absorbed quickly, with a peak level approximately 1 hour after ingestion. The half-life is 5–8 hours and is independent of the dose in patients without hepatic enzyme induction. Absorption and elimination of the drug occur in a linear manner. Intake of food slows down the absorption but does not reduce the extent of absorption. Tiagabine is extensively metabolized by the liver.[66] Almost 95% of the drug is bound to protein. VPA displaces a small amount of tiagabine bound to plasma protein. Twenty-five percent of tiagabine metabolites are excreted in the urine, and 63% are excreted in the feces.[67] Less than 2% is excreted in the urine unchanged. Tiagabine concentrations decrease with hepatic enzyme–inducing AEDs such as CBZ, PHT, phenobarbital, and primidone.[68]

Double-blind, placebo-controlled trials using tiagabine as an add-on therapy in patients with partial seizures with and without secondary generalization have been undertaken with doses of 8 mg qid, 16 mg bid, and 14 mg qid.[69, 70] Results clearly show that tiagabine is superior to placebo in reducing seizure frequency by at least 50% in a significant number of patients with partial complex seizures. Doses of up to 112 mg/day were used in patients who had been also taking enzyme-inducing anticonvulsants. Side effects of tiagabine are dizziness, headache, ataxia, tremor, confusion, and nervousness. In the majority of patients, the side effects were mild to moderate and transient. In some patients with dose adjustments, the side effects resolved.[64, 69] No clinically important alterations in the clinical laboratory values or idiosyncratic reactions have been reported to date. Monotherapy trials are currently underway in United States and Europe.

Topiramate

Topiramate is a new AED with a novel sugar sulfamate structure. It acts as an AED by modulating sodium channels, enhancing GABA activity, and blocking kainate-induced currents at non-NMDA receptors.[71–73] Topiramate is rapidly absorbed after oral ingestion, and its bioavailability is 81–95%. The absorption of topiramate is not affected by food.[74] Protein binding is low (approximately 15% binds with protein), and topiramate readily crosses the blood–brain barrier. Topiramate and its metabolites are excreted through the kidneys; topiramate has no known active metabolites. When administered as adjunctive therapy with hepatic enzyme–inducing drugs such as PHT, CBZ, or phenobarbital, approximately 50% of the ingested dose is metabolized and the remainder excreted as unchanged drug. When topiramate is administrated as monotherapy, 80% is excreted as unchanged drug. The half-life of topiramate, when administered with enzyme-inducing drugs, is 15 hours; when administered as monotherapy or with VPA, its half-life is 22 hours. Therefore, twice daily dosing is recommended. In patients with moderate or severe renal impairment, the half-life is prolonged, and dosing levels should be reduced. Hepatic impairment has little clinically significant effect on topiramate pharmacokinetics.

Topiramate does not affect plasma levels of CBZ, CBZ epoxide, or VPA.[75, 76] It generally has no effect on PHT levels, but in an occasional patient, PHT clearance may be decreased by approximately 20%.[77] If signs of PHT toxicity appear during topiramate therapy, PHT levels should be monitored. In the presence of CBZ, PHT, and phenobarbital, topiramate levels are reduced by approximately 50% from levels obtained during monotherapy, but valproate has no clinically significant effect on topiramate levels. Topiramate lowers serum digoxin levels by approximately 12%.[78] Topiramate has no effect on the progestin component of oral contraceptives but reduces levels of the estrogenic component by approximately 30%.[79]

The efficacy of topiramate as add-on therapy for partial onset seizures in adults with or without secondary generalization has been demonstrated in five placebo-controlled trials using doses of 200–1,000 mg/day.[80–84] Some patients have been treated with doses of up to 1,600 mg/day. A reduction in seizure frequency of approximately 50% was seen at doses of 400–800 mg/day. In one study, 36% of patients treated with 800 mg/day of topiramate had a reduction in seizure frequency of 75–100%.[84] Statistically significant reductions in secondary generalized (76%), complex partial (41%), and simple partial (58%) seizures were found across all studies.[85] A recent study demonstrated that topiramate as adjunctive therapy converted to monotherapy is effective for the treatment of partial onset seizures; almost 50% of subjects treated with 1,000 mg/day in the study had a 50% reduction in seizures.[86] Initial reports suggest that topiramate may be effective for seizures associated with the Lennox-Gastaut syndrome.[87]

The most common side effects are drowsiness; fatigue; dizziness; headache; somnolence; and "thinking abnormally," which refers to slowed thinking and does not include any psychiatric disturbances. Overall, 85% of the central nervous system side effects resolve within several weeks of initiating topiramate therapy.[88] Slowing the titration rate may possibly also reduce the incidence of central nervous system side effects. A recommended titration rate is to start at 50 mg/day and then increase the dosage to 50–100 mg/week. Topiramate is an inhibitor of carbonic anhydrase and is associated with an increased risk of renal stones. Small renal stones occurred in 1.5% of patients in clinical trials, but three-fourths of the patients chose to continue topiramate after passing the stone.[89] Topiramate appears to have significant efficacy and with appropriate titration should represent a valuable addition to the therapeutic armamentarium.

Vigabatrin

VGB is a specific and irreversible inhibitor of GABA-T activity. It induces a dose-dependent increase in brain and cerebrospinal fluid GABA concentrations. Its effect as an anticonvulsant is the result of its effect on the central nervous system GABAergic neuronal system. It does not affect glutamate, aspartate, and taurine levels.[90, 91] VGB is water-soluble, with more than 80% of the oral dose recovered from the urine. Its absorption is not affected by food. Its total volume of distribution is 0.8 liter/kg. VGB has a half-life of approximately 12 hours, which is shorter in children (6–8 hours) and can be up to 14 hours in the elderly. Elimination is dependent on renal function.[92] VGB reduces plasma PHT and phenobarbital levels,[93, 94] but it has no effect on VPA or CBZ levels. Several double-blind studies in patients with partial complex and secondary generalization seizures have clearly shown that

30–60% of patients had at least a 50% reduction in seizures with VGB. This effect was maintained on long-term follow-up of up to 12 months.[94, 95] VGB has been found to be effective in childhood syndromes such as infantile spasms and Lennox-Gastaut syndrome but not in absence or myoclonic seizures.[96, 97] Most side effects are similar to those of other AEDs, the most common ones being drowsiness, irritability, headaches, behavioral changes, unsteady gait, and nervousness. Psychosis has been reported in 3–10% of patients, usually at the initiation of therapy. Most patients with psychosis have no prior history of psychiatric problems.[98] The dosage is 1–3 g/day given in two divided doses. Doses above 3 g do not enhance the efficacy. Because of animal toxicologic findings of microvacuolation in the white matter of the brain, magnetic resonance imaging scans and evoked potentials were performed in most of the clinical trials. No long-term change in the human brain or any indication of neurologic impairment in humans has been reported with VGB as of now.

References

1. Merritt HH, Putnam TJ. A new series of anticonvulsant drugs tested by experiments on animals. Arch Neurol Psychiatry 1938;39:1003.
2. Swinyard EA, Sofia RD, Kupferberg HJ. Comparative anticonvulsant activity and neurotoxicity of felbamate and four prototype antiepileptic drugs in mice and rats. Epilepsia 1986;27:27.
3. Coffin V, Cohen-Williams M, Barnett A. Selective antagonism of the anticonvulsant effects of felbamate by glycine. Eur J Pharmacol 1994;256:R9.
4. White HS, Wolf HH, Swinyard EA, et al. A neuropharmacological evaluation of felbamate as a novel anticonvulsant. Epilepsia 1992;33:564.
5. Rho JM, Donevan SD, Rogawski MA. Mechanism of action of the anticonvulsant felbamate: opposing effects of N-methyl-D-aspartate and g-aminobutyric acid A receptors. Ann Neurol 1994;35:229.
6. Schumaker RC, Fantel C, Kelton E, et al. Evaluation of the elimination of [^{14}C] felbamate in healthy men. Epilepsia 1990;31:642.
7. Ward DL, Schumaker RC. Comparative bioavailability of felbamate in healthy men. Epilepsia 1990;31:642.
8. Wilensky AJ, Friel PN, Ojemann LM, et al. Pharmacokinetics of W-554 (ADD 03055) in epileptic patients. Epilepsia 1985;26:602.
9. Gudipati RM, Raymond RH, Ward DL, et al. Effect of food on the absorption of felbamate in healthy male volunteers. Neurology 1992;42(Suppl 3):332.
10. Adusumalli VE, Yang JT, Wong KK, et al. Felbamate pharmacokinetics in the rat, rabbit, and dog. Drug Metab Dispos 1991;19:1116.

11. Cornford EM, Young D, Paxton JW, Sofia RD. Blood-brain barrier penetration of the new anticonvulsant felbamate. Epilepsia 1992;33:944.
12. Perhach JL, Shumaker RC. Felbamate Absorption, Distribution, and Excretion. In RH Levy, RH Mattson, BS Meldrum (eds), Anti-Epileptic Drugs (4th ed). New York: Raven, 1995;807.
13. Wagner ML, Remmel RP, Graves NM, Leppik IE. Effect of felbamate on carbamazepine and its major metabolites. Clin Pharmacol Ther 1993;53:536.
14. Sachdeo R, Wagner M, Sachdeo S, et al. Steady-state pharmacokinetics of phenytoin when co-administered with Felbatol (felbamate). Epilepsia 1992;33(Suppl 3):84.
15. Sachdeo R, Padela MF. The effect of felbamate on phenobarbital serum concentrations. Epilepsia 1994;35(Suppl 8):94.
16. Wagner ML, Graves NM, Leppik IE, et al. The effect of felbamate on valproic acid disposition. Clin Pharmacol Ther 1994;56:494.
17. Hooper WD, Franklin ME, Glue P, et al. Effect of felbamate on valproic acid disposition in healthy volunteers: inhibition of b-oxidation. Epilepsia 1996;37:91.
18. Colucci R, Glue P, Reidenberg P, et al. Effects of felbamate on the pharmacokinetics of clonazepam. Am J Ther 1996 (in press).
19. Hulsman JARJ, Rentmeester TW, Banfield C, et al. Effects of felbamate on the pharmacokinetics of the monohydroxy and dihydroxy metabolites of oxcarbazepine. Clin Pharmacol Ther 1995;58:383.
20. Reidenberg P, Glue P, Benfield C, et al. Pharmacokinetic interaction studies between felbamate and vigabatrin. Br J Clin Pharmacol 1995;40:157.
21. Taloxa Product Monograph. Kenilworth, NJ: Schering-Plough, 1995.
22. Banfield CR, Zhu GR, Jen JF, et al. The effect of age on the apparent clearance of felbamate: a retrospective analysis using nonlinear mixed-effects modeling. Ther Drug Monit 1996;18:19.
23. Leppik IE, Dreifuss FE, Pledger GW, et al. Felbamate for partial seizures: results of a controlled clinical trial. Neurology 1991;41:1785.
24. Theodore WH, Raubertas RF, Porter RJ, et al. Felbamate: a clinical trial for complex partial seizures. Epilepsia 1991;32:292.
25. Bourgeois B, Leppik IE, Sackellarees JC, et al. Felbamate: a double-blind controlled trial in patients undergoing presurgical evaluation of partial seizures. Neurology 1993;43:693.
26. Sachdeo R, Kramer LD, Rosenberg A, Sachdeo S. Felbamate monotherapy: controlled trial in patients with partial onset seizures. Ann Neurol 1992;32:386.
27. Faught E, Sachdeo RC, Remier MP, et al. Felbamate monotherapy for partial-onset seizures: an active-control trial. Neurology 1993;43:688.
28. Felbamate Study Group in Lennox-Gastaut Syndrome. Efficacy of felbamate in childhood epileptic encephalopathy (Lennox-Gastaut syndrome). N Engl J Med 1993;328:29.
29. Patton WN, Duffull SB. Idiosyncratic drug-induced hematological abnormalities: incidence, pathogenesis, management and avoidance. Drug Safety 1994;11:445.
30. Browne TR, Szabo GK, McEntegart C, et al. Bioavailability studies of drugs with nonlinear pharmacokinetics: II. Absolute bioavailability of

intravenous phenytoin prodrug at therapeutic phenytoin serum concentrations determined by double-stable isotope technique. J Clin Pharmacol 1993;33:89.

31. Andrews CO, Turnbull TL, Paloucek PF, et al. Safety and pharmacokinetics of fosphenytoin following intravenous loading dose administration [abstract]. Pharmacotherapy 1994;14:367.

32. Wilder BJ, Ramsay RE, Marriott J, Loewen G. Safety and tolerance of intramuscular administration of fosphenytoin, a phenytoin prodrug, for 5 days in patients with epilepsy [abstract]. Neurology 1993;43:308.

33. Leppik IE, Boucher BA, Wilder BJ, et al. Pharmacokinetics and safety of a phenytoin prodrug given I.V. or I.M. in patients. Neurology 1990;40(3 pt. i):456.

34. Dean JC, Smith KR, Boucher BA, et al. Safety, tolerance, and pharmacokinetics of intramuscular (IM) fosphenytoin, a phenytoin prodrug in neurosurgery patients. Epilepsia 1993;34(Suppl 6):111.

35. Vollmer K-O, von Hodenberg A, Kolle EU. Pharmacokinetics and metabolism of gabapentin in rat, dog and man. Arzneimittelforschung/Drug Res 1986;36:830.

36. Taylor CP, Rock DM, Weinkauf RJ, Ganong AH. In vitro and in vivo electrophyisological effects of the anticonvulsant gabapentin [abstract]. Soc Neurosci Abstr 1988;14:866.

37. Taylor CP, Vartanian MG, Yuen P-W, et al. Potent and stereospecific anticonvulsant activity of 3-isobutyl GABA relates to in vitro binding at a novel site labeled by tritiated gabapentin. Epilepsy Res 1992;14:11.

38. Taylor CP, Vartanian MG, Andruszkiewiewicz R, Silverman RB. 3-Alkyl GABA and 3-alkylglutamic acid analogues: two new classes of anticonvulsant agents. Epilepsy Res 1992;11:103.

39. Stewart BH, Kluger AR, Thompson PR, Bockbrader HN. A saturable transport mechanism in the intestinal absorption of gabapentin is the underlying cause of the lack of proportionality between increasing dose and drug levels in plasma. Pharmacol Res (in press).

40. Comstock TJ, Sica DA, Bockbrader HN, et al. Gabapentin pharmacokinetics in subjects with various degrees of renal function [abstract]. J Clin Pharmacol 1990;30:862.

41. Browne TR. Efficacy and Safety of Gabapentin. In D Chadwick (ed), New Trends in Epilepsy Management: The Role of Gabapentin. London: Royal Society of Medicine Services, 1993;47.

42. Ojemann LM, Wilensky AJ, Temkin NR, et al. Long-term treatment with gabapentin for partial epilepsy. Epilepsy Res 1992;13:159.

43. Ramsay RE. Clinical efficacy and safety of gabapentin. Neurology 1994;44(Suppl 5):S23.

44. Leach MJ, Marden CM, Miller AA. Pharmacological studies on lamotrigine, a novel potential antiepileptic drug: 2. Neurochemical studies on the mechanism of action. Epilepsia 1986;27:490.

45. Miller AA, Wheatley P, Sawyer DA, et al. Pharmacological studies on lamotrigine, a novel potential antiepileptic drug: 1. Anticonvulsant profile in mice and rats. Epilepsia 1986;27:483.

46. Cohen AF, Land GS, Breimer DD, et al. Lamotrigine, a new anticonvulsant: pharmacokinetics in normal humans. Clin Pharmacol Ther 1987;42:535.

47. Yuen AWC, Peck AW. Lamotrigine pharmacokinetics: oral and I.V. infusion in man. Br J Clin Pharmacol 1988;26:242P.
48. Jawad S, Richens A, Goodwin G, Yuen WC. Controlled trial of lamotrigine (Lamictal) for refractory partial seizures. Epilepsia 1989; 30:356.
49. Yau MK, Wargin WA, Wolf KB, et al. Effect of valproate on the pharmacokinetics of lamotrigine at steady state. Epilepsia 1992;33(Suppl 3):82.
50. Depot M, Powell JR, et al. Kinetic effects of multiple oral doses of acetaminophen on a single oral dose of lamotrigine. Clin Pharmacol Ther 1990;48:346.
51. Messenheimer J, Ramsay RE, Willmore LJ, et al. Lamotrigine therapy for partial seizures: a multicenter, placebo-controlled, double-blind, crossover trial. Epilepsia 1994;35:113.
52. Schapel GJ, Beran RG, Vajda FJE, et al. Double-blind, placebo-controlled, crossover study of lamotrigine in treatment resistant partial seizures. J Neurol Neurosurg Psychiatry 1993;56:448.
53. Matsuo F, Bergen D, Faught E, et al. Placebo-controlled study of the efficacy and safety of lamotrigine in patients with partial seizures. Neurology 1993;43:2284.
54. Sander JWAS, Hart TM, Patsalos PN, et al. Lamotrigine and generalized seizures. Epilepsia 1991;32(Suppl 1):S9.
55. Timmings PL, Richaeps A. Lamotrigine in primary generalized epilepsy. Lancet 1992;339:1300.
56. Faigle JW, Menge GP. Metabolic characteristics of oxcarbazepine (Trileptal) and their beneficial implications for enzyme induction and drug interactions. Behav Neurol 1990;3(Suppl 1):20.
57. Klosterskov JP, Saano V, Haring P, et al. Possible interaction between oxcarbazepine and an oral contraceptive. Epilepsia 1992;33:1149.
58. Dam M, Ekberg R, Loyning Y, et al. A double-blind study comparing oxcarbazepine and carbamazepine in patients with newly diagnosed, previously untreated epilepsy. Epilepsy Res 1989;3:7.
59. Friis ML, Kristensen O, Boas J, et al. Therapeutic experiences with 947 epileptic outpatients in oxcarbazepine treatment. Acta Neurol Scand 1993;87:224.
60. Houtkooper MA, Lammertsma A, Meyer JWA, et al. Oxcarbazepine (GP 47680)—a possible alternative to carbamazepine? Epilepsia 1987;28:693.
61. Jensen NO. Oxcarbazepine in patients hypersensitive to carbamazepine. Presented at the 16th Epilepsy International Congress, Hamburg, 1985.
62. Van Amelsvoort TH, Bakshi R, Devaux CB, et al. Hyponatremia associated with carbamazepine and oxcarbazepine therapy. A review. Epilepsia 1994:35:181.
63. Tegretol Oros Release Delivery System Study Group. Double-blind crossover comparison of Tegretol XR and Tegretol in patients with epilepsy. Neurology 1995;45:1703.
64. Thakker KM, Mangat S, Garnett WR, et al. Comparative bioavailability and steady state fluctuations of Tegretol commercial and carbamazepine oros tablets in adult and pediatric epilepsy patients. Biopharm Drug Dispos 1992;13:559.

65. Croucher MJ, Meldrum BS, Krogsgaard-Larsen P. Anticonvulsant activity of GABA uptake inhibitors and their prodrugs following central or systemic administration. Eur J Pharmacol 1983;89:217.
66. Gustavson LE, Mengel HB, Pierce MW, Chu S-Y. Tiagabine, a new gamma-aminobutyric acid uptake inhibitor antiepileptic drug: pharmacokinetics after single oral doses in man. Epilepsia 1990;31:642.
67. Bopp BA. Abbott-70569 Drug Metabolism Report No. 18. Disposition and metabolism of Abott-70569-14C in rats given a 30 mg/kg dose. Abbott Laboratories Division 46 Report No. R&D/91/114. March, 1991.
68. Richens A, Gustavson LE, McKelvy JF, et al. Pharmacokinetics and safety of single-dose tiagabine HCl in epileptic patients chronically treated with four other antiepileptic drug regimens. Epilepsia 1991; 32(Suppl 3):12.
69. Sachdeo R, Leroy R, Krauss G, et al. Safety and efficacy of bid and qid dosing with tiagabine HCl versus placebo as adjunctive treatment for complex partial seizures [abstract]. Neurology 1995;45(Suppl 4):202.
70. Rowan AJ, Uthmanb B, Ahmann P, et al. Safety and efficacy of three dose levels of tiagabine HCl versus placebo as adjunctive treatment for complex partial seizures. Epilepsia 1994;35(Suppl 8):54.
71. White HS, Brown D, Skeen GA, et al. The anticonvulsant topiramate displays unique ability to potentiate GABA-evoked currents. Epilepsia 1995;36(Suppl 3):S39.
72. Lawrence S, Coulter D, Sombati S, DeLorenzo R. Topiramate selectively blocks kainate currents in cultured hippocampal neurons. Epilepsia 1995;36(Suppl 4):38.
73. Sombati S, Coulter DA, DeLorenzo RJ. Effects of topiramate on sustained repetitive firing and low magnesium induced seizures discharges in cultured hippocampal neurons. Epilepsia 1995;36(Suppl 4):38.
74. Doose DR, Gisclon LG, Stellar SM, et al. The effects of food on the bioavailability of topiramate from 100- and 400-mg tablets in healthy male subjects. Epilepsia 1993;33(Suppl 3):105.
75. Sachdeo RC, Sachdeo SK, Walker SA, et al. Steady-state pharmacokinetics of topiramate and carbamazepine in patients with epilepsy during monotherapy and concomitant therapy. Epilepsia 1996 (in press).
76. Liao S, Rosenfeld WE, Palmer M, et al. Steady state pharmacokinetics of topiramate and valproic acid in patients with epilepsy and during combination therapy. Epilepsia 1994;35(Suppl 4):117.
77. Sachdeo RC, Sachdeo SK, Levy RH, et al. Topiramate and phenytoin pharmacokinetics in patients with epilepsy during monotherapy and combination therapy. Epilepsia 1996 (in press).
78. Liao S, Palmer M. Digoxin and topiramate drug interaction in male volunteers. Pharm Res 1994;10:S405.
79. Doose DR, Rosenfeld WE, Schaefer P, et al. Evaluation of the potential pharmacokinetic interaction between topiramate and the oral contraceptive combination, norethindrone/ethinyl estradiol. J Clin Pharmacol 1994;34:1031.
80. Faught E, Wilder BJ, Ramsay RE, et al. Topiramate dose ranging trial in refractory partial epilepsy. Epilepsia 1995;36(Suppl 4):33.

81. Privitera M, Fincham R, Penry K, et al. Dose ranging trial with higher doses of topiramate in patients with resistant partial seizures. Epilepsia 1995;36(Suppl 4):33.
82. Martinez-Lage J, Ben-Menachem E, Shorvon SD. Double blind, placebo controlled trial of 400 mg/day topiramate as add-on therapy in patients with refractory partial epilepsy. Epilepsia 1995;36(Suppl 3):S149.
83. Tassinari C, Chauvel P, Chodkiewicz J, et al. Double blind, placebo controlled trial of 600 mg/day topiramate as add-on therapy in patients with refractory partial epilepsy. Epilepsia 1995;36(Suppl 3):S150.
84. Ben-Menachem E, Dam M, Henriksen O, et al. Double blind, placebo controlled trial of 800 mg/day topiramate as add-on therapy in patients with refractory partial epilepsy. Epilepsia 1995;36(Suppl 3):S150.
85. Pledger G, Reife R, Lim P, Karim R. Overview of topiramate efficacy from adjunctive therapy trials. Epilepsia 1995;36(Suppl 3);S150.
86. Sachdeo R. Single center topiramate monotherapy trial. Epilepsia 1995;36(Suppl 3):S151.
87. French JA, Bourgeois BFD, Dreifuss FE, et al. An open label multicenter study of topiramate in patients with Lennox-Gastaut syndrome. Neurology 1995;45(Suppl 4):321.
88. Reife R, Lim P, Pledger G. Topiramate: side effect profile in double line studies. Epilepsia 1995;36(Suppl 4):34.
89. Wasserstein AW, Rak I, Reife R. Nephrolithiasis during treatment with topiramate. Epilepsia 1995;36(Suppl 3):S153.
90. Neal MJ, Shah MA. Development of tolerance to the effects of vigabatrin (gamma-vinyl-GABA) on GABA release from rat cerebral cortex, spinal cord and retina. Br J Pharmacol 100:324.
91. Ben-Menachem E, Persson LI, Mumford J, et al. Effect of long-term vigabatrin therapy on selected neurotransmitter concentrations in cerebrospinal fluid. J Child Neurol 1991;6(Suppl 2):2S11.
92. Rey E, Pons G, Richard MO, et al. Pharmacokinetics of the individual enantiomers of vigabatrin (gamma-vinyl GABA) in epileptic children. Br J Clin Pharmacol 1990;30:253.
93. Rimmer EM, Richens A. Interaction between vigabatrin and phenytoin. Br J Clin Pharmacol 1989;27(Suppl 1):S27.
94. Herranz JL, Arteaga R, Farr IN et al. Dose-response study of vigabatrin in children with refractory epilepsy. J Child Neurol 1991;6(Suppl 2):2S45.
95. Livingston JH, Beaumont D, Arzimanoglou AM, Aicardi J. Vigabatrin in the treatment of epilepsy in children. Br J Clin Pharmacol 1989;27(Suppl 1):S109.
96. Chiron C, Dulac O, Beaumont D, et al. Therapeutic trial of vigabatrin in refractory spasms. J Child Neurol 1991;6(Suppl 2):2S52.
97. Dulac O, Chiron C, Luna D, et al. Vigabatrin in childhood epilepsy. J Child Neurol 1991;(Suppl 2):S30.
98. Sander JW, Hart YM, Trimble MD, Shorvon SD. Behavioral disturbance associated with vigabatrin therapy. Epilepsia. 1992;32(Suppl 1):12.

Index